Nervous System

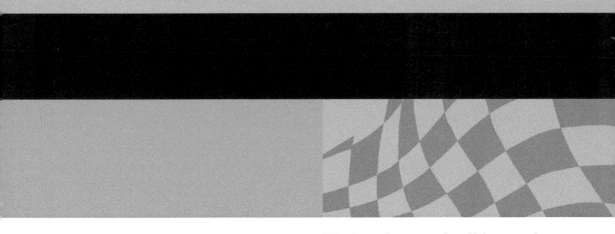

First and second edition authors:

Daniel Lasserson

Carolyn Gabriel

Basil Sharrack

Charlie Briar

Third edition authors:

Mark Hughes

Thomas Miller

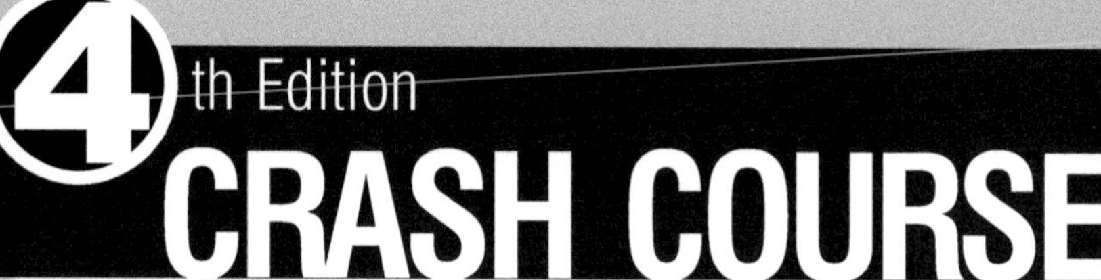

SERIES EDITOR
Dan Horton-Szar
BSc(Hons), MBBS(Hons), MRCGP,
Northgate Medical Practice,
Canterbury,
Kent, UK

FACULTY ADVISOR
Colin Smith
MD FRCPath,
Academic Department of Neuropathology,
Centre for Clinical Brain Sciences,
University of Edinburgh,
Edinburgh, UK

Nervous System

Jenny Ross
MBChB BMedSci
CT1 ACCS Anaesthesia,
Edinburgh, UK

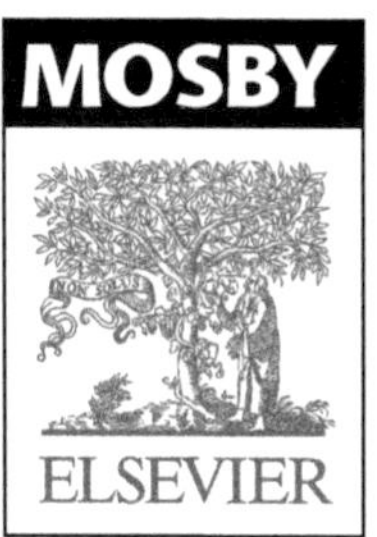

Edinburgh London New York Oxford Philadelphia St Louis Sydney Toronto 2015

ELSEVIER
MOSBY

Commissioning Editor: Jeremy Bowes
Development Editor: Ewan Halley
Project Manager: Andrew Riley
Designer/Design Direction: Stewart Larking
Illustration Manager: Jennifer Rose
Icon Illustrations: Geo Parker

First edition 1998

Second edition 2003

Third edition 2007

Fourth Edition 2012

Updated Fourth edition 2015

ISBN: 978-0-7234-3857-1

British Library Cataloguing in Publication Data
A catalogue record for this book is available from the British Library

Library of Congress Cataloging in Publication Data
A catalog record for this book is available from the Library of Congress

Printed in Great Britain

Last digit is the print line: 10 9 8 7 6 5 4 3

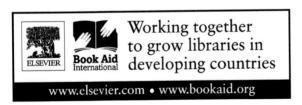

Series editor foreword

The *Crash Course* series first published in 1997 and now, 15 years on, we are still going strong. Medicine never stands still, and the work of keeping this series relevant for today's students is an ongoing process. These fourth editions build on the success of the previous titles and incorporate new and revised material, to keep the series up-to-date with current guidelines for best practice, and recent developments in medical research and pharmacology.

We always listen to feedback from our readers, through focus groups and student reviews of the *Crash Course* titles. For the fourth editions we have completely re-written our self-assessment material to keep up with today's 'single-best answer' and 'extended matching question' formats. The artwork and layout of the titles has also been largely re-worked to make it easier on the eye during long sessions of revision.

Despite fully revising the books with each edition, we hold fast to the principles on which we first developed the series. *Crash Course* will always bring you all the information you need to revise in compact, manageable volumes that integrate basic medical science and clinical practice. The books still maintain the balance between clarity and conciseness, and provide sufficient depth for those aiming at distinction. The authors are medical students and junior doctors who have recent experience of the exams you are now facing, and the accuracy of the material is checked by a team of faculty advisors from across the UK.

I wish you all the best for your future careers!

Dr Dan Horton-Szar

Prefaces

Author

The nervous system is one of our body's most fascinating organ systems. However, the vast literature and seemingly complex concepts surrounding the subject can be an intimidating prospect for medical students. This textbook has been written specifically with medical students in mind and aims to present the nervous system in a way that is accessible and relevant to undergraduates. Not only is the information more than enough to pass your undergraduate exams, more importantly it will provide a strong foundation in the basic neurosciences that will prove invaluable in your study of the clinical neurosciences.

I wish you the best of luck with your exams!

Jenny Ross

Faculty advisor

Since my undergraduate medical training two decades ago, the curriculum has changed greatly. On the negative side formal courses covering neuroanatomy, neurophysiology and neuropharmacology have disappeared. On the positive side they have been replaced by more integrated courses with greater emphasis on clinical relevance. This book is aligned with the ethos of integration. In one single volume the reader is provided with a clinically relevant introduction to neuroanatomy, neurophysiology, neuropathology and neuropharmacology. In addition there is a section covering neuropsychology, an important and developing area of clinical neuroscience. A key element in the success of the book is the section around clinical examination of the nervous system, building on the basic neuroscience discussed in the preceding chapters.

Have the previous editions been successful? The level of sales and the feedback from students would suggest the book is filling an important slot in the crowded marketplace of clinical neuroscience textbooks. An important part of the success of the "Crash Course" books is that they are written by students for students, and that with every new edition comes a new author with the ability to critically evaluate the previous edition. The third edition was written by Tom Miller and Mark Hughes, and both have now graduated and are developing successful careers in clinical neuroscience. The fourth edition has been revised by Jenny Ross, a senior medical student. The layout of the book has been modified and the self assessment section expanded. However, Jenny has retained the ethos of the previous edition and has made my job as faculty advisor of this edition straightforward. I am delighted with the end result.

Clinical neuroscience remains an exciting and rewarding career choice. Study of the nervous system can initially be daunting but for those who take a little time to familiarize themselves with the basic principles the rewards can be great. Clinical neurosciences impact on all aspects of medical care and patients with neurological problems are common and deserve at least a basic standard of care from all doctors they encounter. I hope this book will encourage students to achieve a fundamental understanding of the nervous system and that, for a small number, will be the first step towards a more detailed knowledge and the beginnings of a long and fulfilling career investigating and treating disorders of the nervous system.

Colin Smith

Acknowledgements

FIGURE CREDITS

Fig. 1.1 with permission from AR Crossman and D Neary. Neuroanatomy, 3e. Churchill Livingstone, Elsevier Ltd, 2005

Figs 4.2, 4.10, 4.12 and 6.21 adapted with permission from AR Crossman and D Neary. Neuroanatomy, 4e. Churchill Livingstone, Elsevier Ltd, 2010

Fig. 8.1 adapted with permission from C Page, M Curtis, M Sutter et al. Integrated Pharmacology. Mosby, Elsevier Ltd 1997

Figs 9.1 and 9.3 adapted with permission from A Stevens and J Lowe. Human Histology, 2e. Mosby, Elsevier Ltd 1997

Fig. 12.1 adapted with permission from R Barker, S Baresi, M Neal. Neuroscience at a Glance, 2e. Wiley-Blackwell Publishers, 2003

Fig. 14.3 adapted with permission from K Lindsay, Neurology and Neurosurgery, 5e. Churchill Livingstone, Elsevier Ltd, 2011

Figs 17.4, 17.8, 17.19, 17.23 and 17.24 adapted with permission from O Epstein, D Perkin, D de Bono, et al. Clinical Examination, 3e. Mosby, Elsevier Ltd, 1997

Figs 17.51, 17.52, 17.59 reproduced with permission from J Weir and P Abrahams. Imaging Atlas of Human Anatomy, 2e. Mosby, Elsevier Ltd, 1997

Contents

Introduction and overview of the nervous system

1

Objectives

In this chapter you will learn about:

- The skull and cranial meninges.
- The cerebral hemispheres and cortices and the effects of cortical damage.
- The blood supply to the central nervous system and cerebrovascular disease.
- The production, function and circulation of cerebrospinal fluid.
- The role of glial cells in the central nervous system.
- The structure and function of the blood–brain barrier.
- The metabolic requirements of the central nervous system.

INTRODUCTION

The nervous system is designed to detect features of the internal and external environments, to process this information, and to use it to direct behaviour and body processes. There are three basic mechanisms that work together to achieve this: perception, information transfer and processing and output to the body.

The nervous system is divided into two anatomically different parts:

- Central nervous system – consisting of the brain and spinal cord
- Peripheral nervous system – this includes all the nerves arriving from and going to the brain and spinal cord.

The peripheral nervous system is divided into somatic and autonomic divisions:

- The somatic division consists of the sensory and motor supply to skin, muscles and joints.
- The autonomic division supplies smooth muscle and glands together with some specialized structures such as pacemaker cells of the heart. One of its main functions is control of the internal environment.

Perception

Specialized receptors in the skin respond to touch, pain and temperature. Receptors in muscle respond to muscle length and others in joints respond to the position of the joint. These combine with information gathered by the special sense organs (sight, hearing, smell and taste) and provide the brain with information about the immediate and remote external environment and the body's position in space. Other receptors monitor the state of the internal environment (e.g. baroreceptors for blood pressure).

Information transfer and processing

Neurons (nerve cells) have specialized projections called axons that can conduct electrical impulses over long distances. Information delivered to neurons can be modified by, or integrated with, other inputs from related areas. In the central nervous system, neurons have many complex connections which allow the brain to use information in several different ways simultaneously.

Output to the body

Once information has been collated and processed by the brain, it is used to drive the outputs of the central nervous system. This includes innervation of other excitable cells such as muscles, internal organs and glands. In this way, the brain controls body movement and can modify circulation and respiration.

COVERINGS OF THE CENTRAL NERVOUS SYSTEM

The brain and spinal cord are supported and protected by the bones of the skull and the vertebral column respectively. Additionally, three membranous layers (meninges) envelop the brain and spinal cord within their bony surrondings; the dura mater is the outermost layer, the middle layer is the arachnoid mater, and the innermost layer is the pia mater.

THE SKULL

The brain rests on the floor of the cranial cavity which consists of three fossae; the anterior, middle, and posterior cranial fossa. Each fossae accommodates particular parts of the brain and contains foramina which provide points of entry and exit for important blood vessels and cranial nerves. This is illustrated in Figures 1.1 and 1.2.

Skull fractures

Skull fractures are common in head injury and are of three main types:

- Linear fractures – simple straight fractures
- Comminuted fractures – complex, branching fractures

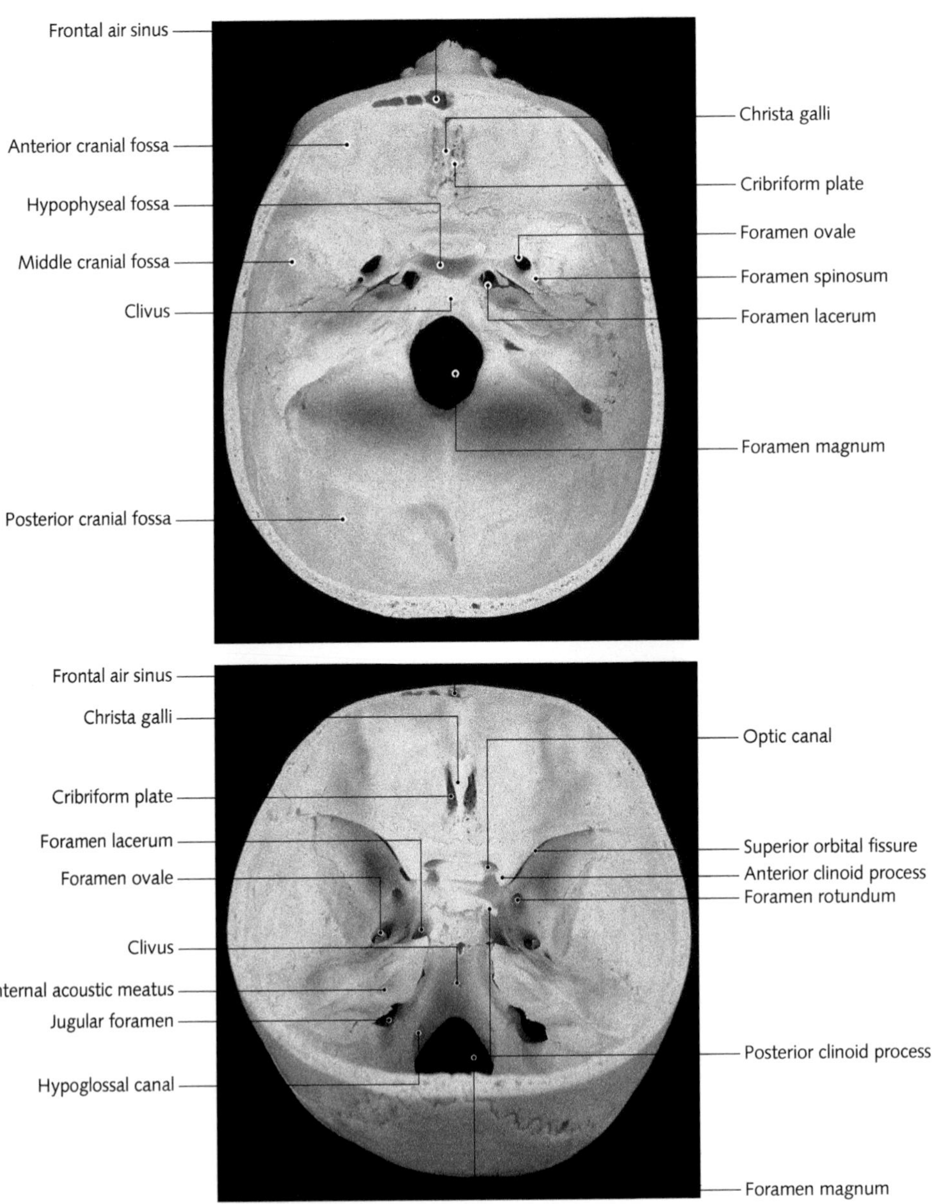

Fig. 1.1 Floor of the cranial cavity.

Fig. 1.2 The three cranial fossae – the parts of the brain they accommodate, the foramina they possess and the nerves and blood vessels entering and leaving the cranial cavity through each

Cranial fossa	Brain structures	Foramina	Nerves/blood vessels
Anterior	Frontal lobe The cribriform plate accommodates the olfactory bulb	Cribriform plate	Olfactory nerve
Middle	Temporal lobe The pituitary gland rests in the hypophyseal fossa	Optic canal	Optic nerve, ophthalmic artery
		Superior orbital fissure	Oculomotor, trochlear, abducens and ophthalmic division of trigeminal nerves
		Foramen rotundum	Maxillary division of trigeminal nerve
		Foramen ovale	Mandibular division of trigeminal nerve
		Foramen lacerum	Internal carotid artery
		Foramen spinosum	Middle meningeal artery
Posterior	Brain stem Cerebellum	Foramen magnum	Medulla oblongata, vertebral arteries, spinal root of accessory nerve
		Hypoglossal canal	Hypoglossal nerve
		Jugular foramen	Internal jugular vein, glossopharyngeal, vagus, accessory nerves
		Internal auditory meatus	Facial, vestibulocochlear nerves

- Depressed fractures – inner table is depressed by at least the thickness of the skull.

When a skull fracture is suspected, a skull radiograph and/or a CT scan should be obtained to confirm the diagnosis. Complications of skull fractures are:

- Extradural haematoma – often caused by linear fractures crossing the middle meningeal groove and causing the rupture of the middle meningeal artery. This may be associated with a 'lucid interval' after the injury as the blood clot expands, with a subsequently decreasing conscious level. Neurosurgical evacuation is required to prevent rising intracranial pressure resulting in brain displacement and death.
- Cerebrospinal fluid rhinorrhoea (cerebrospinal fluid leak from the nose) caused by skull-base fractures tearing the dura in the floor of the anterior fossa and the nasal mucosa. This might occasionally be accompanied by pneumatocoeles and fluid (visible on radiographs), particularly in the sphenoidal sinuses.
- Cerebrospinal fluid otorrhoea (cerebrospinal fluid leak from the ear) caused by fractures of the petrous temporal bone.
- Infection – particularly with compound fractures and persistent cerebrospinal fluid fistulae (cerebrospinal fluid rhinorrhoea and otorrhoea), in which case prophylactic antibiotic cover is needed.

HINTS AND TIPS

Basal skull fractures may not be immediately obvious. Signs include bilateral 'black eyes', bruising over the mastoid process (Battle's sign) and subconjunctival haemorrhage with no clear posterior margin (indicating blood tracking forward). Avoid nasogastric tubes and nasal airways in these patients.

MENINGES

Three concentric membranous layers envelope the brain and spinal cord. The outermost layer, the dura mater, is a tough, fibrous, loose-fitting membrane. Two large relections of dura extend into the cranial cavity; the falx cerebri occupies the great longitudinal fissure between the cerebral hemispheres, while the tentorium cerebelli lies horizontally between the cerebellum and the occipital lobes. The dural venous sinuses, important in the venous drainage of the brain, are described later in the chapter. The arachnoid mater is a translucent membrane that, like the dura mater, loosely surrounds the brain. The subdural space is a virtual space that separates the dura and arachnoid mater, and is transversed by veins en route to the venous sinuses. The pia mater is microscopically thin and closely adherant to the surface of the brain.

Between the pia and arachnoid mater lies the subarachnoid space containing cerebrospinal fluid (CSF) and large blood vessels.

Meningitis

Acute bacterial meningitis

Acute bacterial meningitis is an infection of the pia mater with pus filling the subarachnoid space. Causative organisms vary according to patient age. Three bacteria account for over three-quarters of all cases:

- Neisseria meningitidis (meningococcus)
- Haemophilus influenzae (if very young and unvaccinated)
- Streptococcus pneumoniae (pneumococcus).

Other organisms to consider:

- Neonates: *Escherichia coli*, ß-haemolytic streptococci, *Listeria monocytogenes*
- Elderly and immunocompromised: Listeria, tuberculosis, Gram-negative bacteria
- Hospital-acquired infections: Klebsiella, Escherichia coli, Pseudomonas, *Staphylococcus aureus*.

Clinical features are:

- Fever, headache, photophobia, painful eye movements. Impaired consciousness is a late and ominous feature
- Neck stiffness, positive Kernig's sign
- Occasionally – petechial skin rash (meningococcal meningitis), focal neurological signs, particularly cranial nerve palsies.

Investigations

- In the presence of impaired consciousness or focal neurological signs, a head CT scan should be performed first to exclude a space-occupying lesion.
- Lumbar puncture is the key investigation. CSF will be turbid with a very high polymorphonuclear cell count and low glucose. An immediate Gram stain should be performed and the cerebrospinal fluid should be sent for culture.

Treatment

- Meningitis is a very serious but potentially treatable condition. It is a medical emergency and prompt treatment may save lives and limit morbidity.
- If the lumbar puncture cannot be performed immediately, prompt 'blind' treatment with a broad-spectrum antibiotic could be life saving. General practitioners who suspect meningitis in the community should give benzylpenicillin (1.2 g intramuscularly/intravenously) without delay.
- Prophylactic antibiotics for close contacts (family, school, college, etc.) should be considered.

Prognosis

- Mortality remains high.
- Overall mortality in developed countries ranges between 5% and 30%, depending on the causative organism.

Aseptic meningitis

A large number of viruses (mumps, enteroviruses, coxsackie A and B, Epstein–Barr virus) produce an acute self-limiting aseptic meningitis. Patients are moderately ill with fever, malaise, headache, vomiting and mild neck stiffness. Impaired consciousness is suggestive of an encephalic component.

Cerebrospinal fluid examination shows moderate lymphocytosis. The protein is only slightly elevated and glucose is normal. There is no specific treatment and recovery after a few days is the rule.

Note that an aseptic picture is also seen in partially treated bacterial meningitis.

HINTS AND TIPS

All children should now be vaccinated against haemophilus (B) and meningococcus type C, which were previously the commonest causes of meningitis in children. A good history of vaccinations is important in deciding on appropriate empirical treatment.

THE CEREBRAL HEMISPHERES AND CEREBRAL CORTEX

Anatomy

The fully developed central nervous system is shown in Figure 1.3.

The central nervous system is divided into regions of grey and white matter. In the cerebrum the grey matter may be superficial (cortical ribbon) or deep (deep grey nuclei). Both grey and white matter contain many cell types (astrocytes, oligodendrocytes, microglia, endothelial cells), but only grey matter contains neuronal cell bodies. White matter appears white due to the high myelin content.

The cerebral cortex is divided into four lobes on the basis of the folds (sulci) in the surface, as shown in Figure 1.4:

- The frontal lobe is separated from the parietal lobe by the central sulcus.
- The temporal lobe is separated from these two lobes by the lateral sulcus.
- Demarcation of the occipital lobe is difficult to appreciate from a lateral view but, on the medial (midsagittal) view (Fig. 1.5), the parieto-occipital sulcus can be seen. The leaf-like folia of the cerebellum (sitting behind the midbrain, pons and medulla) can also be seen.

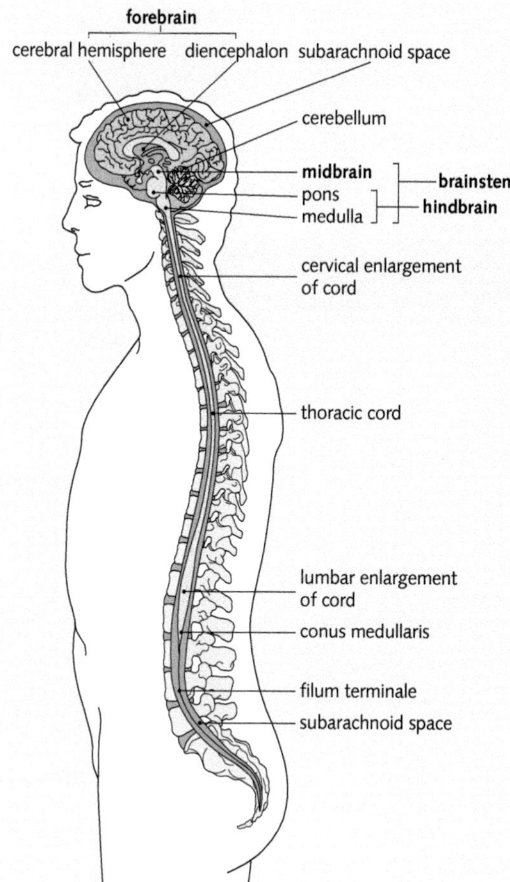

Fig. 1.3 Midsagittal section of the central nervous system showing components of the forebrain, midbrain, hindbrain and spinal cord.

Structure and functional asymmetry

On a macroscopic level the two cerebral hemispheres appear symmetrical and equal. However, on closer examination there are subtle differences between the two hemispheres. For example, the planum temporale (the superior aspect of the temporal lobe lying within the lateral sulcus and forming the junction between the temporal, occipital and parietal lobes) tends to be larger in the left hemisphere of most people. Wernicke's area lies in the posterior part of the planum temporale and is central to the comprehension of speech. Damage here (e.g. following a stroke) results in a lack of language comprehension. Furthermore, when one considers that the left-hand side of the brain controls the right side of the body (which tends to be the dominant hand in most people) it is unsurprising that the left hemisphere is usually described as the dominant hemisphere. However, a small but significant number of left-handed people have a dominant right hemisphere. To screen for this during the history ask which hand the patient writes with.

Despite being joined primarily by the corpus callosum, the two hemispheres carry out different functions. Evidence for this comes from:

- Patients with lesions localized to one hemisphere (e.g. patients who have aphasia following a left hemisphere stroke)
- Patients with severe grand mal epilepsy who have undergone sectioning of the corpus callosum (commissurotomy) to prevent spread of seizures
- 'Split-brain' animal studies, in which a commissurotomy was carried out.

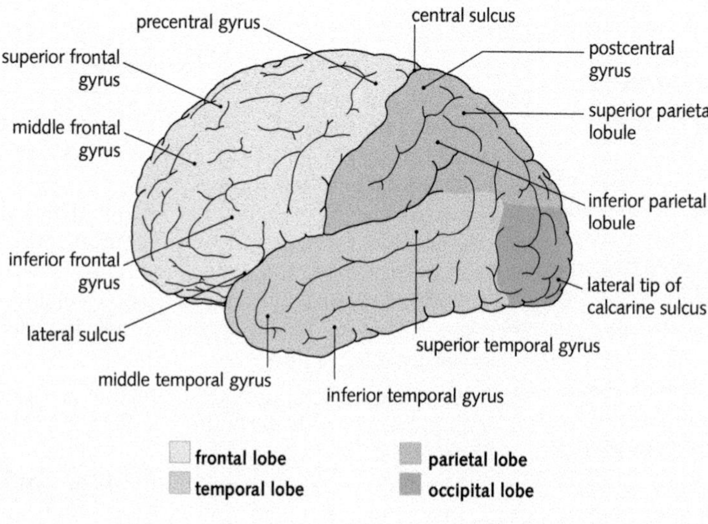

Fig. 1.4 Left cerebral hemisphere, lateral view showing major lobes.

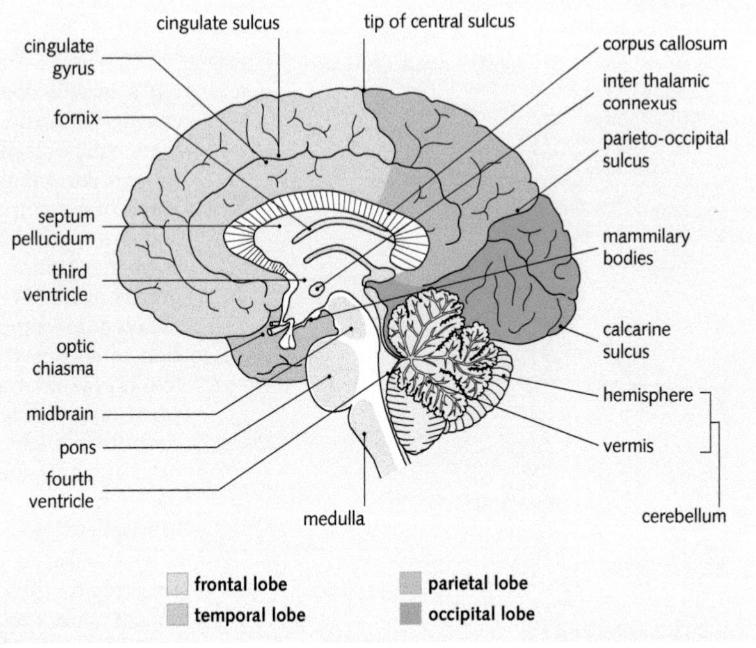

Fig. 1.5 Medial view of the right side of the brain, showing deep structures, midbrain and hindbrain.

An unfortunate fact of neuroscience is that much of our understanding of how the brain works has arisen from 'lesion studies' in which patients have suffered damage (accidental, warfare or iatrogenic) to their brain and as a result developed very specific deficits in particular domains. Furthermore, the localization of functional areas has been experimentally demonstrated by:

- Positron emission tomography (PET) or functional magnetic resonance imaging (fMRI) of normal subjects performing a range of tasks
- Wada's test, in which sodium amobarbital (sodium amytal) is injected into one carotid artery, which temporarily anaesthetizes one hemisphere so that tasks can be processed only by the other one. For example, injection of sodium amobarbital into the left carotid artery will temporarily block speech in most subjects.

Split-brain and other experiments may not give us the whole story, as there is some evidence that the ability of a hemisphere to carry out a task may deteriorate after commissurotomy. In a simplified form, lateralization can be summarized as thus:

- The left hemisphere is involved in intellectual reasoning and language.
- The right hemisphere is more concerned with spatial construction (including depth perception and the internal 'map' of our surroundings) and emotion.

Why should the left and right hemispheres carry out different functions at all? It is believed that to speed up the processing power of the brain, the two hemispheres operate largely independent of each other on their particular functions and hemispheric communication only ensues when more 'processing power' is needed.

There is an element of plasticity in the location of function. In children who sustain damage to one hemisphere, the other one can take over its functions so that there is no appreciable deficit. This is not the case in adults, as shown by the effects of a stroke.

Cortical localization

While reading this book it should become apparent that specific functions are performed solely by different areas of the brain (e.g. visual processing in the occipital lobe, coordination in the cerebellum). The same is true for the other lobes and their cortices.

The lobes can be split up into regions that act as functional units through which information can flow and can be processed. These functional units lie in different cortical regions and their 'functions' depend on their specific input and output connections. In general, lobes can be split up into:

- Primary sensory or motor areas which receive information from outside the brain or project outside the brain.
- Higher-order sensory or motor areas which carry out further processing of information from one

modality (e.g. sight or sound). For example, visual areas V2–V5 segregate information into the colour, form and motion channels. The supplementary motor area has a role in planning movements by integrating inputs from the prefrontal cortex (PFC), basal ganglia and cingulate cortex.
- Association areas where information from different modalities comes together for processing, forming a cohesive representation of the experienced world. For example, the sights, sounds and smells of a rugby match coming together so we can enjoy the 'whole scene'.

However, each lobe is normally ascribed particular functions, forming an anatomical basis for the 'higher functions'.

Frontal lobes

The frontal lobes lie anterior to the central sulcus and contain several functional areas:

- The primary motor cortex (M1) on the precentral gyrus is involved with the initiation of muscle movement (see Ch. 6).
- The premotor and supplementary motor areas just anterior to M1 are involved in the cortical programming and preparation of movement and control of posture (see Ch. 6).
- Broca's area is where the muscle movements that articulate speech are determined before being sent to the bulbar muscles via the cranial nerves. This is the 'how' of speech.
- A frontal eye field (Brodmann's area 8) lying on the middle frontal gyrus controls voluntary conjugate deviation of the eyes while scanning the visual field.
- An extensive area of cortex lying anterior to the motor fields, known as the prefrontal cortex (PFC), is rich in connections from the parietal, temporal and occipital cortices. Association fibres run through the PFC primarily through the subcortical white matter. The PFC is also innervated by several brainstem nuclei (see Ch. 6).

HINTS AND TIPS

Phineas Gage is the most famous patient with frontal lobe damage. Following a railway accident where a tamping rod was forced through Gage's frontal lobes producing a crude frontal lobectomy, Gage went from being a capable, efficient and shrewd business man to being impatient, obstinate and impulsive. His friends said that he was 'no longer Gage'.

HINTS AND TIPS

The prefrontal cortex (PFC) is often seen as the home of higher function, where we plan behaviour and our sequence of response, change our response patterns to the dynamic demands of our environment and where we control our emotional state.

Parietal lobes

The parietal lobes contain:

- A primary somatosensory cortex contained within the postcentral gyrus, the most anterior part of the lobe. Thalamocortical neurons terminate here and this corresponds to the third and final relay elevating general sensation from peripheral receptors to a conscious level.
- The superior parietal lobe receives several sensory modalities and motor inputs. Here these inputs build up a picture of how the body is positioned in the environment.

The parietal lobes in each hemisphere represent the contralateral half of space (the world around us). However, space is not equally represented in the hemispheres. The left hemisphere represents only the right side of space, whereas the right hemisphere represents all of the left side of space and some of the right. This means that the right side of space is 'viewed' by both hemispheres and is slightly over-represented. Clinically, this means that lesions to the left parietal cortex will not completely disrupt processing of the right side of space because the right hemisphere can compensate to some degree. Right-sided lesions will produce more severe effects on the processing of the left half of space, because this is not carried out elsewhere in the brain. This phenomenon is known as neglect (see Ch. 8).

Temporal lobes

The temporal lobes contain:

- An auditory association cortex which lies immediately posterior to the primary auditory cortex. In the dominant hemisphere this is known as Wernicke's area, where language comprehension and responses occurs.
- Other higher-order sensory areas involved in visual object recognition.
- The inferomedial part of the temporal lobe curls inwards to form the hippocampus which lies in the floor of the inferior horn of the lateral ventricle deep to the parahippocampal gyrus. Both structures are involved in learning and memory (see Ch. 13)
- Towards the anterior end of the hippocampus and temporal lobes lies a collection of subcortical grey matter known as the amygdala.

Occipital lobes

Chapter 8 describes more fully the function and roles of the occipital lobes and cortex in the construction of the visual world.

HINTS AND TIPS

Anton's syndrome is characterized by a delusion of reality in which a blind person denies their blindness. Despite the complete blindness, the patient confabulates and denies any loss of visual perception. This is usually due to bilateral medial occipital cortex damage producing cortical blindness. This usually follows stroke or haemorrhage.

Figure 1.6 demonstrates roughly what happens where in the cortex.

CORTICAL DAMAGE

The various functions of the different lobes have already been covered. What remains is to understand the effects of damage to these areas.

Frontal lobes

Damage to the frontal lobes can produce particular neurological deficits such as:

- An inability to organize responses and to solve problems.
- Motor weakness if lesions involve primary motor cortex.
- 'Perseveration'. This occurs when one is unable to change a response pattern when required to. The Wisconsin card-sorting test is based on the ability of a subject to sort cards according to one rule (e.g. same colour) and then according to another rule (e.g. to sort the cards into the same pattern). The subject determines the new rule by feedback from the examiner about correct or incorrect card sorting. Perseveration occurs when subjects do not stop using a previously correct rule that is now incorrect. In other words they persevere with the old rule despite it being wrong.
- Personality changes in emotional states referred to as disinhibition. People no longer behave appropriately in social situations (they do whatever they want whenever they want).
- Disordered eye movements while scanning a visual field.
- Damage to Broca's area produces expressive dysphasia which is hesitant and limited (described as telegrammatic). Patients may not be able to say particular words.
- Disordered working memory with distractability (see later).

It is rare for these patients to have insight into their condition.

HINTS AND TIPS

Perseveration may be an important feature in dementia. When asked their name, patients may answer correctly, but subsequent (different) questions will elicit the same answer.

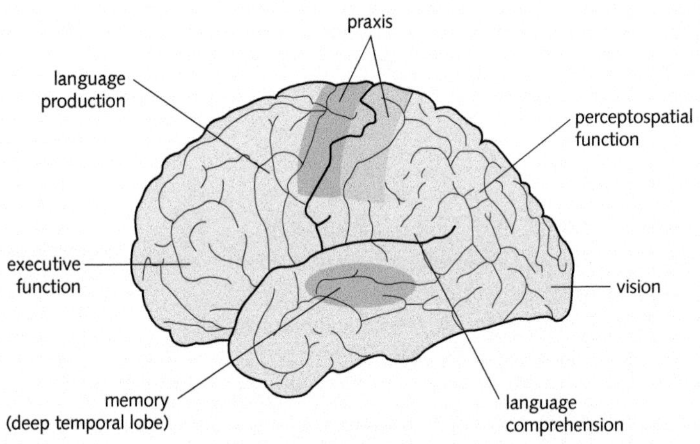

Fig. 1.6 The functional topography of the cerebral cortex by areas.

Parietal lobes

Lesions of the parietal cortex will produce:

- Lack of conscious sensation in the contralateral half of the body
- Attentional defects presenting as neglect
- Inability to make voluntary eye movements and optic ataxia after bilateral parieto-occipital damage (Balint's syndrome)
- Constructional apraxia: an inability to organize movement in space with right-sided lesions (remembering the general function of the right hemisphere). This is tested with the Mini-Mental State Examination (MMSE) by asking the patient to draw two interlocking pentagons
- Disorder of spatial awareness (usually right-sided) presenting with defects in route finding
- Disorder of language (especially if dominant hemispheric damage)
- Agnosia: an inability to perceive and recognize objects normally (see Ch. 7). Patients with parietal damage may also have astereognosia – an inability to recognize objects by touch. For example, they could not pick out a particular coin from a selection in a pocket by touch alone.

Temporal lobes

Temporal lobes lesions produce the following deficits:

- Disorders of verbal information learning in left-sided lesions and visuospatial information learning in right-sided lesions (remembering the general roles of each hemisphere).
- Problems in understanding spoken and written language but no reduction seen in the fluency of language (receptive aphasia; compare with expressive dysphasia). This results in meaningless and irrelevant speech, with little understanding.
- Object agnosia, whereby patients cannot recognize objects from visual information but can do so via other modalities of sense (e.g. touch).

Connections

Commissural fibres connect neurons in different hemispheres. Association fibres connect neurons in the same hemisphere. Projection fibres connect the cerebral cortex with lower levels of the brain and spinal cord. There are vast numbers of connections in the central nervous system and there are many inputs modulating the effects of all connections.

THE BLOOD SUPPLY TO THE CENTRAL NERVOUS SYSTEM

Figure 1.7 shows the arteries which supply blood to the brain. These form an anastomosis known as the circle of Willis. Figure 1.8 shows the territories of the major arteries supplying the cortex. Knowledge of these is required when assessing a person with a stroke. Four vessels supply the brain: right and left internal carotid and vertebral arteries:

- The internal carotid arteries send off two branches (the anterior and posterior communicating arteries)

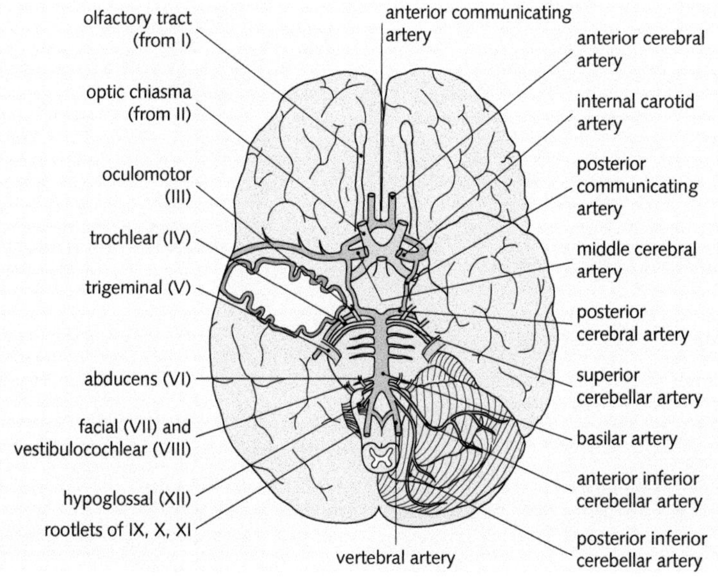

Fig. 1.7 Blood supply to the brain, showing the circle of Willis and its relation to the cranial nerves.

Fig. 1.8 Territories of the cerebral arteries. (A) Lateral and (B) medial views of the left and right cerebral hemispheres. (C) Coronal (transverse) section through the cerebral hemispheres.

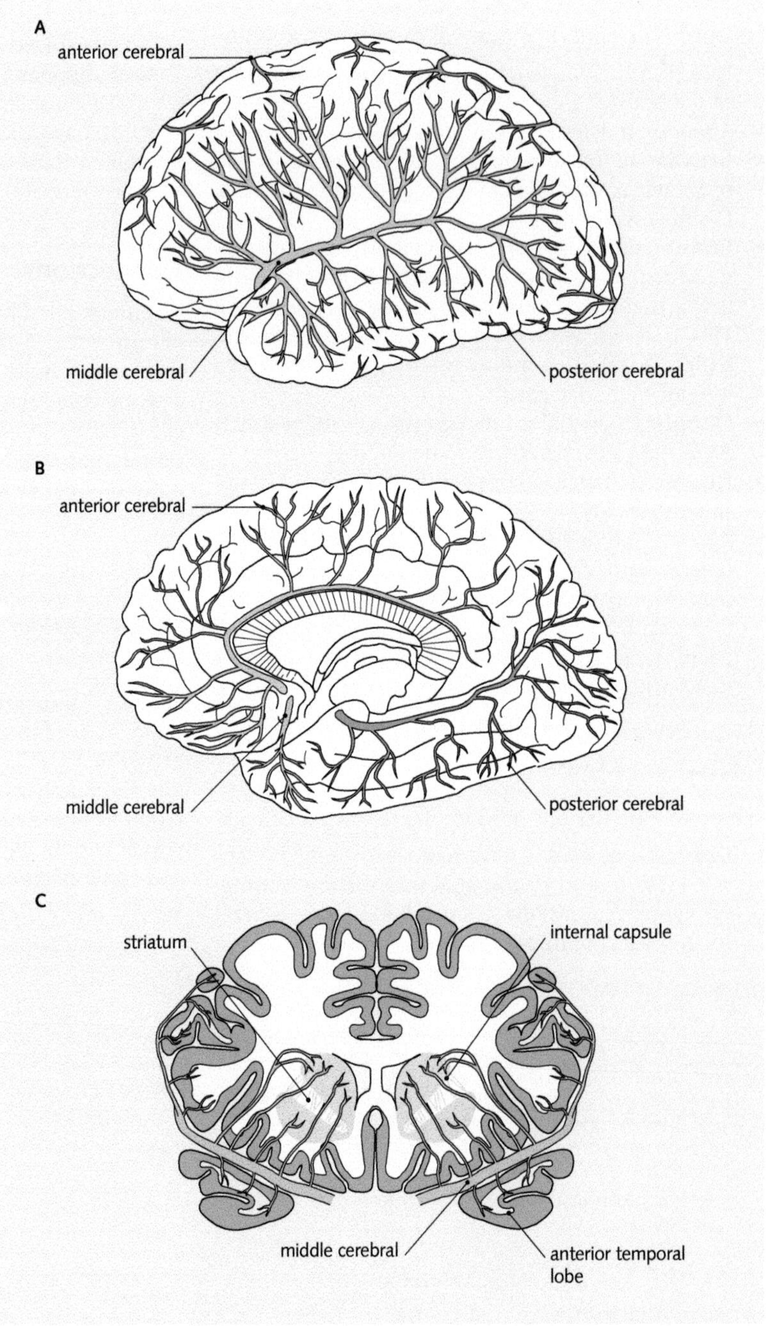

before becoming the middle cerebral artery. This artery has an extensive territory, supplying most of the surface of the brain and some of the basal ganglia.

- The anterior cerebral arteries travel forward on either side of the longitudinal fissure to supply the medial surface of each cerebral hemisphere.
- The vertebral arteries join at the inferior border of the pons to form the single basilar artery. Branches of the vertebral arteries and the basilar artery supply the medulla, pons and cerebellum.
- The posterior cerebral arteries supply the occipital and temporal lobes. Most of their input is derived

from the basilar artery, with a contribution from the carotid vessels via the posterior communicating arteries.

The loop formed between the basilar artery and the internal carotid vessels (via the anterior and posterior communicating arteries) is known as the circle of Willis.

Venous drainage from the cortex is via the superior sagittal sinus which runs in the longitudinal fissure. This drains into the transverse sinuses where it joins the blood coming from the cerebellum and brainstem (Fig. 1.9).

Optic, olfactory and some facial structures drain into the cavernous sinus, which contains many important structures including:

- Internal carotid artery
- Cranial nerves III, IV, VI and the ophthalmic and maxillary divisions of cranial nerve V.

Blood travels from the cavernous sinus to the transverse sinus via the superior petrosal sinus and directly to the internal jugular via the inferior petrosal sinus.

The inferior sagittal sinus and the internal cerebral vein drain the deep structures of the cortex into the straight sinus, which later joins with the transverse sinus. Together, they drain into the internal jugular vein.

HINTS AND TIPS

Spread of infection from the face or orbit may result in cavernous sinus thrombosis. As the infection tracts posteriorly, the patient complains of orbital pain, periorbital oedema and visual disturbances. Common signs are a red swollen eye, exophthalmos and palsies of the nerves that run through the cavernous sinus (III, IV, V, VI). On funduscopy, papilloedema may be seen.

CEREBROVASCULAR DISEASE

Hypoxia, ischaemia and infarction

There are almost no tissue stores of oxygen or glucose in the brain. When blood supply fails, the brain ceases to function and cerebral ischaemia ensues resulting in tissue infarction. Cerebral blood flow is maintained by a number of homeostatic mechanisms at approximately 54 mL/100 g per minute, a process termed autoregulation. This begins to fail when the mean arterial blood pressure falls below a level of 60–70 mm Hg. Cerebral

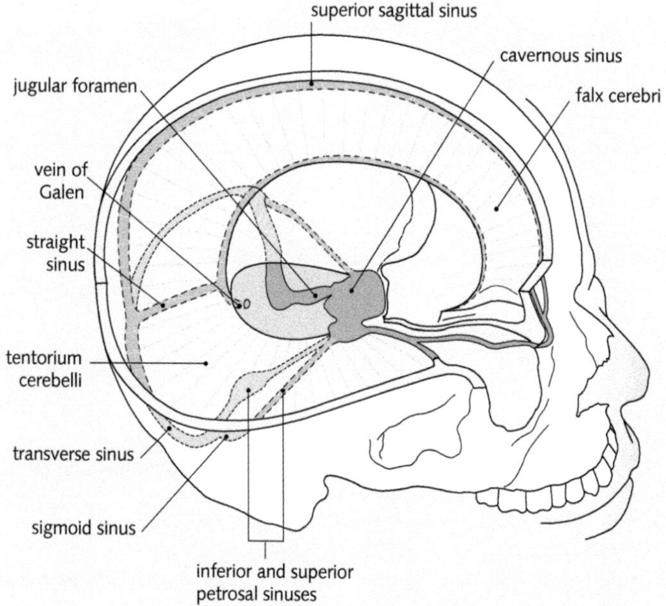

Fig. 1.9 The venous sinuses.

perfusion pressure (CPP) is the difference between systemic blood pressure (SBP) and intracranial pressure (ICP) - CPP= SBP−ICP.

HINTS AND TIPS

Patients with intracranial mass lesions causing raised ICP will have systemic hypertension and bradycardia (Cushing reponse).

Progression from reversible ischaemia to infarction depends on degree and duration of reduced blood flow. Cerebral blood flow below 28 mL/100 g per minute results in development of the morphological changes of infarction (tissue pan-necrosis). The central necrotic zone of an infarct is surrounded by an 'ischaemic penumbra' - an area of tissue which is damaged, but remains viable for a given time period. Restoration of blood flow may, therefore, give a clinical improvement.

Mechanisms of stroke

Strokes can be either thromboembolic or haemorrhagic. Thromboembolic infarcts are predominantly secondary to atheroma or cardiogenic emboli, although very rarely infarcts may be seen secondary to embolic material such as fat (fractured long bones) or malignancy. Haemorrhagic infarcts are mostly seen in the setting of hypertension, although other causes include underlying malignancy or vascular malformation, trauma, vasculitis, recreational drugs and iatrogenic causes.

Hypertensive infarcts occur most frequently in the following sites:

- The putamen and the internal capsule
- Central white matter
- Thalamus
- Cerebellar hemisphere
- Pons.

It is often very difficult to differentiate clinically between primary cerebral haemorrhage and thromboembolic infarction, and pathologically between thrombotic and embolic infarctions.

Transient ischaemic attack

Transient ischaemic attack is a focal neurological deficit of a presumed vascular origin from which a full clinical recovery occurs within 24 hours. They are thromboembolic in nature and should be recognized and managed promptly because they are an indication that a full stroke may be imminent. Carotid territory transient ischaemic attacks present with:

- Transient monocular blindness (amaurosis fugax)
- Transient sensory or motor symptoms of the face, arm or leg
- Transient aphasia.

Vertebrobasilar transient ischaemic attacks present with a combination of:

- Dysarthria
- Vertigo and unsteadiness
- Diplopia
- Circumoral paraesthesiae
- Sensory or motor symptoms affecting the limbs singly or in combination
- Cranial nerve palsies.

HINTS AND TIPS

Patients often describe amaurosis fugax as 'a black curtain descending over one eye'.

Ischaemic stroke

Thromboembolic infarctions constitute approximately 85% of all strokes. The clinical features are extremely variable and depend on the site and the extent of the lesion (Fig. 1.10).

Haemorrhagic stroke

Haemorrhagic strokes constitute 15% of all strokes. They are usually hypertensive (Fig. 1.11). In the majority of cases, the symptoms develop while the patient is awake and active. Headache is a prominent feature. Clinical features depend on the site of bleeding:

- Capsular haemorrhage - hemiplegia (face, arm and leg) and depressed consciousness
- Pontine haemorrhage - tetraplegia, small pupils and coma
- Cerebellar haemorrhage - severe headache, ipsilateral ataxia and depressed consciousness.

Investigations

Investigations should be directed towards confirming the diagnosis (CT, MRI) and addressing the aetiological factors (electrocardiogram, carotid Doppler, echocardiogram).

Management

Acutely, use the 'BRAIN ATTACK' mnemonic:

- B - Blood pressure. Do not treat acutely (discuss with senior if > 200/120 mmHg)
- R - Respiration. Keep O_2 saturation > 95%
- A - Airway management
- I - Intravenous saline. Keep hydrated
- N - Normoglycaemia. Avoid dextrose
- A - Aspirin. As soon as haemorrhage excluded on CT scan

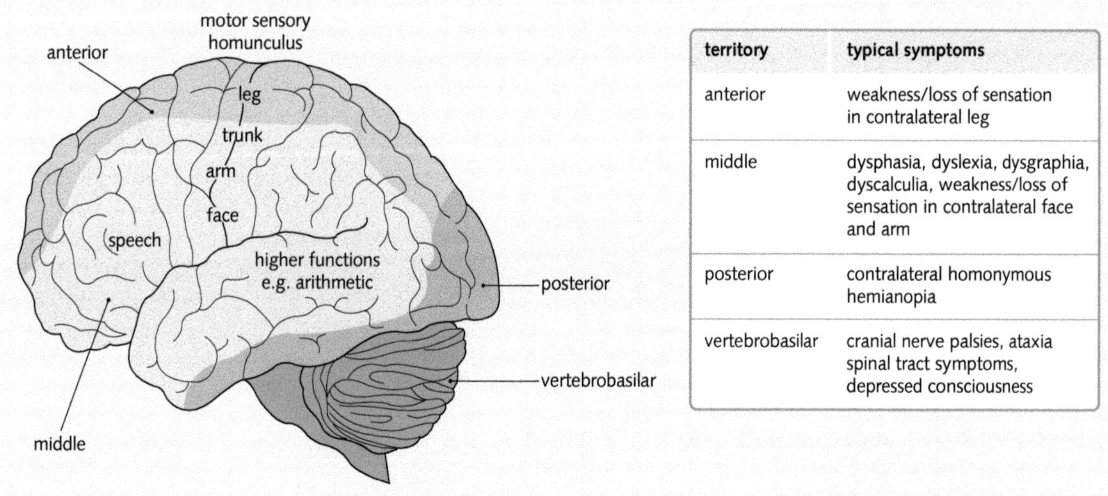

territory	typical symptoms
anterior	weakness/loss of sensation in contralateral leg
middle	dysphasia, dyslexia, dysgraphia, dyscalculia, weakness/loss of sensation in contralateral face and arm
posterior	contralateral homonymous hemianopia
vertebrobasilar	cranial nerve palsies, ataxia spinal tract symptoms, depressed consciousness

Fig. 1.10 Cerebral artery territories and symptoms of strokes in those areas.

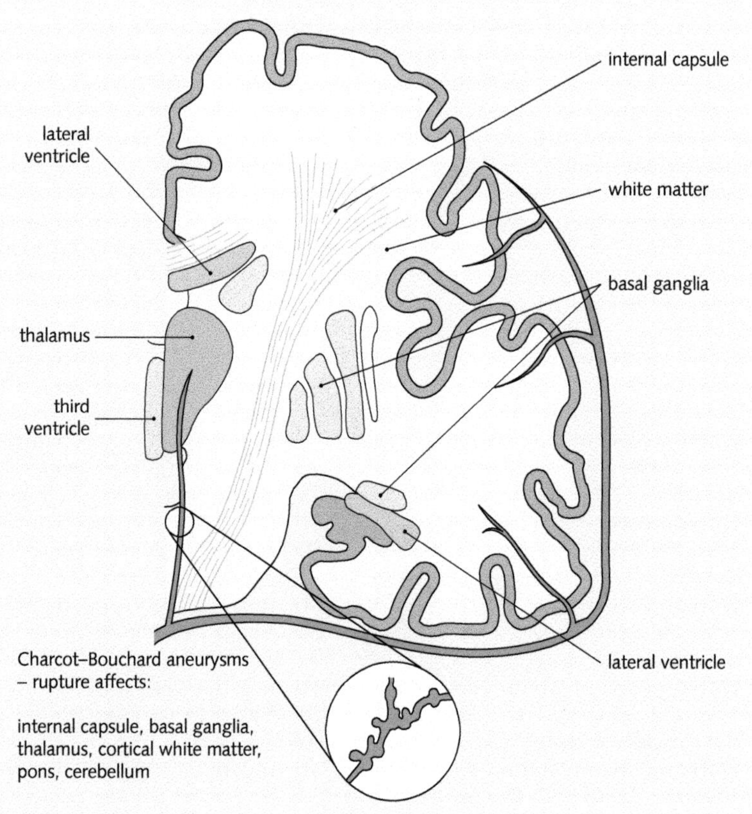

Fig. 1.11 Charcot–Bouchard aneurysms and the structures with rupture effects.

- T – Temperature. Keep $< 37\,^{\circ}C$ and treat pyrexia urgently
- T – TEDS (compression stockings) for all to prevent deep vein thrombosis
- A – Assess water swallow test
- C – CT scan as soon as possible
- K – Keep 30° head-up tilt.

In an established stroke, skilled nursing and physiotherapy are the main pillars of treatment. Specialist stroke units have lower mortality than standard hospital care. For secondary prevention, all potentially modifiable risk factors should be addressed. Aspirin or warfarin and endarterectomy (for severe symptomatic carotid stenosis) should be considered. Evidence suggests that all people with proven atheromatous disease should be on lifelong lipid-lowering drugs (statins).

Subarachnoid haemorrhage

Subarachnoid haemorrhage is relatively uncommon and typically occurs in people between the ages of 35 and 65 years. Rupture of a cerebral berry aneurysm is the commonest cause (70%), with arteriovenous malformations accounting for 15% of cases. Berry aneurysms result from a defect in the media and elastica of the cerebral arteries, causing the media to bulge outward covered only by the adventitia. Genetic factors are important, particularly polycystic kidney disease and coarctation of the aorta.

Berry aneurysms vary in size (average 1 cm) and shape, and are commonly located at bifurcations of the cerebral arteries (Fig. 1.12). The severity of symptoms is related to the severity of the bleed with:

- Severe headache 'as if hit on the head with a sledgehammer'
- Nausea and vomiting.

The signs of subarachnoid haemorrhage are:

- Neck stiffness, positive Kernig's sign (pain on passively extending the knee when the hip is flexed to 90°) – both are signs of meningeal irritation, which develop 6 hours after the bleed
- Focal neurological signs (particularly III nerve palsy in posterior communicating artery aneurysms)
- Drowsiness, depressed consciousness
- Retinal haemorrhages.

Patients should be investigated with head CT scanning. A lumbar puncture should be performed if the scan is normal. This may show frank blood or xanthochromia (indicative of previous blood in the cerebrospinal fluid). CT angiography and/or digital subtraction angiography are used to locate the aneurysm(s). Patients should be kept in bed and given adequate analgesia. The aneurysm(s) should be clipped or coiled at an appropriate time.

Mortality is related to the severity of the bleed and is particularly high in patients with depressed consciousness.

THE VENTRICULAR SYSTEM AND CEREBROSPINAL FLUID

The ventricles of the brain contain cerebrospinal fluid and are joined together to allow the fluid to circulate. The paired lateral ventricles (Fig. 1.13) have frontal, occipital and temporal horns and communicate with the third ventricle (which lies posterior and inferior) through the interventricular foramen of Monro.

HINTS AND TIPS

The ventricles may become distorted by a space-occupying lesion. CT or MRI allow this 'mass effect' to be visualized.

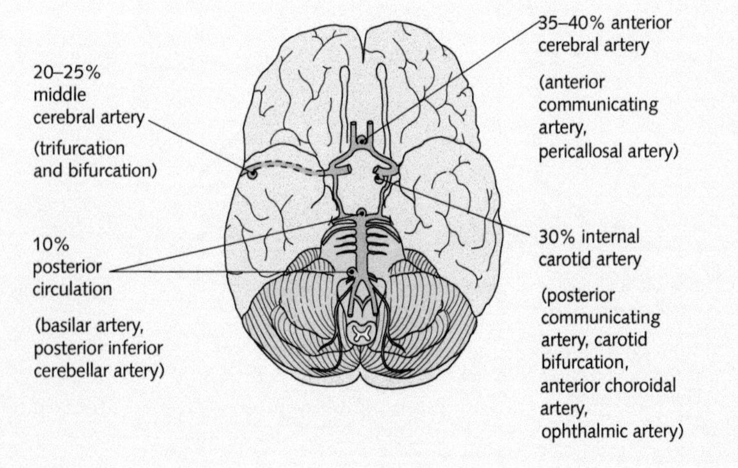

Fig. 1.12 Common sites of aneurysms of the intracranial vessels.

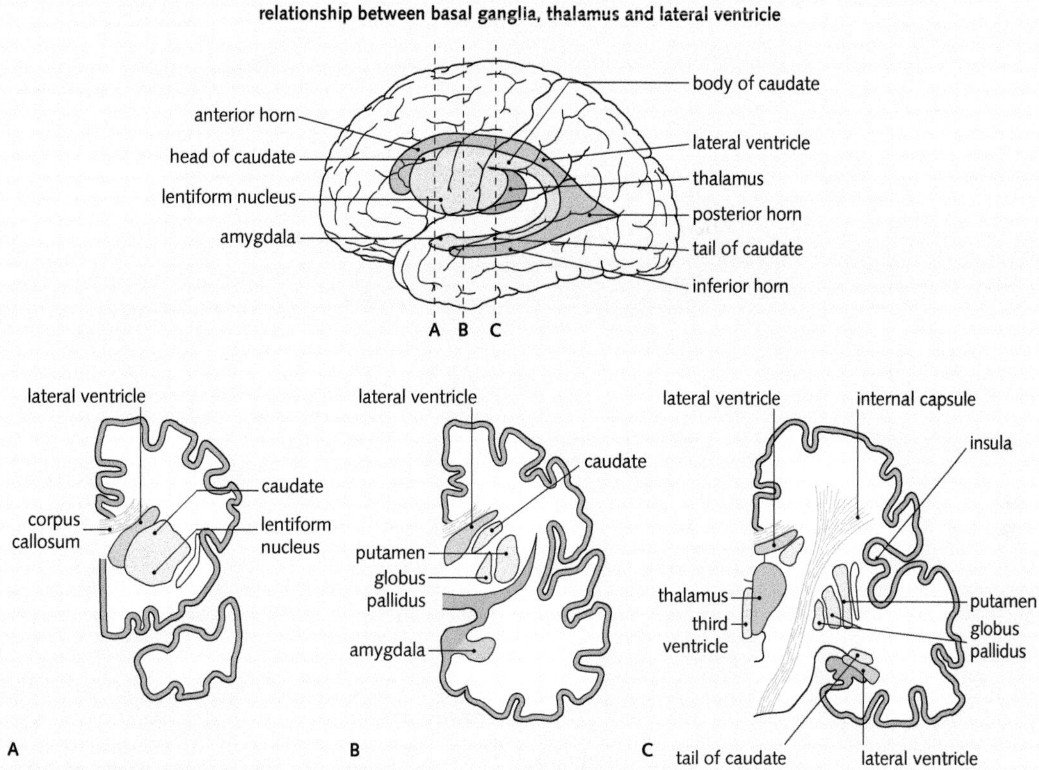

Fig. 1.13 The lateral ventricle, and its relationship to the basal ganglia and thalamus.

The cerebrospinal fluid circulates in the ventricles, spinal canal and subarachnoid space. It provides a cushion to prevent the delicate nervous tissue from being damaged by surrounding bones. The CSF also plays an active role in providing nutrition to the central nervous system and in removing waste products.

Most of the CSF is formed by the choroid plexi of the lateral, third and fourth ventricles. The CSF is produced at a rate of approximately 500 mL/day in an adult. As the total CSF space is 100–150 mL (30 mL in the ventricles and the remainder in the subarachnoid space) this volume must be turned over approximately three times a day. Groups of choroid plexus epithelial cells project into the ventricles, giving a folded appearance. These folds contain a leaky fenestrated capillary in the centre, and on their surface have microvilli which project into the ventricles. Figure 1.14 depicts the flow of CSF.

The CSF is produced by a combination of capillary filtration and active transport of solutes. Blood and CSF are in osmotic equilibrium because water follows the gradients created. Despite the protein content of CSF being approximately 1000-fold lower than that of blood plasma, its higher ionic concentration results in the two fluids having the same osmolality. Figure 1.15 shows the differences between blood and CSF. These parameters can be measured on lumbar puncture.

The CSF flows from the lateral ventricles into the third ventricle (through the foramen of Munro) and then through the aqueduct of Sylvius into the fourth ventricle. From here it gains access to the subarachnoid space via three orifices: a medial foramen of Magendie and two lateral foramina of Luschka. It reaches the nervous tissue by travelling along blood vessels in the perivascular (Virchow–Robin) space (Fig. 1.16) where it equilibrates with extracellular fluid. By equilibrating with brain extracellular fluid, unwanted metabolites are excreted into the blood. As the choroid plexus is able to absorb material from CSF (choline, dopamine, serotonin metabolites, urea, creatinine, K^+) it can be considered an excretory organ of the brain.

CSF is taken back into the circulation by:

- Arachnoid granulations, which are protrusions of the arachnoid space covered by a thin layer of cells that line the venous sinuses
- Perineural lymph vessels of the cranial and spinal nerves.

CSF surrounding the brain confers three primary mechanical benefits:

- By floating the brain in a fluid-filled compartment its effective weight is reduced from approximately 1.4 kg to just 50 g.

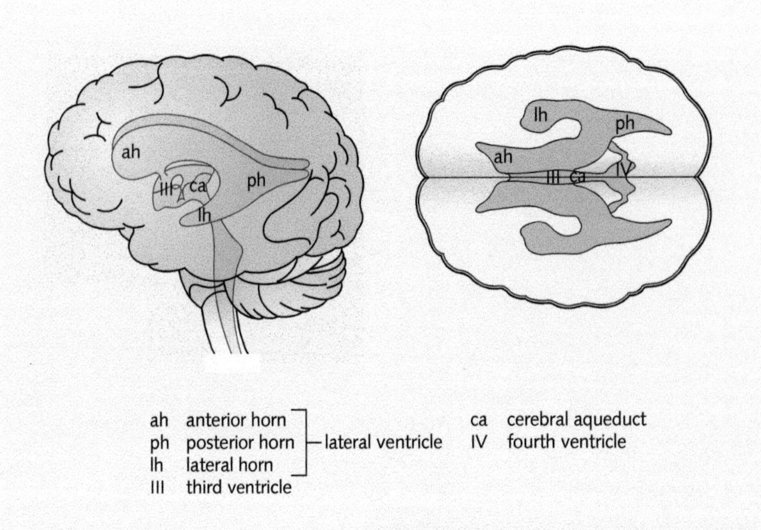

Fig. 1.14 The ventricular system. Fluid produced in the lateral ventricles drains via the interventricular foramina into the third ventricle, where more cerebrospinal fluid (CSF) is added by choroid plexus tissue of the third ventricle. Flow continues via the aqueduct of the midbrain to the fourth ventricle. From here fluid escapes into the subarachnoid space via two lateral apertures.

Fig. 1.15 Differences between blood plasma and cerebrospinal fluid (CSF)

	Plasma	CSF
Protein (mg/dl)	7000	35
Glucose (mg/dl)	90	60
Na (mmol/l)	138	138
K (mmol/l)	4.5	2.8
Osmolarity (mOsm/l)	295	295
pH	7.41	7.33

- Adjustments to CSF and meninges compensate for transient changes in intracranial pressure caused by alterations in cerebral blood flow. As cerebral blood flow increases, CSF is pushed from the ventricles into the subarachnoid space surrounding the spinal cord (locally increased elasticity of the dura mater accommodates for the increase in volume). Long-term increases in intracranial pressure can be compensated by increasing CSF flow to the venous sinuses.
- The CSF decreases the force with which the brain impacts the cranium when the head moves.

Hydrocephalus

This condition is caused by an increase in cranial CSF volume resulting in increased pressure within the ventricular system. It can be divided into three types:

- Obstructive (non-communicating) hydrocephalus – caused by a congenital or acquired obstruction in the CSF pathway resulting in the accumulation of fluid proximal to the block (Fig 1.17). Blockage is most likely to occur at the outlets of the fourth ventricle (the foramina of Luschka and Magendie) but may also occur at the level of the cerebral aqueduct (of Sylvius). Ventricles rostral to a blockage dilate and put pressure on the brain tissue. This increases intracranial pressure and in the newborn can distort the skull bones (as the sutures have not fused). It may be relieved surgically by shunting (e.g. ventriculoperitoneal shunt) or by endoscopic ventriculostomy.
- Communicating hydrocephalus – caused by reduced absorption, excessive production or increased viscosity of CSF (Fig 1.18).
- Normal pressure hydrocephalus – gross ventricular enlargement is seen without cortical atrophy on a CT scan. The pathogenesis is unknown but may be due to a partial obstruction of CSF flow from the subarachnoid space. The classic clinical triad is dementia, gait disturbance and early urinary incontinence.

Useful investigations in hydrocephalus include:

- Head CT/MRI – this shows the pattern of ventricular dilatation and excludes the presence of space-occupying lesions.
- Transfontanelle ultrasonography – this is a useful non-invasive test in newborn babies.
- Intracranial pressure monitoring – a pressure transducer inserted into the lateral ventricle, brain or subdural space.

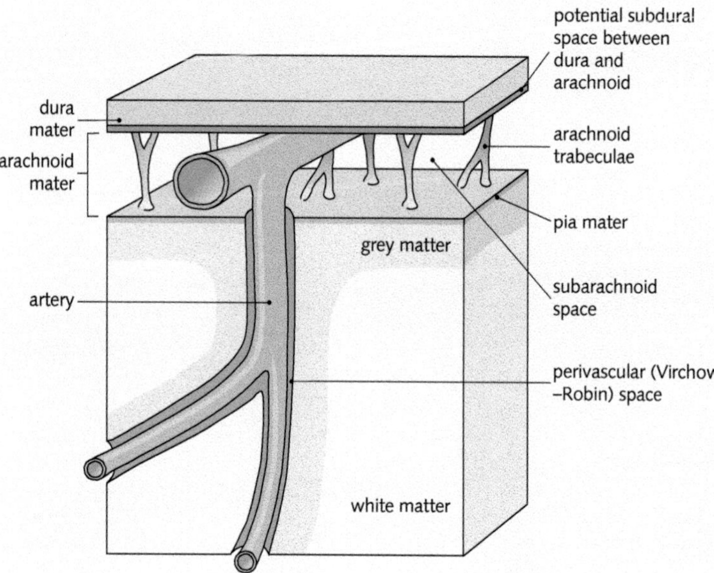

Fig. 1.16 Spaces filled with cerebrospinal fluid – subarachnoid and perivascular.

Fig. 1.17 Causes of obstructive hydrocephalus

Congenital	Acquired
Aqueduct stenosis	Acquired aqueduct stenosis (adhesion following infection or haemorrhage)
Dandy–Walker syndrome	Intraventricular tumours (colloid cyst, ependymoma)
Arnold–Chiari malformation	parenchymal tumours (pineal gland, posterior fossa)
Vein of Galen aneurysm	Space-occupying lesion causing tentorial herniation
Atresia of fourth ventricle foraminae	

Fig. 1.18 Causes of communicating hydrocephalus

Pathogenesis	Causes
Reduced absorption by arachnoid granulations	Infection (especially TB), subarachnoid haemorrhage, trauma, carcinomatous meningitis
Excessive cerebrospinal fluid (CSF) production	Choroid plexus papilloma
Increased CSF viscosity	High protein content

SUPPORTIVE CELLS

Glial cells

Glial cells are the supporting cells for the neurons of the nervous system. There are 5–10 times more glial cells than neurons in the nervous system.

Macroglia

- Schwann cells are found only in the peripheral nervous system, where they surround axonal processes of neurons. They wrap around individual cells like a Swiss roll, and insulate the axon with myelin. One Schwann cell insulates just one axon. Schwann cells also play an important role in the regeneration of damaged peripheral axons.
- Oligodendrocytes are the equivalent of Schwann cells in the central nervous system, providing myelin insulation. Unlike Schwann cells, each oligodendrocyte can myelinate many axons. Oligodendrocytes are also associated with several molecules that are inhibitory to axonal growth, therefore contributing to the failure of adult central nervous system neurons to regenerate after injury.
- Astrocytes are small stellate cells with long branching processes that provide the framework for the surrounding neurons and capillaries (Fig. 1.19). They provide a 'scaffold' which prevents axons of different nerve cells from coming into contact with one

Fig. 1.19 Astrocytes, and their relation to neurons and capillaries.

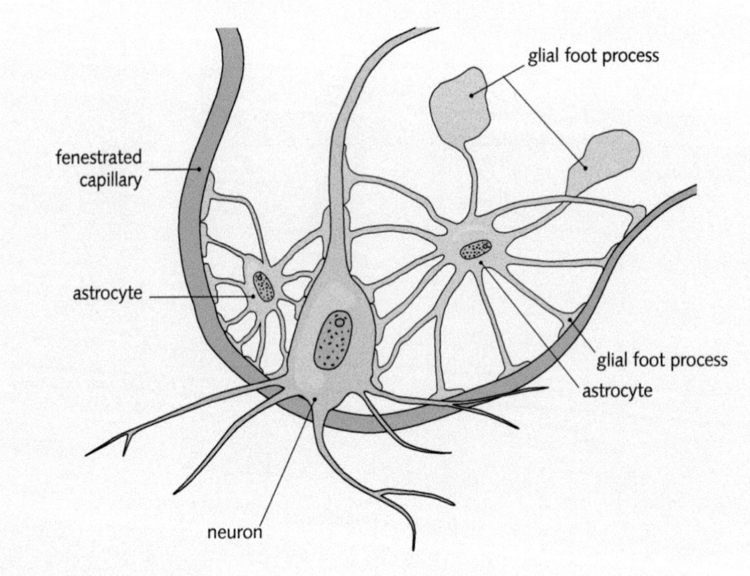

another, and their signals suffering interference. Astrocytes can also take up, store and release some neurotransmitters (such as γ-aminobutyric acid (GABA) and glutamate), preventing them from constantly activating postsynaptic neurons and also potentially playing an adjunctive role in chemical neurotransmission. Astrocytes store glycogen (which can be broken down to glucose at times of high metabolic demand) and help to regulate interstitial fluid potassium concentration. They can act as phagocytes and play a role in scar formation.

- Ependymal cells line the ventricles of the brain and the central canal of the spinal cord. Ependymocytes have cilia on their surface which project into the fluid-filled cavities and contribute to the flow of CSF. They may also have a role in absorbing solutes from the CSF. Choroidal epithelial cells, which produce and secrete CSF, also come in this group.

Microglia

These are resident macrophages which are derived from monocytes outside the nervous system (in the reticuloendothelial system). Under normal circumstances they appear to be inactive. When there is tissue damage or inflammation they multiply and act as phagocytes. Similar to macrophages elsewhere, they are antigen-presenting cells and can, therefore, interact with other elements of the immune system. Macrophages from the periphery can be recruited to the central nervous system to supplement the function of microglia when required.

THE BLOOD–BRAIN BARRIER

The blood–brain barrier exists to maintain the environment of the brain in a steady state, protected from extracellular ion changes, peripheral hormones (such as adrenaline (epinephrine)) and drugs. It also prevents neurotransmitters from the central nervous system entering the peripheral circulation.

Two factors combine to maintain the balance between plasma and CSF:

- The endothelial cells of the cerebral capillaries have very high resistance tight junctions between them. As a result, even small ions will not permeate between endothelial cells in brain capillaries. Brain capillary endothelial cells also lack the methods of transcellular transport which are present in peripheral capillaries (fluid-phase and carrier-mediated endocytosis).
- Astrocytes have foot processes which adhere to the capillary endothelial cells such that they are entirely enclosed. Astrocytic foot processes also secrete factors that help to maintain the tight junctions between endothelial cells.

Small lipid-soluble molecules, such as diamorphine, cross this barrier easily, but hydrophilic molecules rely on specific transporter systems. D-glucose, for example, has a stereospecific membrane transporter that facilitates diffusion from the circulation to the CSF at high rates because the brain relies heavily on glucose for energy. However, in situations where there is a dramatic fall in plasma glucose levels (e.g. in diabetic hypoglycaemic states), glucose may diffuse back out of the CSF into the plasma. This is a medical emergency as the neurons needs glucose to survive.

Other transport systems include those for amino acids – one each for basic (e.g. arginine), neutral (e.g. phenylalanine) and acidic (e.g. glutamate) amino acids. Clinically, the neutral transporter is important as it will transport L-dopa (used to replace dopamine lost from the substantia nigra in Parkinson's disease). However, dopamine cannot be given as a treatment because it does not have a transporter.

In certain regions of the brain (including the posterior pituitary and choroid plexus) the capillaries are fenestrated and so there is no blood–brain barrier. Specialized ependymal cells (tanycytes) isolate these areas from the rest of the brain. The absence of the blood–brain barrier at the posterior pituitary allows oxytocin and vasopressin to be secreted directly into the systemic circulation. At other sites, it enables the brain to analyse the concentrations of water and ions for homeostatic functions.

Abrupt changes in the ionic concentration can be damaging to neurons. The blood–brain barrier not only helps to protect the brain from such changes in plasma levels, but also helps to remove excess ions from the CSF. For example, intense neuronal activity can increase the CSF potassium concentration. A high concentration of K^+ channels on endothelial cells clears the excess.

Brain ischaemia, brain tumours, haemorrhage, systemic acidosis or infections such as bacterial meningitis can break down the blood–brain barrier.

HINTS AND TIPS

In cerebral ischaemia the blood–brain barrier opens, resulting in cytotoxic cerebral oedema: paucity of oxygen causes a decline in endothelial cell ATP which secondarily disrupts the function of the NA^+/K^+ATPase pump. As a result Na^+ accumulates in the cell, water follows osmotically and the cell swells. This swelling compromises the integrity of the tight functions, allowing an influx of ions and water into the brain extracellular space.

HINTS AND TIPS

In diabetic ketoacidosis (where plasma glucose concentration becomes excessively high), pH of the plasma may fall below 7, at which point the blood–brain barrier is compromised and neuronal death occurs.

METABOLIC REQUIREMENTS OF THE CENTRAL NERVOUS SYSTEM

Mechanisms within the blood–brain barrier provide the substrates for cellular metabolism in the brain via the CSF.

The brain is vulnerable to interruptions in its blood supply because it can store neither oxygen nor glucose, and cannot normally undergo anaerobic metabolism. It has a high metabolic rate due to the energy demand of Na^+/K^+ ATPase pumps in the neuronal membranes. Brain metabolism accounts for 20% of the body's oxygen and 60% of its glucose requirement. Cranial blood vessels are controlled by autoregulation to maintain a constant blood supply.

Under conditions of starvation for several days, the central nervous system can adapt to use ketones (fat derivatives acetoacetate and hydroxybutyrate) as its main energy source. These compounds normally make up approximately 30% of the fuel for the brain in adults but, after fasting for 40 days, this can rise to 70%.

In infants, the blood–brain barrier transport of glucose is 30% of the adult level, whereas ketone transport is approximately seven times as high. Amino acid transport in children is also higher than in adults, reflecting a higher rate of protein synthesis in the developing brain.

HINTS AND TIPS

Cerebral blood flow (CBF) is determined by the difference in systemic blood pressure (SBP) and intracranial pressure (ICP): CBF = SBP – ICP. Therefore, patients with raised intracranial pressure will be hypertensive.

The development of the nervous system and disorders of development

Objectives

In this chapter you will learn about:

- The embryological development of the brain and spinal cord.
- The development of the brainstem, cranial nerves, forebrain, pituitary gland and choroid plexuses.
- The different types of neural tube defects and their prenatal diagnosis.
- Holoprosencephaly, neuronal migration disorders and other congenital diseases.
- The pre-, peri- and postnatal causes of cerebral palsy.

THE DEVELOPMENT OF THE NERVOUS SYSTEM

Development of the nervous system begins at approximately 3 weeks' gestation. At this point the embryo consists of three layers:

- Endoderm (forms the gastrointestinal tract among other things)
- Mesoderm (forms muscles, connective tissues and blood vessels)
- Ectoderm (forms the entire nervous system and the skin).

Neurulation

At around day 22 of gestation, an area of ectoderm on the dorsal surface of the embryo, called the neural plate, thickens and folds to form the neural groove. The ridges on either side of the groove expand and begin to fuse in the midline approximately halfway along its length (at the level of the fourth somite). Somites are paired blocks of mesoderm, segmentally arranged alongside the neural groove of the embryo. The very tips of these ridges become the neural crest, and the fused neural tube gives rise to the brain and spinal cord. The tube at the cranial (rostral or head-end) neuropore fuses on day 25, and the caudal (or tail-end) neuropore on day 27. The stages of neurulation are shown in Figure 2.1.

HINTS AND TIPS

If the cranial neuropore fails to close, the fatal condition of anencephaly results – the embryo continues to develop but the brain does not, and the structures which would normally overlie the brain are prevented from forming. This usually results in spontaneous abortion. Failure of the caudal neuropore to close results in disruption of the lumbar and sacral segments of the cord. Structures that lie superficial to the cord are also involved (e.g. meninges, vertebral arch, paravertebral muscles and skin) because their development relies on closure of the neural tube. Malformation involving the vertebral arch and the cord is called spina bifida.

The neural crest cells give rise to most of the cells in the peripheral nervous system (including the dorsal root ganglia) along with cells of the autonomic ganglia, adrenal medulla and melanocytes in the skin. Dorsal root ganglia send their developing axons into the developing spinal cord and also towards the periphery. The advancing growth cones of these neuronal processes are guided to their appropriate central and peripheral targets by means of diffusible neurotrophic factors and cell adhesion molecules.

By the end of development, the segmental arrangement of the nervous system (as determined by the somites) is retained only in the spinal cord.

Embryology of the spinal cord

The neural tube contains neuroblast cells. Its hollow centre becomes the spinal canal. Neuroblasts adjacent to the canal divide and travel to the outer mantle layer, ultimately forming the neurons of the grey matter of the spinal cord. These neuroblasts/neurons project nerve fibres that grow outwards into the marginal zone, ultimately forming the white matter of the spinal cord.

The neuroblasts in the primitive grey matter form two discrete populations – a dorsal alar plate and a

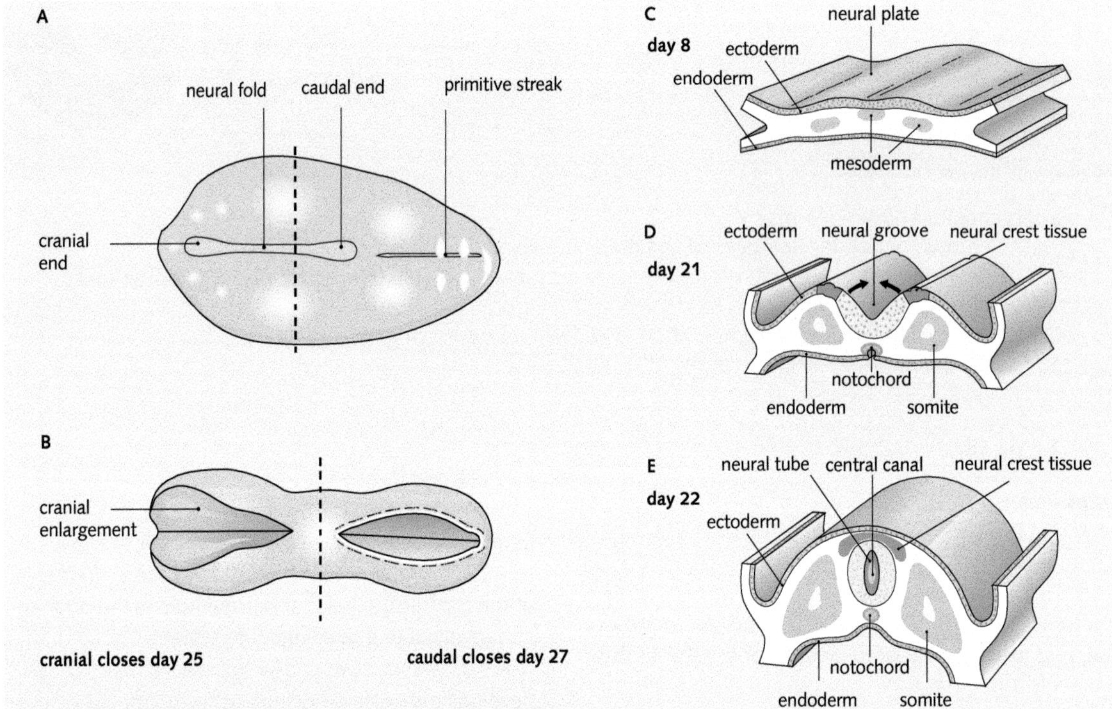

Fig. 2.1 Stages of neurulation. A, Early embryonic disc. B, Progression to formation of brain vesicles and spinal canal. C–E, Transverse sections of neural tube taken at different stages of development.

ventral basal plate separated by a shallow groove (sulcus limitans):

- The alar plate cells form the sensory cells of the posterior (dorsal) horn.
- The basal plate cells form the motor cells of the anterior (ventral) horn along with sympathetic (in the thoracic region) and parasympathetic (in the lumbar and sacral regions) preganglionic neurons.

Figure 2.2 shows the formation and development of the alar and basal plates.

The mesenchymal tissue around the neural tube forms the coverings of the brain and spinal cord.

In the first 8 weeks of gestation, the spinal cord is the same length as the vertebral column. After 8 weeks the vertebral column grows at a faster rate. By 40 weeks of gestation (term), the spinal cord stops at the level of L3 and, in adults, it ends at L1. The spinal nerve roots below this level descend within the vertebral canal until they reach the appropriate exit foramen. The pia mater remains attached to the coccyx and, therefore, elongates with respect to the spinal cord. The strand of pia mater between the coccyx and the lower end of the spinal cord is known as the filum terminale, and collectively with the individual nerve roots below L1, as the cauda equina (literally 'horse's tail').

Lumbar puncture

The spinal cord ends at the level of L1 in adults. Therefore, below this level the spinal canal does not contain the spinal cord. Consequently, a needle can be inserted safely between the L3/L4 vertebrae into the subarachnoid space in order to remove cerebrospinal fluid (CSF) for diagnostic purposes.

Cauda equina syndrome

A prolapsed intervertebral disc or fracture can cause compression of the cauda equina. The symptoms of this include pain in the nerve distribution of the root affected, saddle anaesthesia (around the anus) and disturbance of bladder/bowel function. It is a neurosurgical emergency and the pressure must be relieved to preserve the function of the nerves.

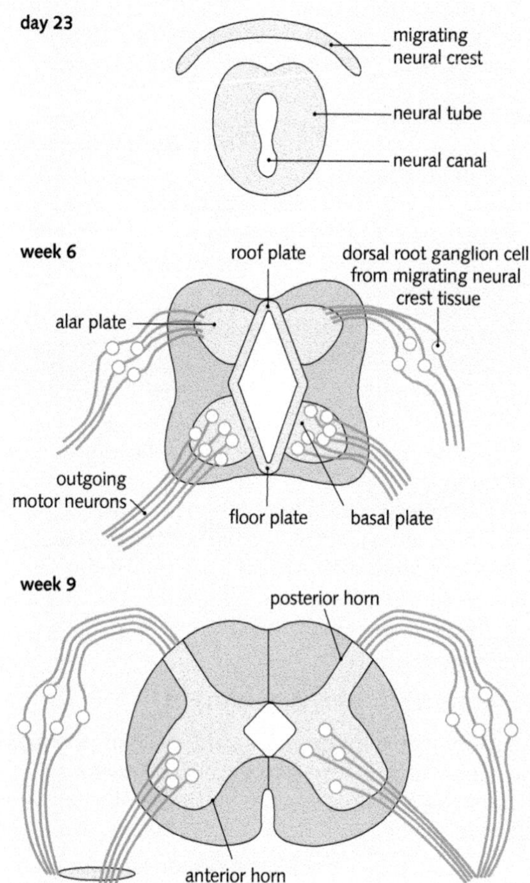

Fig. 2.2 Cross-sections through the developing spinal cord, showing development of alar and basal plates and the primitive beginnings of inflow and outflow tracts.

Embryology of the brain

General arrangement

The neural groove rostral to the fourth pair of somites enlarges before it fuses to form three primary brain vesicles or swellings:

- The first brain vesicle becomes the prosencephalon or forebrain.
- The second becomes the mesencephalon or midbrain.
- The third becomes the rhombencephalon or hindbrain.

Figure 2.3 shows the fate of these vesicles. Before the 5th week of gestation, the first and third vesicles divide in two:

- The forebrain vesicle forms the telencephalon and diencephalon.
- The hindbrain vesicle forms the metencephalon and myelencephalon (or medulla).

The central canal of the neural tube enlarges to form:

- Lateral ventricles in the primitive cerebral hemispheres
- Third ventricle in the diencephalon
- Cerebral aqueduct (of Sylvius) in the midbrain
- Fourth ventricle in the hindbrain.

The neural tube bends to form:

- The cervical flexure (between the primitive spinal cord and the third vesicle)
- The cephalic flexure (between the first and second vesicles).

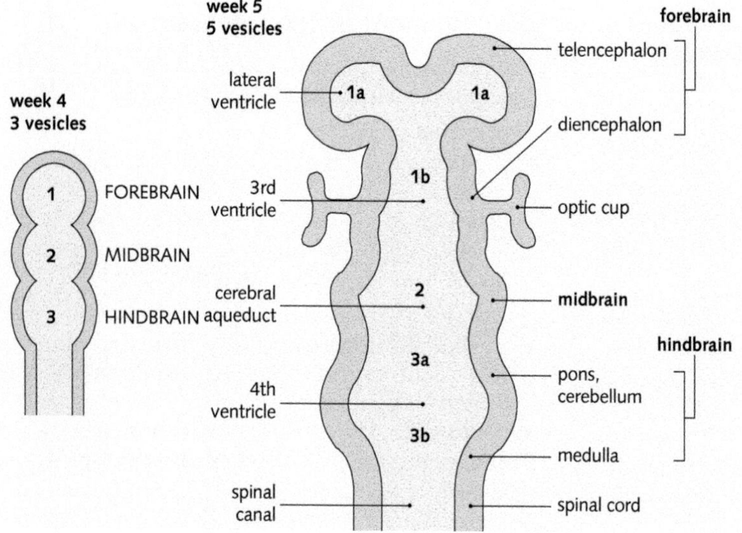

Fig. 2.3 Development of the brain from the three-vesicle stage to adult areas.

Development of the brainstem

The brainstem has the same basic structure as the spinal cord, except that it has to accommodate the large motor and sensory tracts that run between the spinal cord and the brain.

The medulla

Initially, the myelencephalon or medulla is organized like the primitive spinal cord with alar and basal plates. As it flattens out further up, forming the floor of the fourth ventricle, the alar plates (sensory cell groups) move outwards until they lie lateral to the basal plates (motor cell groups). Other cells from the alar plate migrate ventrolaterally to form the olivary nuclei. This process is shown in Figure 2.4.

The cells of the alar and basal plates are arranged in columns according to whether they innervate somatic (body wall) or visceral (internal organ) structures:

- The basal plate forms the motor nuclei for cranial nerves IX, X, XI, XII.
- The alar plate forms sensory nuclei for cranial nerves V, VIII, IX, X along with the gracile and cuneate nuclei (receiving inputs from the spinal cord).

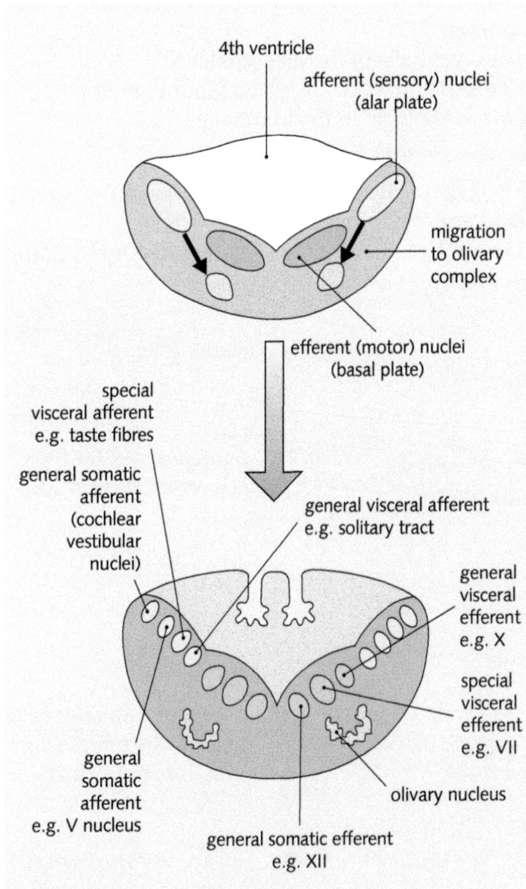

Fig. 2.4 Development of the medulla, with grouping of sensory and motor nuclei.

Pons and cerebellum

The pons is formed by the anterior part of the metencephalon and part of the alar plate of the medulla. It contains a thick band of fibres (important in motor processing) which connect the forebrain with the cerebellum. The neurons of the ventromedial alar plate at this level form:

- The main sensory nucleus of V
- A sensory nucleus of VII
- Vestibular and cochlear nuclei of VIII
- Pontine nuclei.

The neurons of the basal plate form the motor nuclei of V, VI and VII.

The cerebellum develops from the most posterior parts of the alar plates, above the level of the medulla. Cerebellar growths project over the top of the fourth ventricle and fuse in the midline, with migrating cells from the alar plates becoming the cerebellar cortex.

Development of the midbrain

The midbrain retains the basic alar/basal plate structure. The neural canal narrows to form the aqueduct of the midbrain (also known as the aqueduct of Sylvius) as shown in Figure 2.5:

- The cells of the basal plate form the pure motor nuclei of the third and fourth cranial nerves, and possibly the red nucleus, substantia nigra and reticular formation (involved in motor processing).
- The cells of the alar plates become the sensory neurons of the superior and inferior colliculi (involved in visual and auditory reflexes, respectively).

Development of the forebrain

The forebrain situated rostral to the optic vesicles becomes the telencephalon and contains:

- Cerebral cortex
- Commissures – made up of cortico-cortical connections
- Basal ganglia – which develop as swellings that protrude into the cavity of the lateral ventricles, along with the developing hippocampus.

The telencephalon (hemispheres) expands much more than the other parts of the brain and ultimately covers the diencephalon and midbrain. The two swellings meet in the midline, trapping a small amount of mesenchymal tissue which forms the falx cerebri. Similarly, the occipital lobes of the hemispheres are separated from the cerebellum by mesenchyme (which becomes the tentorium cerebelli).

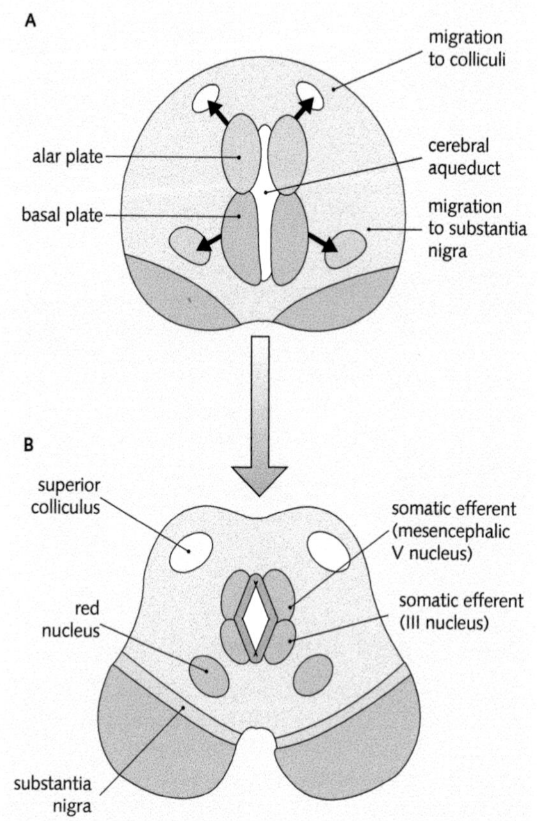

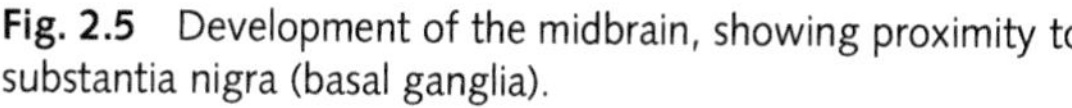

Fig. 2.5 Development of the midbrain, showing proximity to substantia nigra (basal ganglia).

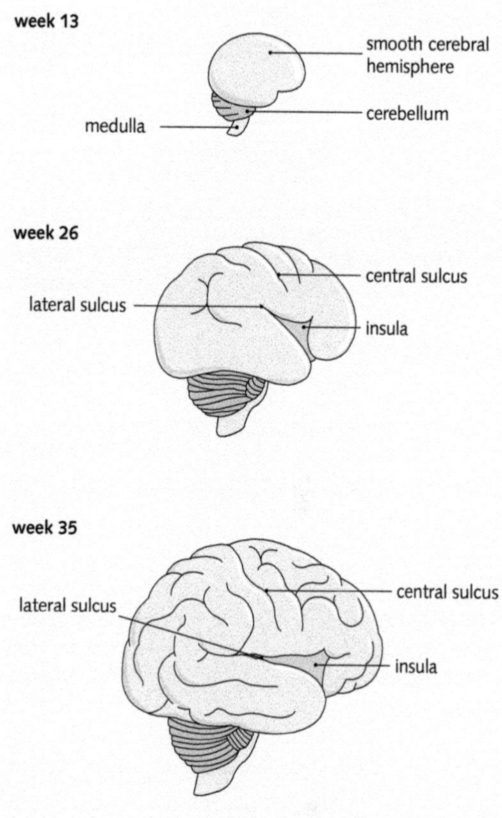

Fig. 2.6 Growth of the cerebral cortex over the insula and the development of gyri.

Grooves gradually appear on the smooth surface of the hemispheres and become the sulci. The gyri thus formed allow a much greater volume of cortex (folded up) to be packed into the cranium. The cortex that covers part of the corpus striatum (lentiform nucleus) is called the insula. It remains fixed while the temporal, parietal and frontal lobes grow rapidly to bury it within the lateral sulcus. This process is shown in Figure 2.6.

The rest of the forebrain becomes the diencephalon (Fig. 2.7) and consists of:

- Hypothalamus (most rostral/ventral)
- Posterior pituitary gland and its stalk (the infundibulum)
- Thalamus
- Epithalamus (most caudal/dorsal).

Pituitary gland

The pituitary gland is composed of two parts:

- A posterior (neural) part that develops from a downward growth (the infundibulum) from the floor of the hypothalamus.
- An anterior (glandular) part that develops as an inward growth (Rathke's pouch) from the oral cavity towards the brain. It passes through the developing sphenoid bone to reach the downgrowth from the hypothalamus.

Development of the cranial nerves

There are three developmentally distinct groups of cranial nerves:

- Somatic efferents. These innervate muscles that develop from the parts of the rostral somites which become the head myotomes. This group includes cranial nerves III, IV, VI to the ocular muscles, and XII to the tongue muscles.
- Pharyngeal arch (branchial) nerves. These supply motor and sensory innervation to the embryological pharyngeal arches that formed the primitive oral cavity and pharynx. This group includes cranial nerves V (from the first arch), VII (second arch),

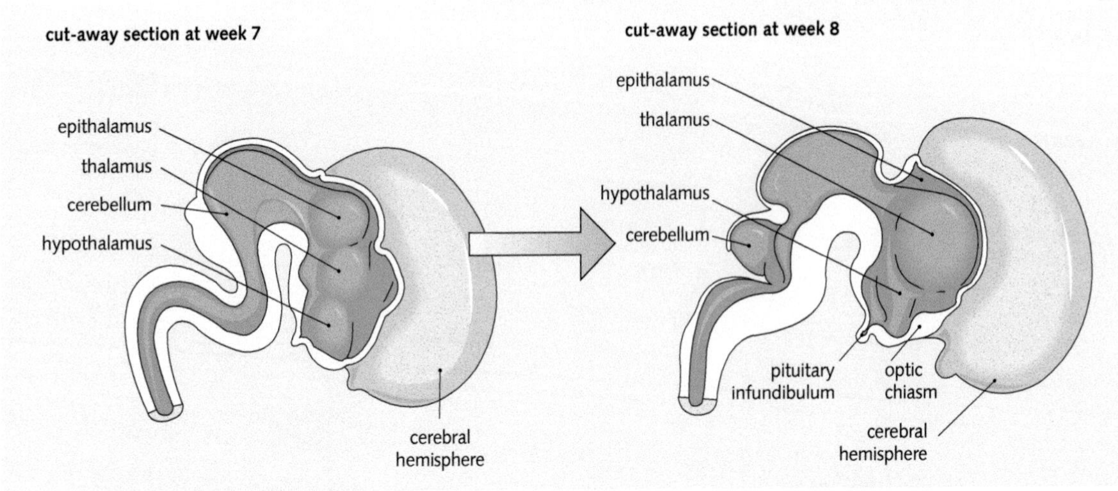

Fig. 2.7 Development of the diencephalon, showing cervical and cranial flexures.

IX (third arch) and X (fused fourth and sixth arches with the cranial branch of XI, the accessory nerve). The relationship of these nerves is shown in Figure 2.8.

- Special sensory nerves. These afferent nerves relay information from special sense receptors to the appropriate central pathway. This group includes cranial nerves I (olfaction), II (vision) and VIII (hearing and balance).

Development of the choroid plexi

The cerebrospinal fluid producing choroid plexus is formed from two layers (the pia mater and the ependymal lining of the cavities of the ventricles) which together are called the tela choroidea. This surrounds a core of vascular connective tissue. The tela choroidea push into the ventricles and develop into the choroid plexi.

Fig. 2.8 Pharyngeal arch nerves in the embryo and adult.

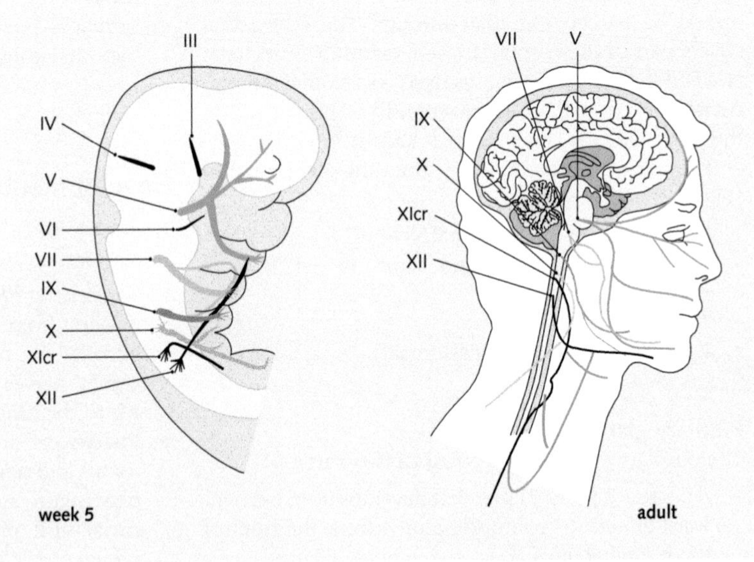

MALFORMATIONS, DEVELOPMENTAL DISEASE AND PERINATAL INJURY

Neural tube defects

HINTS AND TIPS

Prenatal diagnosis of neural tube defects: Open spina bifida and anencephaly are detectable prenatally by a raised α-fetoprotein (AFP). The top 3% of maternal serum AFP levels will include most neural tube defects (as well as many normal fetuses and most twin pregnancies). One in 10 pregnant women with a high serum AFP level will have an abnormal baby. Confirmation is with ultrasonography and amniocentesis.

Neural tube defects are caused by varying degrees of failure of fusion of the posterior neural arch. The pathogenesis of the disorders is thought to be due to a mixture of:

- Environmental factors – folic acid (folate) taken at the time of conception and in the first trimester of pregnancy reduces the incidence of neural tube defects. Other factors have not been proved, but it is interesting to note that the incidence in the UK is 10 times higher than in Japan, despite comparable education about the importance of folate supplements.
- Genetic factors – subsequent children born to a mother with an affected child have a 10-fold increased risk, but in monozygotic twins rarely are both affected.

Spina bifida

The lumbosacral site is most common (80%). Spina bifida is caused by local defects in the development and closure of the neural tube and vertebral arches. The main types are shown in Figure 2.9. Deficiency of the meninges in these patients predisposes to meningitis. Bladder problems are also common due to a partial cauda equina syndrome.

The spinal cord may be tethered by a fibrous band or tight filum terminale, associated with increasing deficit as the child grows and the cord stretches. Surgery to release the tethered cord may be indicated.

Rachischisis

This is the most severe defect in which the entire neural tube fails to close. It is not compatable with life.

Anencephaly

Anencephaly represents failure of fusion at the cephalic end of the neural tube. Almost no forebrain structures develop, usually with absence of the skull vault. This condition is not compatible with long-term survival.

Arnold–Chiari malformation

Arnold–Chiari malformation is caused by failure of fusion at the craniocervical junction, and is often associated with a lumbar meningocoele or myelomeningocoele. The brainstem is displaced downwards, with the cerebellar tonsils and medulla herniating through the foramen magnum. It is associated with hydrocephalus, especially dilatation of the third and fourth ventricles. Defects may include mental retardation, lower (ocular) cranial nerve palsies and cerebellar/brainstem signs. Complications include syringomyelia.

Forebrain disorders

Holoprosencephaly

Holoprosencephaly is a congenital disorder in which the prosencephalon (the forebrain of the embryo) fails to develop into two hemispheres. Genes, called Hox genes, that normally guide the placement of embryonic structures, fail to activate along the midline of the brain. Therefore, structures that are normally paired on the left and right merge. In most cases of holoprosencephaly, the malformations are so severe that babies die before birth. In less severe cases, babies are born with normal or near-normal brain development and facial deformities that may affect the eyes, nose and upper lip.

HINTS AND TIPS

Cyclopia is a rare form of holoprosencephaly characterized by the failure of the embryonic prosencephalon to properly divide the orbits of the eye into two cavities.

Neuronal migration disorders

Neuronal migration disorders (NMDs) are a group of birth defects caused by the abnormal migration of neurons in the developing nervous system. In the developing brain, neurons must migrate from their place of origin adjacent to the ventricles to the areas where they will finally settle into their correct neural circuits. Neuronal migration, which occurs as early as the 2nd month of gestation, is guided by a complex assortment of chemical signals. When these signals are absent or incorrect, neurons do not end up where they belong. This can result in structurally abnormal or missing areas of

Fig. 2.9 Neural tube defects.

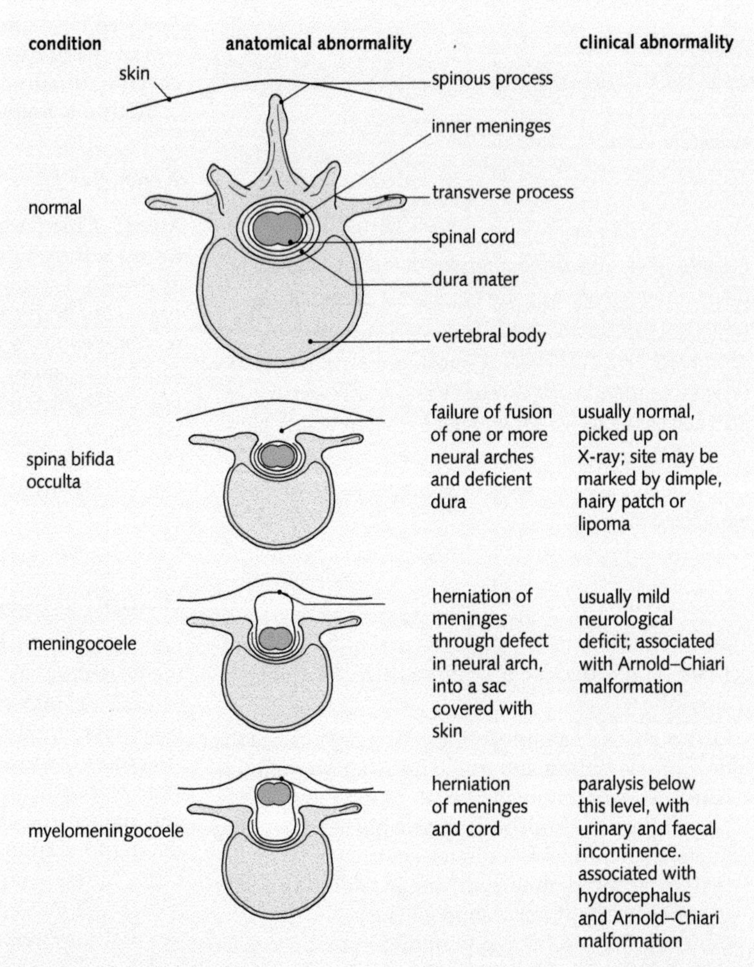

the brain in the cerebral hemispheres, cerebellum, brainstem, or hippocampus. The structural abnormalities found in NMDs include:

- Lissencephaly – which literally means 'smooth brain', is characterized by the absence of normal convolutions in the cerebral cortex and an abnormally small head (microcephaly)
- Agyria, macrogyria, microgyria and pachygyria ('thick' gyri)
- Agenesis of the cranial nerves.

Symptoms vary according to the abnormality, but often feature poor muscle tone and motor function, seizures, developmental delays, mental retardation, failure to thrive, feeding difficulties, swelling in the extremities and microcephaly. Treatment is symptomatic, and may include anti-seizure medication and physical, occupational, and speech therapies.

Other congenital diseases

Some other congenital diseases are listed below:

- Microcephaly – can be developmental or caused by intrauterine infection (e.g. with maternal chickenpox in pregnancy).
- Arteriovenous malformations – may be associated with epilepsy or subarachnoid haemorrhage.
- Syringomyelia – a fluid-filled cavity within the cord, sometimes extending to the brainstem (syringobulbia) is probably due to many different causes. Usually asymptomatic until adulthood when it expands, sometimes after provocation by a sudden increase in intracranial pressure (e.g. a fit of coughing). This is rare but anatomically interesting. The symptoms of syringomyelia are shown in Figure 2.10.

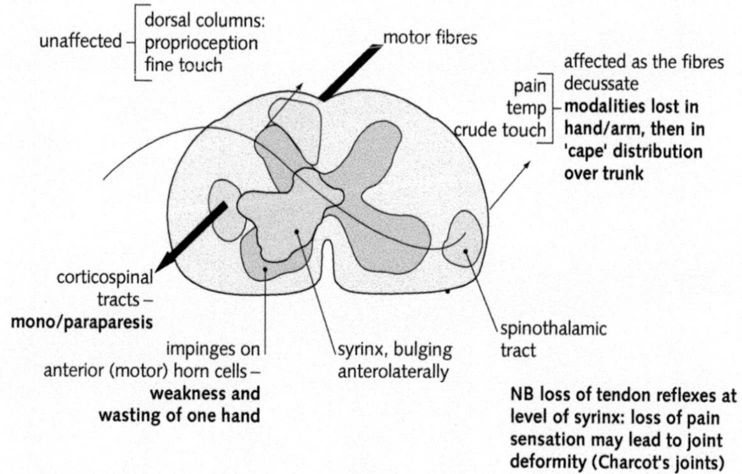

Fig. 2.10 Diagrammatic representation of the cervical cord to explain the symptoms of syringomyelia. Sensory loss is described as dissociated, because pain and temperature sensations are affected, but not joint position and vibration senses. If the cavity extends to the brainstem (syringobulbia), dysarthria, dysphagia, tongue wasting, ataxia and nystagmus may occur.

- Diastematomyelia – the spinal cord is split in two by a fibrous or cartilaginous spur. It presents as a slowly progressive cord syndrome.

HINTS AND TIPS

With an arteriovenous malformation, auscultation over the cranium (especially over the eyeball) may reveal a bruit.

HINTS AND TIPS

Patients who have had a spinal cord injury or neoplasm are at increased risk of developing syringomyelia.

Cerebral palsy

Cerebral palsy is a heterogeneous group of childhood disorders in which injury to the brain early in life results in a non-progressive neurological disorder of movement and tone (Fig. 2.11). Birth trauma, although the most widely known cause, actually only accounts for approximately 10% of cases. Spastic diplegia is the most common presentation, sometimes with ataxia, hemiplegia, tetraplegia and dyskinetic syndrome. Other modalities may also be affected, and there may be associated learning difficulties (although intelligence is preserved in up to 70% of patients), visual problems and epilepsy (30%). Prevalence is approximately 2 per 1000 live births.

Fig. 2.11 Prenatal, perinatal and postnatal causes of cerebral palsy

Type	Cause
Prenatal	Intrauterine infection (particularly TORCH), intracranial haemorrhage, brain malformations
Perinatal	Asphyxia during a difficult birth
Postnatal	Infection e.g., meningitis Traumatic head injury

Cellular physiology of the nervous system and introduction to pharmacology

Objectives

In this chapter you will learn about:

- The basic structure of the neuron and understand the functions of the individual elements.
- The anatomical and functional difference between projection neurons and interneurons.
- What is meant by the resting potential of a cell.
- The sequence of events involved in an action potential.
- How the action potential is propagated along the axon.
- The differences between electrical and chemical synapses.
- The series of events involved in chemical synaptic transmission.
- The difference between temporal and spatial summation and the concept of facilitation.
- The properties of the major types of neurotransmitters and their receptors.

NEURONAL STRUCTURE AND FUNCTION

The nervous system is highly complex but the basic principles which underlie its function are fairly simple. Understanding these concepts is the first stage in appreciating the way in which the whole system works.

Neurons

Neurons are excitable cells that can conduct electrical impulses. They communicate with other excitable cells via specialized junctions called synapses. They vary considerably in structure according to location and function. Figure 3.1 shows a typical neuron.

The cell body (soma) has a series of branching processes called dendrites which collect information from surrounding excitable cells and conduct it to the cell body. The principal role of dendrites is to increase the potential for synapse formation. Accordingly, the number of dendrites reflects the way information is processed in that pathway. A cell with many inputs may condense information from several pathways, whereas a cell with few inputs may be part of a highly conserved parallel pathway.

The output of the nerve cell is a binary signal (meaning that it is an all-or-nothing impulse or train of impulses). The output is generated at the axon hillock when the cell's electrical threshold potential is reached. The output travels down another process extending from the cell body – the axon. In contrast to dendrites, there is only one axon per neuron (although the axon may divide into numerous branches).

The axon transmits the output of the neuron (the action potential) to the terminal boutons (presynaptic swellings containing vesicles of neurotransmitter). Different arrangements of the cell body and its processes are shown in Figure 3.2.

Neurons are surrounded by a lipid bilayer (cell membrane) within which proteins are embedded. Some proteins form ion channels, some form receptors to specific chemicals and others function as ion pumps (e.g. Na^+–K^+ exchange pumps). Ion channels within the axolemma (axonal surface membrane) enable the axon to conduct action potentials. The axoplasm (cytoplasm within the axon) contains microtubules, mitochondria and neurofilaments. These organelles play a key role in maintaining the ionic gradients necessary for action potential production and also enable the transport and recycling of proteins away from and, to a lesser extent, towards the cell body.

HINTS AND TIPS

Certain viruses exploit the retrograde transport of transmitter fragments (from axon to cell body) to gain access to the nervous system. These include the herpes simplex viruses, herpes zoster, rabies and the polio virus. This mechanism is also being evaluated as a possible means of delivering therapeutic interventions in diseases such as motor neuron disease.

Arrangement of neurons

According to the function of the area, neurons can be arranged as:

- Layers (e.g. as in cerebral and cerebellar cortices) (Fig. 3.3)
- Rods (e.g. motor neurons in the spinal cord)

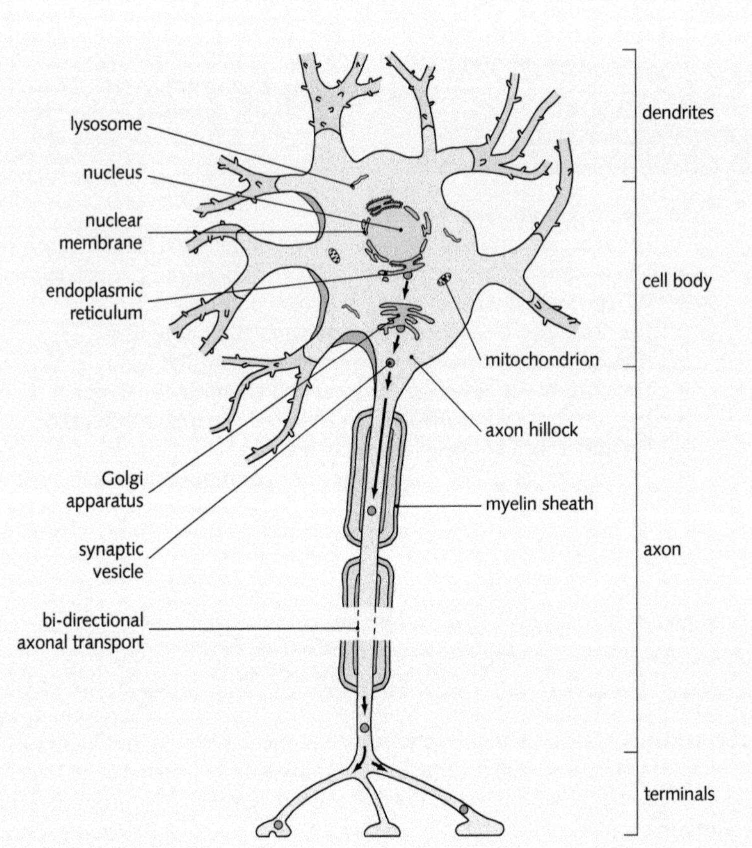

Fig. 3.1 Features of a typical neuron. Note that, although only anterograde transmitter transport is shown, retrograde movement of molecules also occurs.

- Clumps or nuclei (e.g. cranial nerve nuclei in the brainstem).

There are two classes of neuron:

- Projection neurons (Golgi type-1 neurons) influence cells located in a different part of the nervous system and so have long axons (e.g. cortical motor neurons). The long axons often project small collateral branches that help to spread information further in the central nervous system. These are distinct from projection neurons which have connections outside the nervous system. Such neurons may be either afferent (sensory) axons (e.g. from skin receptors) or efferent (motor) axons (e.g. to muscles or glands).
- Local interneurons (Golgi type-II neurons) have shorter axons that do not leave their cell group. They provide more opportunities for cells within a group or circuit to communicate with one another. Their axons often give off many collateral branches. This increases the ability of cells in the circuit to process information. Humans possess far larger numbers of these neurons compared with their closest evolutionary relatives.

Ion channels

Ion channels are protein macromolecules which span the lipid bilayer and allow ions to move from one side of the cell membrane to the other. It is ion channels which imbue the neuron with the fundamental quality of electrical excitability.

The electrochemical gradient across the membrane determines the direction of ion movement. Generally ions flow from regions of high concentration to regions of low concentration. However, in the presence of a voltage gradient, there may be no flow of ions even with non-equilibrated concentrations.

Ion channels can be open or closed. Their status in this respect is determined either by altering the voltage across the membrane (voltage-gated ion channels) or by the binding of a chemical messenger (ligand-gated ion

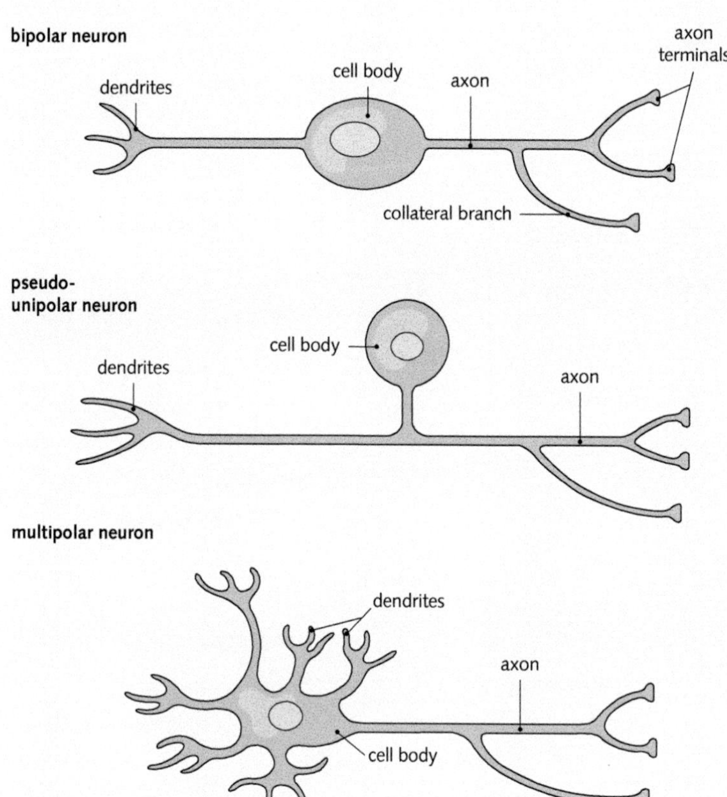

Fig. 3.2 Neurons with different morphology.

channels). In addition, some ion channels respond not to voltage changes or chemical messengers, but to mechanical stretch or pressure.

NEURONAL EXCITATION AND INHIBITION

All nerve cells are electrically polarized. This means that there is an electrical potential gradient across their membranes. The value of this potential determines whether a cell will or will not generate an action potential and depends on the relative membrane permeability to the ions in the extracellular fluid (mainly Na^+ and Cl^-) and intracellular fluid (mainly K^+).

The signal to alter permeability comes either from neurotransmitter interaction with receptors at the synapse or direct electrical excitation of the neuron. Similarly, a neuron may be inhibited from firing when the membrane potential is moved further away from the threshold value (usually achieved by increasing permeability to Cl^-).

Ionic basis of resting potentials

In the resting neuron there is far more potassium within the cell than outside and far less sodium. The cell membrane is relatively impermeable to ions (although there is some leak of K^+). If there were no active channels at work, and no other ions crossed the membrane, potassium ions would tend to move out of the cell (down their concentration gradient) leaving a relatively negative charge behind. This would continue until the electrical force attracting the positive K^+ ions into the cell is equal (and opposite) to the chemical force of the concentration gradient. The electrical potential at which this equilibrium is reached is calculated using the Nernst equation:

$$E_X \cong \frac{RT}{zF} ln \frac{[X_O]}{[X_i]}$$

where E_x is the equilibrium potential for ion X, R is the international gas constant, T is the temperature in degrees Kelvin, z is the valency of X, F is Faraday's constant, X_o is the concentration of X outside the cell, X_i is the concentration of X within the cell.

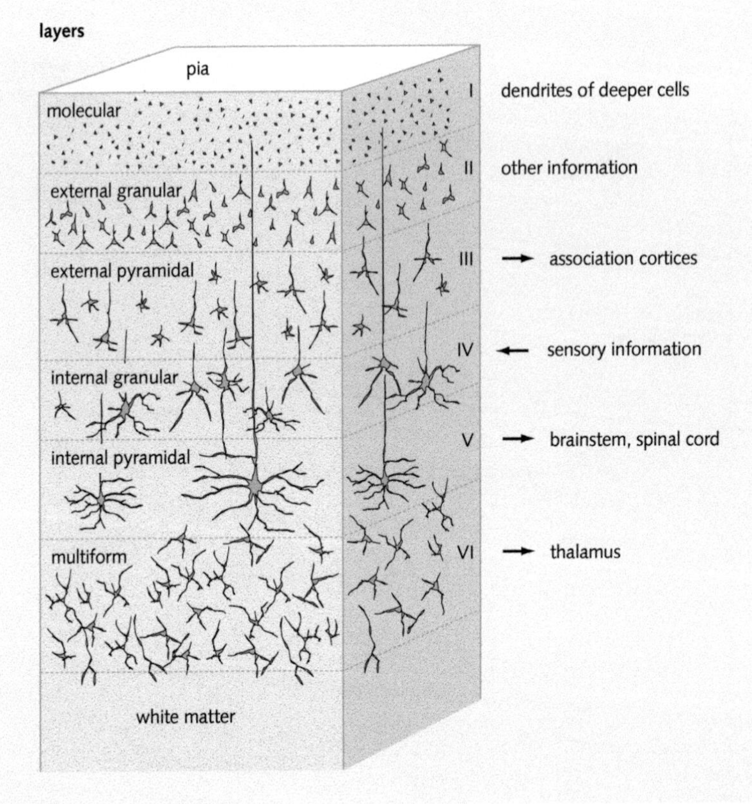

Fig. 3.3 Schematic diagram showing the layers in a typical area of cerebral cortex.

The equilibrium potential for potassium is -74.8 mV. However, the overall potential difference across a resting neuronal membrane is slightly more positive (around -65 mV) due to a small sodium leak in the membrane (the equilibrium potential for sodium is around +55 mV). The Goldman equation is a modified version of the Nernst equation. It takes into account the relative permeabilities of all the ions involved in generating the membrane potential. Figure 3.4 shows how the Goldman equation predicts the actual membrane potential more accurately than the Nernst equation.

Because of the small inward leak of sodium ions one might think that the potential would eventually equilibrate halfway between -74.8 mV and +55 mV. This does not occur because the membrane contains a Na^+–K^+ ATPase exchange pump. This pump moves Na^+ ions out of the cell (against both their electrical and chemical gradient) at a ratio of three Na^+ ions out in exchange for two K^+ ions in. This is an energy-requiring process. Many of these pumps are found in the membranes of all excitable cells and they are largely responsible for the high metabolic requirements of neurons.

Generation and propagation of the action potential

In the 1950s Hodgkin and Huxley discovered the ionic mechanism of action potential propagation by studying the squid giant axon. A neuronal action potential may be induced by inputs from other nerve cells or inputs from sensory neurons. An excitatory input causes an influx of Na^+ ions which pass down their electrical and chemical gradients through voltage-gated Na^+ channels – bringing the membrane potential closer to zero. This is known as depolarization.

If the influx of Na^+ is sufficient to reach the threshold potential for the membrane (generally around -55 mV), a sudden and massive increase in the number of open voltage-gated Na^+ channels occurs. This causes the membrane potential to shift towards the value of the Nernst equation for sodium (+55 mV):

- An action potential is an all-or-nothing reaction of the cell to an influx of positively charged ions.
- Because the size of the action potential is constant, intensity of the stimulus is coded by the frequency of firing of a neuron.

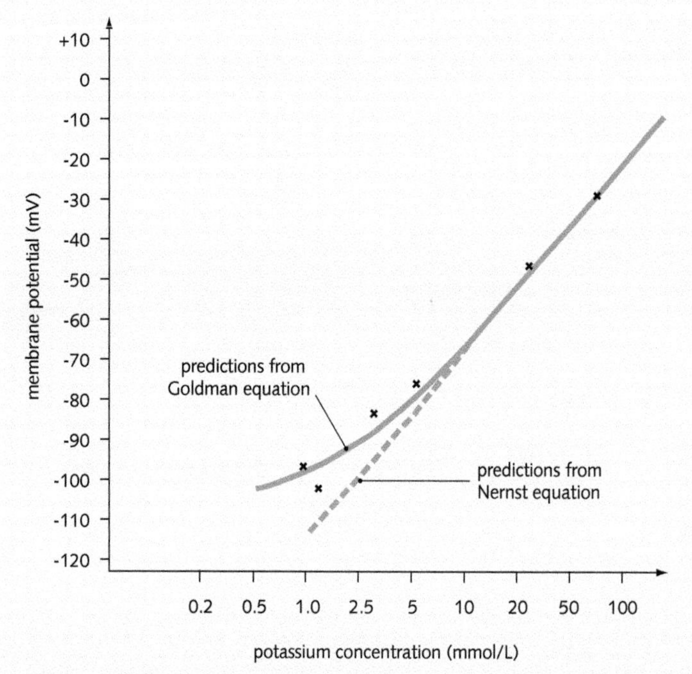

Fig. 3.4 Effect of changing external potassium concentration on the resting potential of a neuron (as determined by experimental electrophysiology). The predictions made by the Goldman equation are more accurate because it takes into account more of the ions involved than the Nernst equation does.

The sodium channels are only open briefly and will not reopen until the membrane potential is restored to its resting level. This causes an absolute refractory period in which the cell cannot fire again.

Potassium channels also open at the time of depolarization, but are much slower. Once open they begin to return the membrane potential to the Nernst equation value for potassium (as the Na^+ channels have now shut). These channels are also slow to close and, consequently, the resting potential of −65 mV is 'overshot'. This results in a brief period of hyperpolarization. The slow closing of the K^+ channels causes a relative refractory period. During this time the neuron will only fire in response to greater than normal stimulation; the efflux of K^+ offsets the influx of Na^+. Figure 3.5 shows the contributions of the Na^+ and K^+ channels to the action potential:

- The action potential is generated at the axon hillock as it has a high concentration of Na^+ channels and a reduced threshold for action potential generation.
- Current passes along the axon from the active region to the neighbouring resting region (which has a more negative membrane potential). At this site current flows outwards across the membrane causing the axon to depolarize. This causes opening of voltage-gated Na^+ channels in that region and consequent depolarization. This mechanism allows the action potential to be propagated down the length of the axon.
- Current does not move backwards as the recently depolarized membrane is in a refractory state. Current is therefore unidirectional.

Myelin is an electrical insulator which surrounds the axons of many neurons and reduces axon contact with extracellular fluid. Each glial cell (oligodendroglia in the central nervous system (CNS) and Schwann cells in the peripheral nervous system) produces the myelin sheath over only a short segment of axon. Therefore, a long axon will be surrounded by the membranes of many glial cells. Adjacent segments of myelin are separated by a small gap – the node of Ranvier. In myelinated cells depolarization occurs only at nodes of Ranvier (where the majority of the sodium channels are located). Current therefore travels along between nodes. This mechanism is known as 'saltatory' (literally jumping or leaping) conduction and is illustrated in Figure 3.6. Conduction in myelinated neurons is approximately six times faster than in non-myelinated neurons.

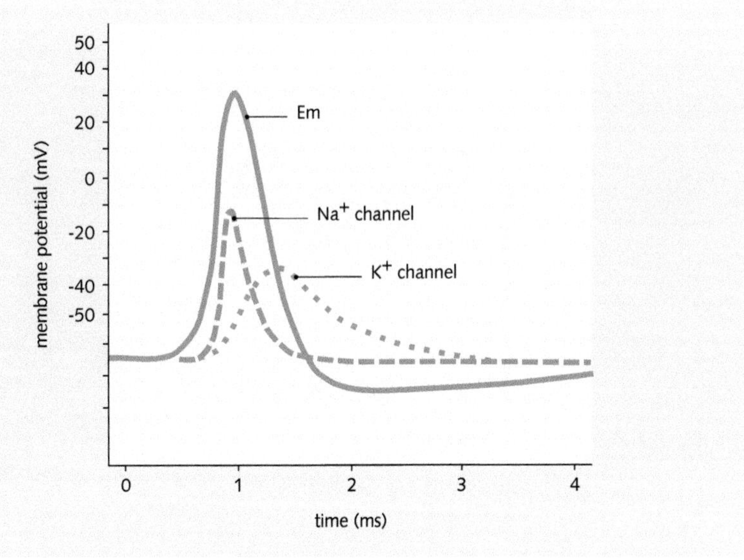

Fig. 3.5 Relation between the opening of ion channels and the timing of the action potential (Em, membrane potential).

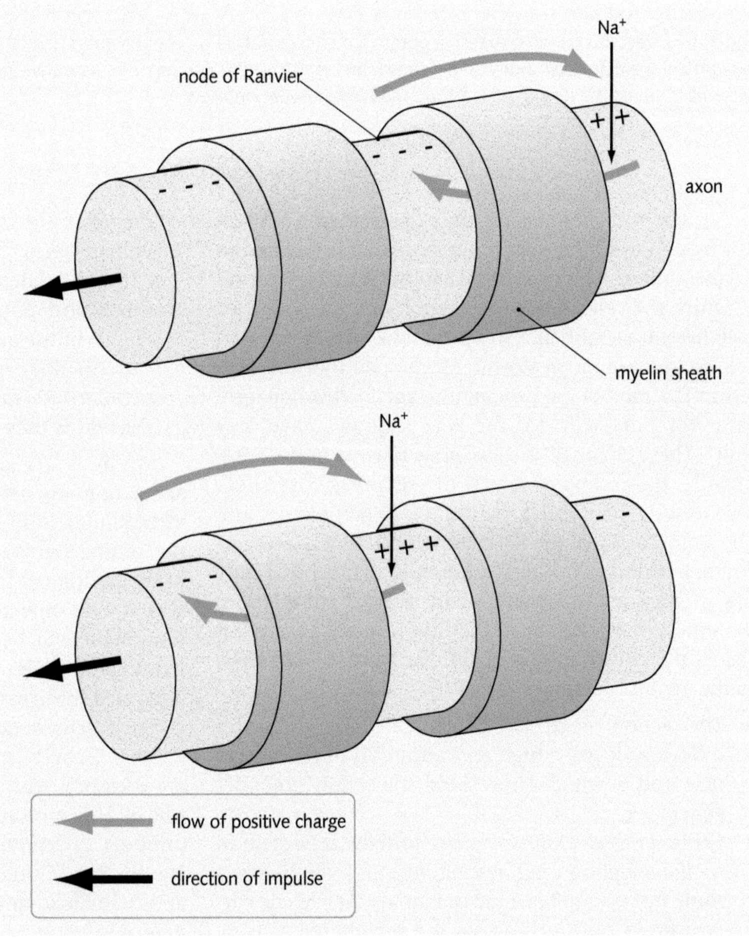

Fig. 3.6 Saltatory conduction in a myelinated axon.

HINTS AND TIPS

Nerves can be tested by stimulating at their distal end and recording the action potential at a more proximal part of the axon. For example, nerves in the fingers can be electrically stimulated and the action potential in the median nerve at the wrist assessed to evaluate function. This is useful in median nerve compression, as occurs in carpal tunnel syndrome.

Velocity of action potentials

Factors limiting the movement of the action potential along the axon are:

- Axonal diameter – the larger the diameter, the lower the internal resistance
- Membrane conductance – if poorly insulated, the axon leaks charge
- Membrane capacitance – current is used up charging the membrane.

Myelin reduces both membrane conductance and membrane capacitance. Less charge is lost through the membrane if the axon is myelinated.

The velocity (in metres per second) of an action potential in a myelinated axon is approximately six times the diameter (in micrometres).

HINTS AND TIPS

Neurons can be demyelinated in diseases such as Guillain–Barré syndrome and multiple sclerosis. In both cases demyelination is immune mediated and causes slowing (or even cessation) of nerve conduction. Changes are reversible in Guillain–Barré syndrome but permanent and progressive in multiple sclerosis.

SYNAPTIC TRANSMISSION

Synapses are junctions between the terminal boutons of neurons and target cells (which may be another nerve, muscle or gland cell). The presynaptic membrane is separated from the postsynaptic membrane by the synaptic cleft. Synapses alter the membrane potential of the postsynaptic cell. They may be:

- Chemical (where a neurotransmitter is required)
- Electrical (where there is a cytoplasmic connection between the cells).

Figure 3.7 shows the differences between these types.

Fig. 3.7 Comparison of electrical and chemical synapses

Feature	Electrical	Chemical
Cytoplasmic continuity	Yes	No
Delay	None	0.8–1.5 ms
Agent	Ion	Neurotransmitter
Space between cells	2 nm	30–50 nm
Direction of signal	One way or both ways	One way
Variation in function	Either on or off	Modifiable activity levels

For chemically operated synapses (which make up the vast majority of junctions in the nervous system), the postsynaptic site contains specific receptor proteins that bind the released chemical. This is essential for amplifying the signal from the neuron, as the extracellular current generated in the presynaptic neuron is not sufficient to cause a significant depolarization of the postsynaptic cell. Electrical synapses are rare in the human central nervous system because they allow only minimal synaptic integration. They *are* found in astrocytes and cardiac myocytes where the presence of fast-conducting gap junctions enables rapid and extensive depolarization.

Types and location of synapses

Synapses (Fig. 3.8) may be:

- Excitatory (depolarizing – increasing the membrane permeability to Na^+ (E_x = +55 mV) and hence dragging the membrane potential towards threshold level).
- Inhibitory (hyperpolarizing – increasing the membrane permeability to Cl^- (E_x = −65 mV) or K^+ (E_x = −75 mV) thereby taking the membrane potential further from the threshold).

Location can enhance action – the closer a synapse to the axon hillock, the greater its effect.

The most common sites for synapses are:

- Axodendritic – 'standard' form of synapse between neurons
- Axosomatic – usually inhibitory synapse. When placed close to the axon hillock these synapses inhibit cell firing more effectively than an axodendritic synapse
- Axoaxonic synapses – can modulate the release of transmitter from the presynaptic cell.

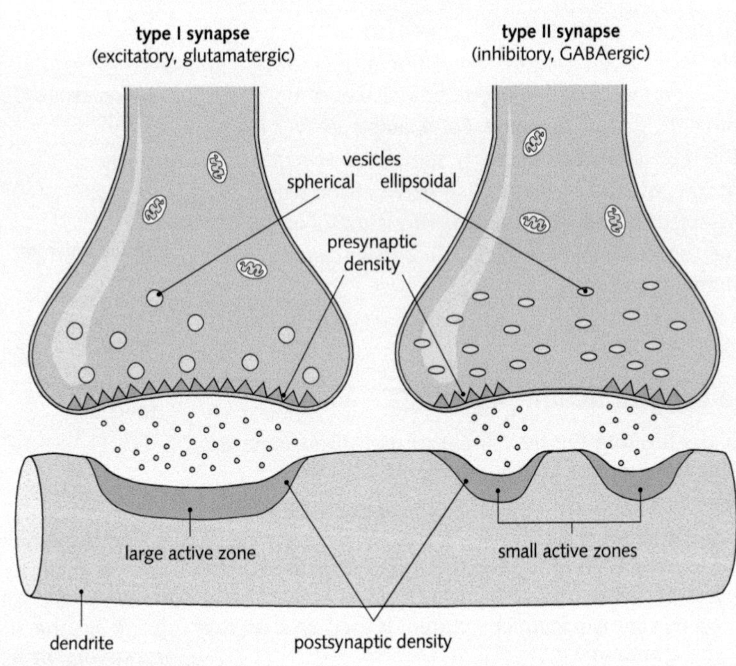

Fig. 3.8 Excitatory (depolarizing) and inhibitory (hyperpolarizing) synapses.

Process of transmission

Figure 3.9 shows the sequence of events from arrival of the action potential to termination of transmitter effect:

Step 1: Action potential arrives at the terminal bouton and the depolarization opens voltage-gated calcium channels in the presynaptic terminal.

Step 2: Calcium ions enter the terminal bouton. Ca^{2+} influx results in the phosphorylation and alteration of several presynaptic calcium-binding proteins. This process liberates vesicles from their presynaptic actin network.

Step 3: The vesicle membrane then fuses with the presynaptic membrane and the contents are released into the synaptic cleft. The vesicle membrane is then invaginated back into the presynaptic terminal and recycled to form more vesicles which are filled with transmitter for re-use. This process is used by some viruses to gain access to the interior of the cell (e.g. poliovirus or herpes virus).

Step 4: The transmitter diffuses across the cleft to postsynaptic receptors and, in some systems, to presynaptic receptors to regulate transmitter release. Once the transmitter has bound to the postsynaptic receptors it causes a change in the postsynaptic membrane potential (either an excitatory or inhibitory postsynaptic potential (EPSP or IPSP)). The size of change attributable to a single vesicle is very small. However, if many vesicles are released, these EPSPs are summed. This may cause a change in membrane

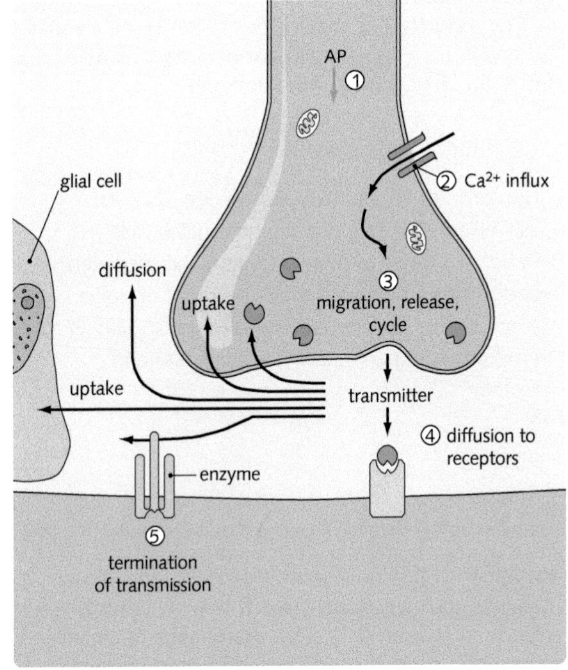

Fig. 3.9 Synaptic transmission.

potential which is sufficient to reach the postsynaptic cell's threshold. This theory of small, identical EPSPs corresponding to individual vesicle release is known as the quantum hypothesis (the amount of

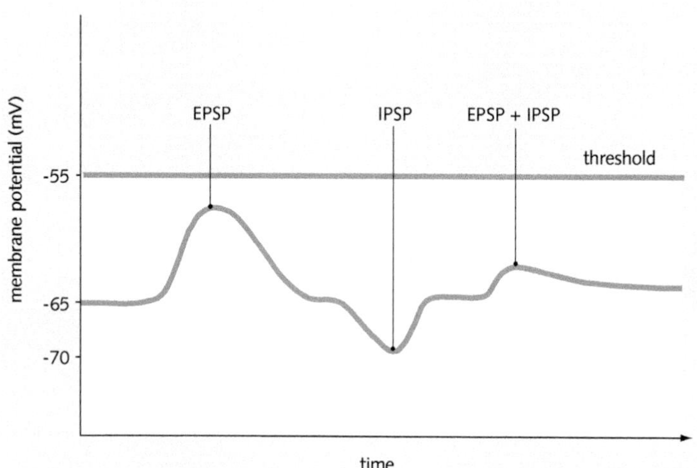

Fig. 3.10 Effects of excitatory postsynaptic potential (EPSP) and inhibitory postsynaptic potential (IPSP) on the membrane potential.

transmitter in each vesicle being the quantum). The effects of EPSPs and IPSPs on the membrane potential are shown in Figure 3.10.

Step 5: the effect of the chemical transmitter is terminated by one or more of the following mechanisms:

- Enzymatic destruction of the transmitter in the cleft (e.g. acetylcholinesterase in cholinergic neurons)
- Re-uptake of the transmitter into the terminal bouton
- Uptake of transmitter into glial cells
- Diffusion out of the cleft.

Modulation of these mechanisms forms the basis of central nervous system therapeutics.

Temporal and spatial summation

Temporal summation occurs when numerous EPSPs at one synapse combine to bring the membrane potential to threshold. These EPSPs must occur in rapid succession as the fluctuations they cause individually fade away rapidly.

Spatial summation occurs when several different synapses located on the same neuron transmit a signal for an EPSP at approximately the same time. All the EPSPs combine to bring the membrane potential to threshold. Figure 3.11 shows the difference between temporal and spatial summation. The same principles apply to IPSPs, except that the membrane potential moves away from its threshold level.

Facilitation

If a sequence of action potentials reaches the terminal bouton within a short space of time, the effect of the transmitter on the postsynaptic cell is enhanced (i.e. either more excitation or more inhibition occurs). This may be due to accumulation of Ca^{2+} within the presynaptic bouton causing increased exocytosis. Facilitation can only be sustained as long as there is a transmitter in the vesicles. The enzymes that generate transmitter molecules and peptide transmitters are synthesized in the cell body and must be transported along the axon, which takes time. The facilitatory effect is therefore not sustained indefinitely.

Neurotransmitters and their receptors

There are several neurotransmitters at work in the brain. Most have a central nucleus of neurons within which their actions tend to predominate. These neurons often serve particular roles and when activated they alter the representation of information in the brain. Some neurotransmitter synthetic pathways are shown in Figure 3.12. The effect of a neurotransmitter depends on the type of receptor that is present at the synapse. One neurotransmitter can have different effects throughout the central nervous system, depending on the receptors it acts upon.

Receptors can be classified according to the second messenger system that they use to alter the membrane potential. The two main classes of receptor are outlined in Figure 3.13:

- The ionotrophic receptor is coupled with an ion channel for cations or anions. When simulated, these receptors have a direct effect on membrane potential.
- The metabotrophic receptor is coupled to a G-protein and uses cAMP (cyclic adenosine

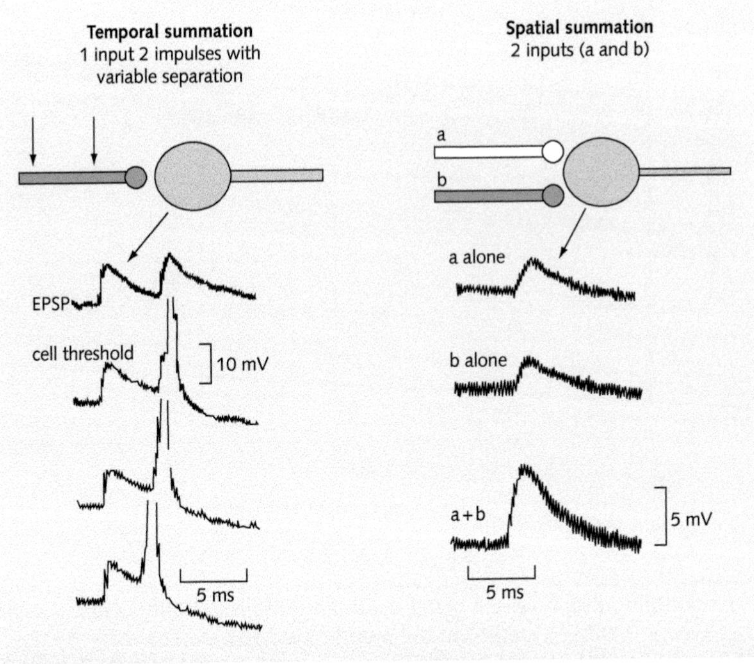

Fig. 3.11 Temporal and spatial summation.

monophosphate) or IP3 (inositol 1,4,5-triphosphate) as a second messenger. Subsequent intracellular effects bring about changes to ion channels and alter the membrane potential.

Glutamate

Glutamate is the main excitatory neurotransmitter of the brain. Other neurotransmitters tend to modulate or augment glutamate transmission. Three glutamate receptors exist:

- AMPA (α-amino-5-hydroxy-3-methyl-4-isoxazole propionic acid) receptors: this is a glutamate-gated Na^+- and K^+-ion channel. Activation of AMPA receptors at normal negative membrane potentials permits passage of Na^+ into the cell, permitting a rapid and large depolarization. AMPA receptors are thus the principal receptor through which neuronal transmission occurs.
- NMDA (*N*-methyl-D-aspartate) receptors: NMDA receptors require two conditions for activation. One is the presence of glutamate and the second is the removal of a Mg^{2+} ion block in the channel. This occurs when the membrane potential of the neuron is raised usually following AMPA activation. NMDA receptor activation permits movement of large amounts of both Na^+ and Ca^{2+} into the cell. Passage of large amounts of Ca^{2+} activates the cellular machinery and is likely to be involved with learning and memory (see Ch. 13).
- Metabotropic glutamate receptors (mGluR). This is a G-protein coupled receptor.

GABA

γ-Aminobutyric acid (GABA) is the principal inhibitory neurotransmitter in the brain. It works to oppose the action of the excitatory neurotransmitters. Two major types of GABA receptor exist: $GABA_A$ and $GABA_B$ receptors. Both modulate synaptic function by permiting movement of Cl^- ions into the postsynaptic cell thereby hyperpolarizing the cell (increasing the negative charge of the cell) and preventing depolarization.

Noradrenaline (norepinephrine)

Noradrenergic neurons originate in the locus coeruleus of the pons, of which in humans there are two, one on either side. Noradrenergic neurons project extensively throughout the brain and the peripheral autonomic nervous system. There are four adrenoreceptors of note: α_1, α_2, β_1 and β_2. These receptors are more recognizable in the context of peripheral effects. α_1 and β_2 receptors tend to oppose each other: α_1-receptors increase noradrenergic function and β_2-receptors decrease noradrenergic function.

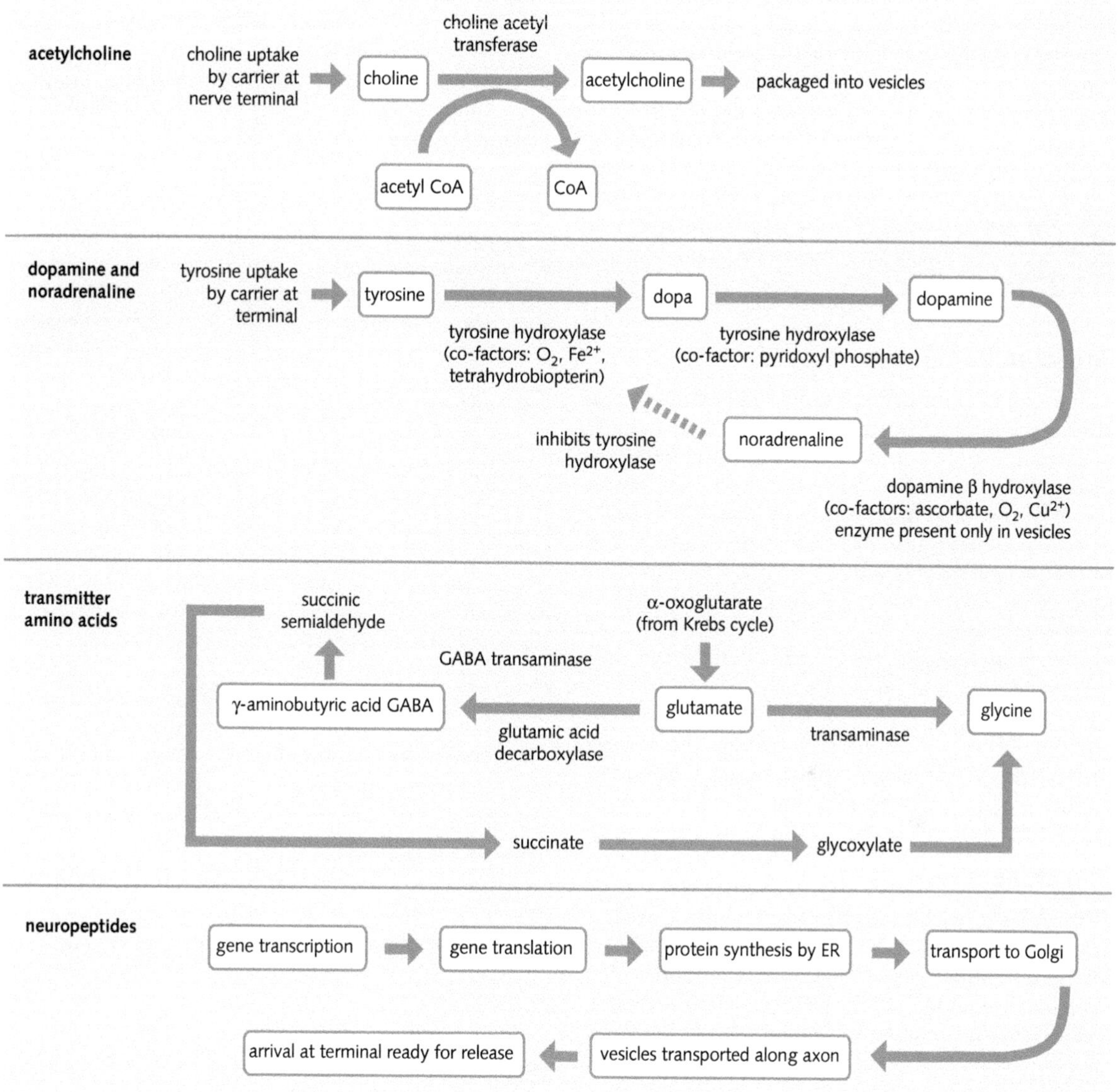

Fig. 3.12 Neurotransmitter synthetic pathways.

Fig. 3.13 Comparison between the two main types of neurotransmitter receptor – ionotrophic and metabotrophic		
	Ionotropic	**Metabotrophic**
Structure	Transmembrane ion channel composed of five subunits, binding sites for ligand and modulators outside cell	Single transmembrane protein with sites for interaction with ligand outside cell and interaction with G-protein inside cell
Functional units	Each subunit has four transmembrane domains and subunits create a charge field to attract either cations or anions, e.g. AChα subunit attracts Na^+, $GABA_B$ subunit attracts Cl^-	Seven transmembrane domains with specific amino-acid residues within domains important for ligand binding, e.g. D_1 receptor has aspartate in domain 3 for dopamine binding

It seems that as a global role, noradrenaline is responsible for modulating arousal, the sleep–wake cycle and cognitive function (such as attention, working memory and anxiety). To do this noradrenaline acts to increase the flow of Ca^{2+} through neurons, making neurons more responsive to stimuli. Electrophysiological recordings from noradrenergic neurons show they are best activated by new, unexpected stimuli. Noradrenaline can make neurons of the cortex more responsive, speed up information processing and make the brain function more efficiently.

Serotonin (5-HT)

Serotonin neurons are mostly clustered within the nine raphe nuclei, each of which projects to different regions of the brain. Caudal nuclei in the medulla innervate the spinal cord to modulate pain-related sensory signals. Rostral nuclei in the pons and midbrain innervate the cortex in a similar way to locus coeruleus neurons. Over twenty 5-hydroxytryptamine (5-HT) receptors exist, all of which modulate neuronal firing via different second messenger systems.

5-HT is implicated in the control of mood and emotional behaviour and low levels of serotonin are associated with many mood disorders. Cortical serotonin activity is believed to promote a positive world view, counteracting the tendency of the amygdala to produce negative emotions and world views.

Dopamine

There are two nuclei from which dopaminergic neurons arise: the substantia nigra of the midbrain and the ventral tegmental area (VTA). The substantia nigra projects to the striatum of the basal ganglia (the caudate nucleus and the putamen) to facilitate the induction of voluntary movement (see Ch. 6). The VTA neurons innervate much of the telencephalon including the cortex of the frontal lobe and limbic system.

Traditionally dopamine has been associated with 'reward' in animals and humans, such that an animal will seek out activities that increase dopaminergic transmission. In reality it is more likely that dopamine increases brain awareness of stimuli that will increase survival. Dopamine also plays role in attention; application of dopamine to prefrontal cortex neurons strengthens transmission of information.

Acetylcholine

Acetylcholine is found at the neuromuscular junction and at postganglionic parasympathetic synapses. Central cholinergic neurons also exist in the striatum and the cortex. The cholinergic pathways in the brain may be important for memory formation; anticholinesterase drugs seem to help people with Alzheimer's disease and anticholinergics make their symptoms worse.

Two acetylcholine receptors exist:

- Nicotinic receptors: these are ion channels receptors involved in the fast transmission of acetylcholine transmission.
- Muscarinic receptors: these are G-protein-coupled receptors and transmit more slowly.

Cortex-bound neurons appear to mediate attention. When undertaking tasks that require long durations of attention, large amounts of acetylcholine (ACh) efflux have been measured. It appears that ACh can change neuronal firing by reducing the signal-to-noise ratio of the neuron. Imagine listening to two stereos playing two different albums. Should you wish to listen to your favourite album, you would turn down the stereo that is not playing your favourite. The same is true of the signal-to-noise ratio: the signal is your favourite album and the noise is the other, less favourite, album. Post-synaptic cells are bombarded by transmission not only from the cell it is interested in, but also transmission from several other neurons. ACh helps to increase the strength of the signal that the post-synaptic cell is interested in.

HINTS AND TIPS

Myasthenia gravis is an autoimmune condition caused by antibodies to the postsynaptic acetylcholine receptor. It is characterized by muscle weakness which becomes progressively worse with exercise (fatigability). Reduction in symptoms after intravenous injection of a short-acting anticholinesterase (edrophonium bromide) confirms the diagnosis (the Tensilon test).

Peptides

Peptides (opioids, neuropeptide-Y, substance-P, somatostatin) are an extremely diverse group, with equally wide-ranging functions. Some have hormone activity (somatostatin, insulin), others modulate nociceptive pathways in the spinal cord and brainstem (opioids). They are commonly released along with small molecules which themselves have neurotransmitter-like actions (e.g. ATP). Peptides are commonly referred to as neuromodulators because they are thought to modulate the release and postsynaptic effects of other neurotransmitters.

Regulation of transmitter synthesis

Transmitter synthesis is regulated in the short term by the intracellular calcium level at the terminal bouton. If the neuron fires many action potentials, Ca^{2+} builds

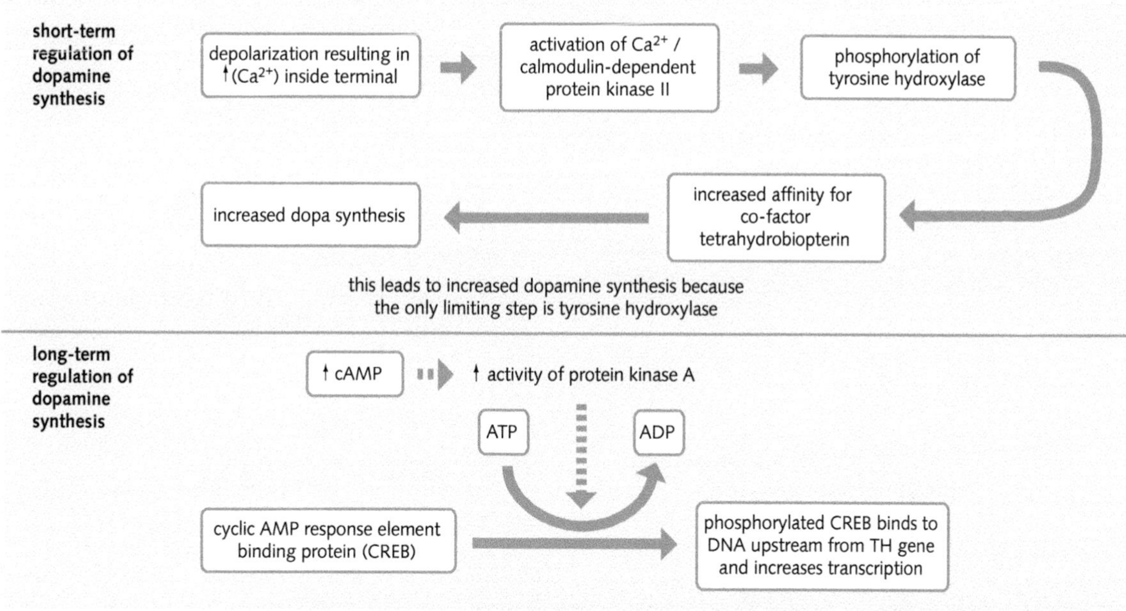

Fig. 3.14 Short- and long-term regulation of dopamine synthesis (TH, tyrosine hydroxylase).

up at the bouton. This increases the activity of Ca^{2+}-dependent protein kinases and in turn influences the enzymes in the transmitter pathway.

In the longer term, regulation occurs by second messenger action on gene transcription of the rate-limiting enzyme. Figure 3.14 shows these processes for dopamine regulation.

Neural networks

Different kinds of processing require different arrangements of connections in a neuronal circuit. Neurons that form the output from a particular circuit integrate information from that circuit and send it elsewhere. An example is the cortical motor neuron that projects its axon in the corticospinal tract. A large number of neuronal contacts influence the cells because many different circuits govern voluntary movement. This is an example of convergence.

Sensory information entering the brain needs to go to different areas for processing. Pain, for example, has components of localization, intensity and emotion, yet only a few receptors send this information to the central nervous system. The neurons in this circuit show a diverging pattern of connections. Similar information goes to different areas that are responsible for different aspects of pain perception.

Visual information is initially processed in isolation in the central nervous system in parallel pathways. Consequently, when certain neuronal groups are active the brain appreciates that information is coming in from a restricted part of 3D space and this increases our perceptual abilities. At higher levels, this information is integrated so that we consciously perceive a picture rather than a collection of lines and colours in different areas of the visual field.

Noise is background neuronal activity that is unconnected with information carried in the circuit. Noise makes the information in a circuit less well defined. At the cellular level, arrangements of inhibitory connections can reduce 'noise'.

Different patterns of inhibition serve different functions:

- Recurrent inhibition is shown in Figure 3.15. It permits a stable discharge without sudden (potentially damaging) surges in activity. An example is in the spinal cord where spinal motor neurons are prevented from firing too often by connections with Renshaw cells. The most active cells activate the Renshaw cells maximally, thereby causing a global inhibitory feedback onto the group of cells they belong to. In this way, only the most stimulated cells continue to fire and the output of the group of cells becomes more focused.
- Lateral inhibition is shown in Figure 3.16. Inhibitory interneurons can be used to 'sharpen' a response, to give a distinct border between the 'on' and 'off' part of a receptive field.
- Presynaptic inhibition is shown in Figure 3.17. An inhibitory synapse placed on a terminal bouton can reduce the membrane depolarization caused

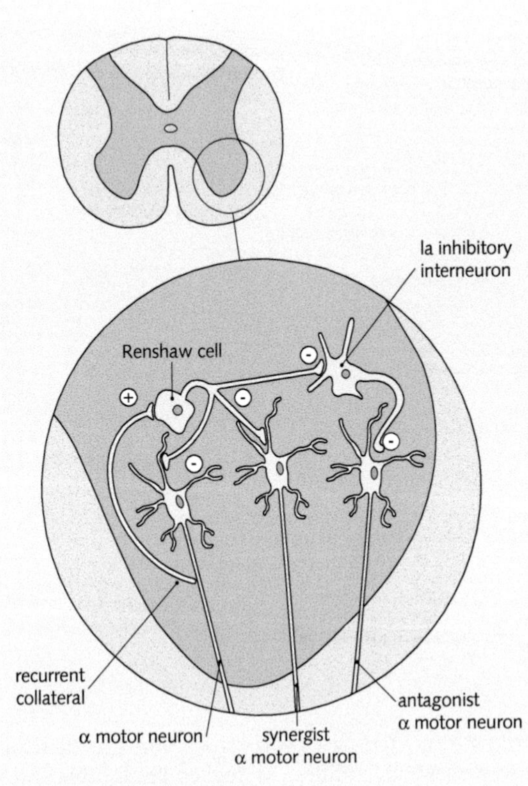

Fig. 3.15 Recurrent inhibition. When the α motor neuron is activated, it also activates the Renshaw cell, which in turn inhibits the motor neuron and synergistic motor neurons. It also relieves antagonistic motor neurons of their inhibition.

by an incoming action potential. By increasing permeability to Cl^-, when the inside of the cell becomes more positive with Na^+ current, Cl" starts to move into the bouton. This reduces the inward flow of Ca^{2+} and therefore reduces exocytosis.

Inhibition is used in the creation of receptive fields, as shown in Figure 3.16. A receptive field is the area which, when stimulated, causes a particular neuron to fire. It can be altered by inhibitory connections with neighbouring sensory units. This can produce a receptive field where the receptor responds to stimulation in one area but is inhibited by stimulation immediately adjacent to that area, a so-called 'on' centre and an 'off' surround (e.g. in retinal ganglion cells).

Considering higher level processing, there are connections between large groups of cells. Feedback loops between circuits encourage stable patterns of firing within individual circuits. Parallel pathways occur where there is more than one route between two groups of cells. This arrangement may serve to allow different processing to occur along a pathway (e.g. in relay nuclei), or may simply be an example of redundancy (useful if one pathway is damaged).

HINTS AND TIPS

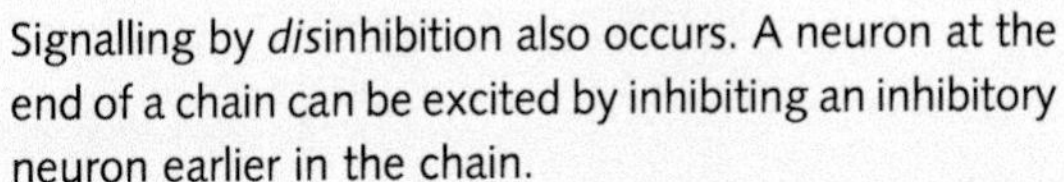

Signalling by *dis*inhibition also occurs. A neuron at the end of a chain can be excited by inhibiting an inhibitory neuron earlier in the chain.

INTRODUCTION TO PHARMACOLOGY OF THE NERVOUS SYSTEM

Manipulation of neurotransmission forms the basis for CNS pharmacology and therapetics. Chapter 16 brings together some of the concepts introduced earlier and outlines the mechanism of action of certain drugs that modulate the nervous system.

Delivering drugs to the brain is problematic due to the presence of the blood–brain barrier. The cells of the cerebral vessel walls are bound tightly with intercellular junctions such that diffusion between cells becomes negligible. There are very few gap junctions to help with paracellular drug transport. Lipid-soluble molecules diffuse readily through the lipid layer, however, water soluble molecules diffuse much more slowly. This relative impermeability underlies the stable internal environment needed for optimal neural function; fluctuations in the concentration of nutrients, hormones or ions do not affect synaptic or neuron cell function. Molecular transport mechanisms do exist for the delivery of molecules neurons are unable to produce themselves (e.g. glucose, neutral proteins).

This impermeability represents an obstacle for drug delivery. Drugs which are lipophilic find passage into the brain relatively easy (e.g. chloramphenicol), whereas hydrophilic drugs find the passage much more difficult (e.g. penicillin). There are four options for overcoming this problem:

1. High-dose drug administration to overcome poor membrane permeability. This is only feasible if the drug is non-toxic in high doses.
2. Intrathecal (i.e. into the spinal cord) delivery of drugs. This requires that the drug or vehicle is not neurotoxic when delivered in high doses, as well as appropriate training.
3. Change the shape or structure of a drug to make it more lipophilic.

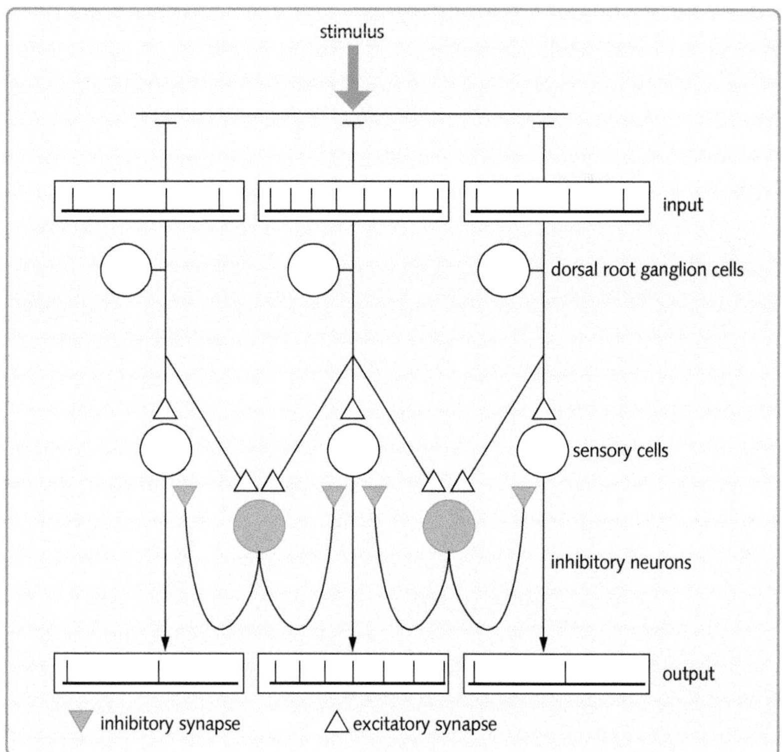

Fig. 3.16 Lateral inhibition. A stimulus causes a response in one receptor maximally and, to a lesser extent, in neighbouring receptors. If solely excitatory neurons link the inputs (level one), the signal becomes blurred. However, if inhibitory interneurons are introduced, then the cells which are not maximally stimulated will cease to fire. This sharpens the border between 'off and 'on' (level 2) in a receptive field.

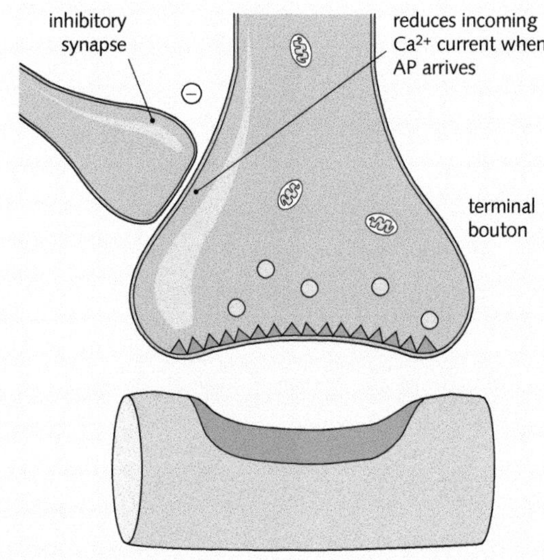

Fig. 3.17 Presynaptic inhibition preventing vesicle mobilization and release by decreasing calcium influx.

4. Engage a transport system used to deliver proteins to the central nervous system from the blood (e.g. L-dopa; see below) or develop a drug that can be combined with a molecule that is transported across the blood–brain barrier.

A classic example of this is the delivery of dopamine to patients with Parkinson's disease. It is not possible to give dopamine itself in the treatment of Parkinson's disease because of its vasopressive systemic effects. The precursor of dopamine is levodopa (L-dopa). This is inert in the periphery and only produces 'active' dopamine once decarboxylated by amino acid decarboxylase, which is found in the endothelial cells of the brain vasculature. L-dopa enters the endothelial cells via an active carrier system on the luminal membrane or via a passive transport channel located on the abluminal side. This example demonstrates how it is possible to use the intrinsic nature of the blood–brain barrier to ensure safe and adequate delivery of drugs to the CNS.

The spinal cord and peripheral nerves

4

Objectives

In this chapter you will learn about:

- The anatomy of the spinal cord.
- The tracts within the cord and the modalities they subserve.
- The effect of damage to the spinal cord.
- Peripheral nerve structure and function.
- Peripheral nerve pathology.

THE SPINAL CORD

The spinal cord and its associated spinal nerves provide sensory, motor and autonomic innervation for the limbs and trunk. It occupies the vertebral canal within the vertebral column and is continuous rostrally with the medulla oblongata. The cord is approximately cylindrical and arranged segmentally with a central cellular area (grey matter) surrounded by nerve-fibre tracts (white matter). The tracts carry information between different levels of the spinal cord (thereby permitting reflex actions), and also to and from the supraspinal structures. In adults, the cord ends at vertebral body level L1/L2 (Fig. 4.1).

The spinal cord bears two enlargements – the cervical (C3–T1) and lumbar (L1–S3) enlargements – which provide innervation of upper and lower limbs respectively. There are 31 bilaterally paired spinal nerves (Fig. 4.2). They attach to the spinal cord via dorsal and ventral roots which contain primary afferent and efferent neurons respectively (afferent neurons carry information to the central nervous system (CNS); efferent neurons carry impulses away from the CNS). Dorsal and ventral roots join to form the spinal nerve proper near to the intervertebral foramen where spinal nerves exit the vertebral canal. Here, small enlagements can also be seen on the dorsal roots. These are the dorsal root ganglia containing the cell bodies of the primary afferent neurons.

HINTS AND TIPS

The cord terminates at the level of the intervertebral disc between L1/L2 in adults. Therefore a lumbar puncture needle can be inserted into the subarachnoid space below this level (e.g. L3/L4) without damaging the cord.

Below the termination of the cord (L1/L2), the lumbar and sacral nerve roots descend as the cauda equina.

HINTS AND TIPS

Spinal nerve roots are vulnerable to injury, particularly compression, caused either by degenerative changes in the spine (e.g. spondylosis) or by prolapsed intervertebral discs.

Grey matter of the spinal cord

Cells in the central grey matter can be divided into a series of layers in the dorsal horn and as a series of columns in the ventral horn (Fig. 4.3). These layers and columns are known as Rexed's laminae (numbered I–X) and are based on groupings of similarly shaped cell bodies:

- The dorsal horn layers are involved in sensory pathways and are the target sites for some sensory afferent nerves, particularly for pain, temperature and crude touch.
- The ventral columns are made up of pools of motor neurons innervating skeletal muscle. Medial motor columns supply proximal muscles and lateral motor columns supply distal muscles.
- In between the dorsal and ventral horns lies the interomediolateral column where the cell bodies of preganglionic sympathetic neurons are found.

THE SPINAL TRACTS

White matter of the spinal cord

The white matter of the spinal cord consists of ascending and descending nerve fibres and completely surrounds the grey matter. As a general rule, the ascending sensory tracts run at the periphery and descending motor tracts

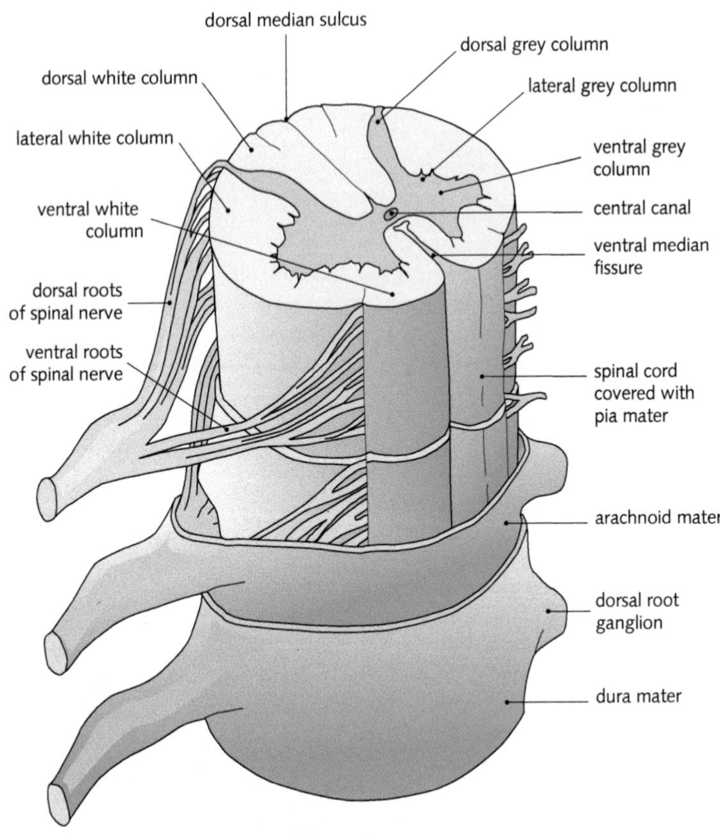

Fig. 4.1 Spinal cord above the level of L1, showing the meningeal coverings (dura mater, arachnoid mater and pia mater).

occupy a more central position, as shown in Figure 4.4. Sensory inputs from the skin terminate in laminae I–IV, with some fibres travelling to the segments above and below in Lissauer's tract.

Ascending tracts

The major difference between the main sensory tracts is that fine touch and vibration information (dorsal column tract) is conveyed up the cord on the same side as it enters, whereas pain, temperature and crude touch (spinothalamic tract) immediately cross and travel upwards on the opposite side of the cord. The point at which the spinothalamic tract crosses to the contralateral side is known as the decussation.

A sequence of three neurons conveys signals between the peripheral receptor and the cerebral cortex:

- First-order neurons (or primary afferent neurons) enter the spinal cord via the dorsal roots of spinal nerves (their cell body lies in the dorsal root ganglion). They make synaptic contact with second order neurons either in the spinal cord grey matter or the medulla.
- The cell bodies of second-order neurons lie in the cord or medulla. Their axons decussate (cross to the contralteral side of the CNS) and ascend to the thalamus where they synapse with third-order neurons.
- Third-order neuron cell bodies lie in thalamus. Their axons project to the somatosensory cortex in the parietal lobe.

Both sensory tracts are arranged segmentally (i.e. fibres from the same level run upwards together in the tract). At the top of the dorsal columns, the segments are arranged in a coherent pattern from medial (sacral) to lateral (cervical), maintaining the body pattern from which they arise.

Dorsal columns

There are two tracts located within the dorsal columns; the fasciculus gracilis (medially) and the fasciculus cuneatus (laterally). One of the functions of the dorsal columns is to rearrange the dermatomal input of the primary sensory fibres into the map of the body surface seen in the primary sensory cortex (the sensory homunculus). Here, the body surface is seen as grossly distorted

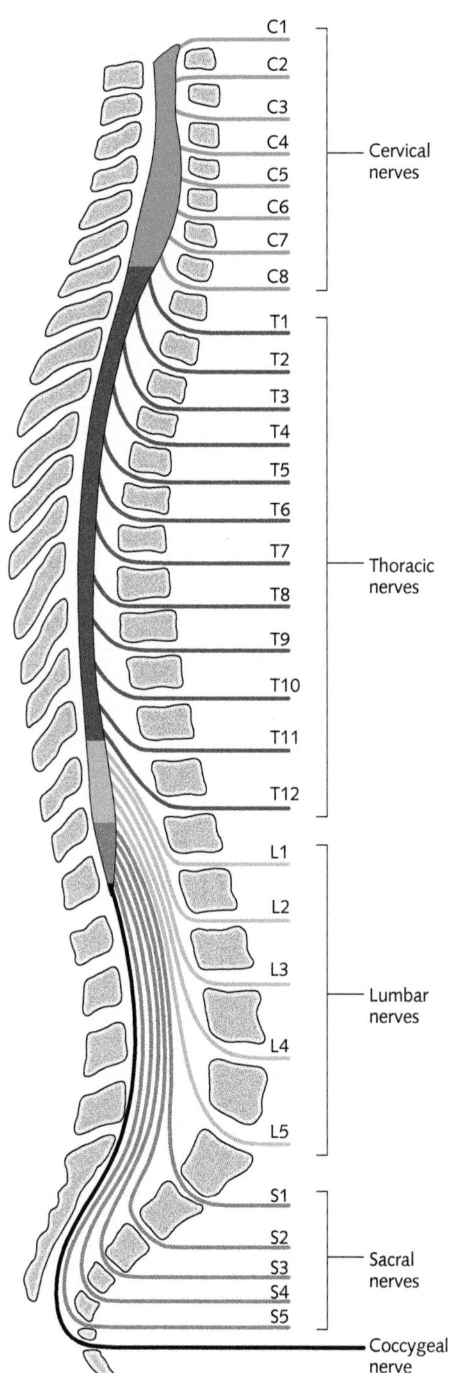

Fig. 4.2 The spinal nerves. The C1–C7 spinal nerves exit the vertebral canal above the first seven cervical vertebrae; C8 exits below the 7th cervical vertebrae; the remainder exit below their corresponding vertebrae.

and is based on the number of receptors originating from any given structure. As such, most of the cortical cells respond to sensory exploratory structures such as the hands, feet and lips, all of which have high numbers of sensory receptors. This pathway:

- Segregates information into modality-specific pathways for touch, hair movement, pressure, vibration and joint rotation
- Contains feedback mechanisms to gate the amount of incoming information to the cortex.

These functions are carried out in the areas where the pathway is interrupted by synapses, which allow for reorganization, segregation and suppression of the ascending sensory signals. Figure 4.5 shows the three-neuron sequence of the dorsal columns. Large sensory axons (Aα) enter the spinal cord and ascend ipsilaterally. The first order neuronal cell bodies lie in the dorsal root ganglia. They synapse with the dorsal column nuclei (gracile and cuneate) of the medulla in the pattern shown below:

- Sensory input from the leg and lower trunk travels to the gracile nucleus
- Sensory input from the arm, upper trunk and neck to the cuneate nucleus
- Sensory input from the face goes via the trigeminal nerve (cranial nerve V) to the trigeminal nucleus.

At this point the fibres are still ipsilateral to the side they have arisen from.

Axons from the cells in the gracile and cuneate nuclei then travel towards the ventral medulla where they decussate and continue toward the thalamus via the medial lemniscus. At the point of the decussation, all somatic sensory systems arising from one side of the body will be processed by the opposite (i.e. contralateral) side of the brain. The next synapse is in the contralateral ventroposterolateral nucleus of the thalamus (or VPL) or the contralateral ventroposteromedial nucleus (VPM) for trigeminal inputs (which have travelled in a separate trigeminothalamic tract).

The homuncular organization which began in the dorsal columns and trigeminal nuclei is amplified in the thalamus and the sensory cortex. The neurons from the VPL and VPM nuclei project to the cortex (the primary somatosensory cortex, S1) via the thalamocortical radiations.

Information travelling along the dorsal column does not arrive at S1 in the same form it has when it enters the spinal cord. Information changes occur at both synapses (in the medulla and thalamus). For instance, lateral inhibition occurs between adjacent sets of inputs in the dorsal column pathway, allowing the distinction between background and 'true' sensory information to be increased and processed accordingly.

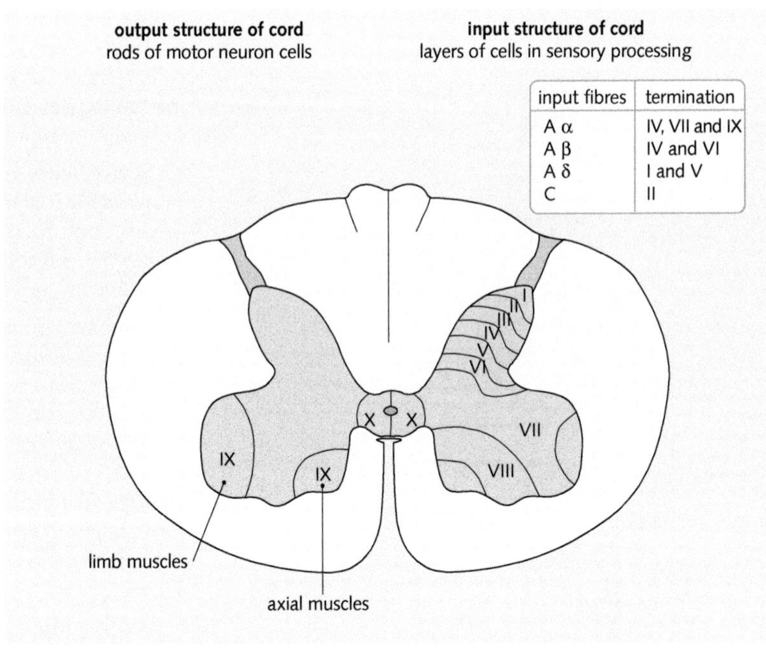

Fig. 4.3 Rexed's laminae. The different termination patterns of afferent fibres are shown.

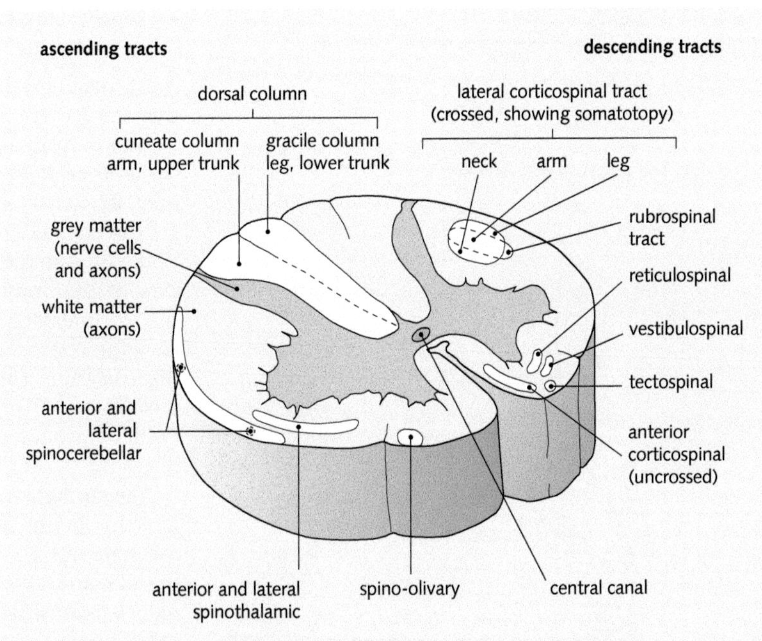

Fig. 4.4 Ascending and descending spinal tracts.

Lesions of the dorsal columns

Tabes dorsalis

This is a late manifestion of syphilis. It predominately affects the dorsal columns and lumbosacral dorsal spinal roots. The loss of proprioception leads to an unsteady high-stepping gait (sensory ataxia), which is exaggerated when the eyes are closed (positive Romberg's sign). Other symptoms and signs include sensory disturbance (legs, chest and bridge of nose), episodes of sudden-onset intense pain, diminished reflexes and joint deformities (Charcot's joints).

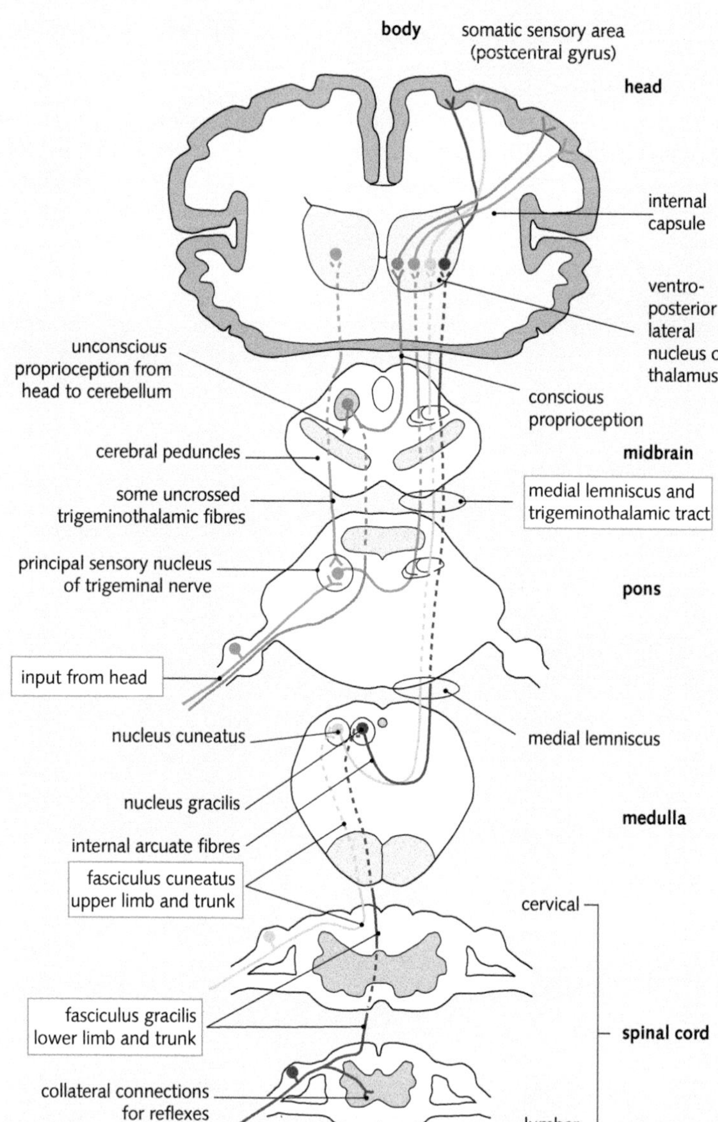

Fig. 4.5 The dorsal column pathway for touch and proprioception. The system is a three-neuron pathway with synapses in the medulla, thalamus and cortex. Note the decussation in the medulla.

Subacute combined degeneration of the spinal cord

Here there is a combination of dorsal column and corticospinal tract loss resulting from a deficiancy of vitamin B_{12} (hence the name 'combined'), although a similar pattern may be seen in copper deficiency. The degeneration of the dorsal columns produces sensory ataxia and lower motor neuron (LMN) signs while the involvement of the corticospinal tract leads to weakness and spasticity of the limbs (upper motor neuron (UMN) signs). Often patients present with falls at night due to ataxia and impaired vision (also seen in B_{12} deficiency). On examination, the classic triad is extensor plantars (UMN), absent knee jerks and absent ankle jerks (LMN). Treatment with B_{12} can lead to a complete recovery.

Spinothalamic tract

In addition to pain, the spinothalamic tract also carries crude touch and thermal information. Pain information is also carried in the spinoreticular and spinomesencephalic tracts.

Noxious and thermal information is carried into the dorsal horn by fast myelinated Aδ fibres (conveying sharp, stabbing pain) and slower unmyelinated C fibres (conveying dull, nagging pain as well as thermal information).

Aδ fibres terminate in laminae I and V. The axons from these cells immediately cross over to the opposite side of the cord (decussate) through the ventral white commissure and ascend in the anterolateral white matter, forming the spinothalamic tract. Note this immediate decussation is different from that of the dorsal column pathway, as it occurs in the spinal cord as opposed to the medulla. The spinothalamic tract is, however, similar to the dorsal column pathway in that there are three orders of neurons; first-order neurons in dorsal root ganglia, second-order neurons in dorsal grey matter and third-order neurons in the thalamus.

C fibres influence the firing of the spinothalamic dorsal horn cells via interneurons, because they terminate in a different layer of the cord-lamina II. This provides further synaptic steps in the pain pathway, which may comprise targets for modulation of pain signal transmission by higher centres. This pathway will be discussed in greater detail in Chapter 5.

Figure 4.6 shows that the spinothalamic fibres join the medial lemniscus in the medulla and project to

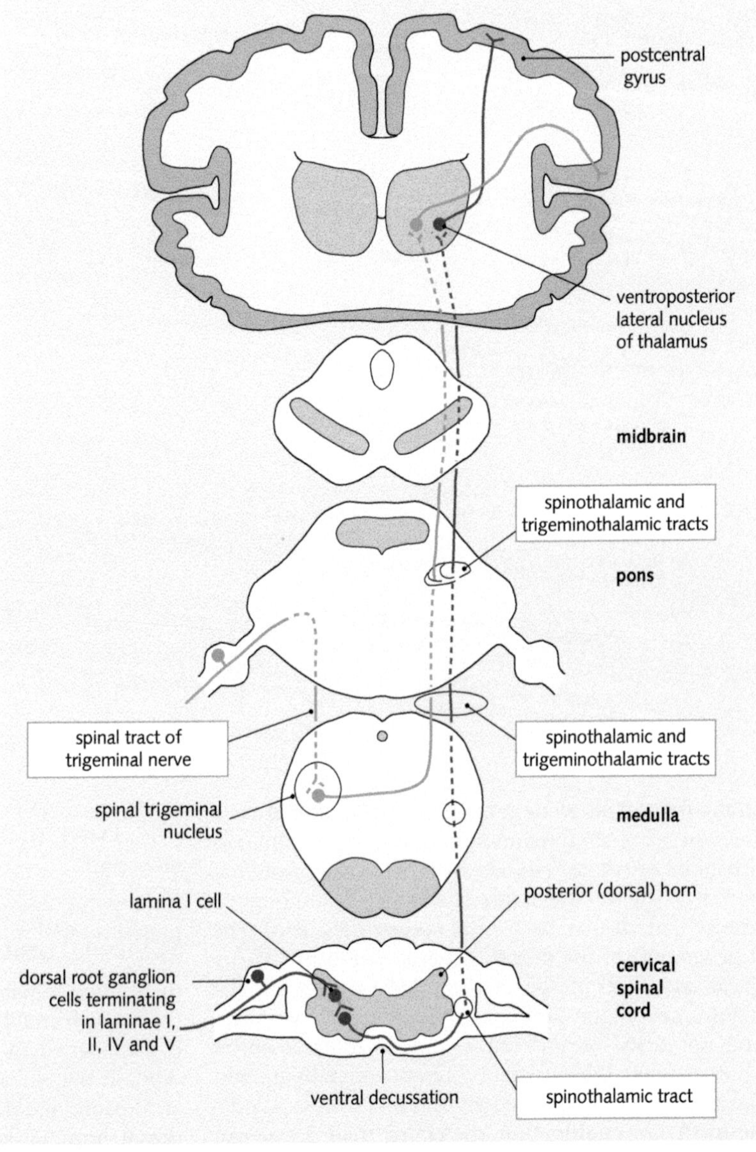

Fig. 4.6 The spinothalamic tract. Note the decussation at the same spinal level as the afferent fibres enter the cord.

the thalamus. The thalamic termination of the tract is in the ventroposterior nuclei and also in the intralaminar nuclei, from which there is a relay to the cortex.

As with fine touch, nociceptive afferent nerves from the face are carried in the trigeminal (V) nerve to the spinal trigeminal nucleus (which takes over the function of dorsal horn laminae I and II). The ascending fibres from the spinal nucleus of V cross over to the other side of the medulla and pass up to the thalamus to join the nociceptive spinothalamic inputs from the rest of the body.

Noxious input also projects to a variety of brainstem structures, some of which are implicated in generating sensations of agonizing pain (spinomesencephalic) whereas others are involved in arousal mechanisms (spinoreticular).

Spinothalamic tract lesions

Syringomyelia

In syringomyelia the central canal becomes enlarged, forming a cavity that compresses adjacent nerve fibres. The spinothalamic tracts can be selectively damaged; second-order neurons subserving temperature and pain may be damaged as they decussate in the ventral white commissure (close to the central canal) causing loss of pain and temperature sensation in the upper limbs ('cape' distribution or 'suspended' sensory loss) with preserved light touch and proprioception sensation, i.e. a dissociated sensory loss. Anterior horn cells are similarly vulnerable (see Fig. 2.10).

Spinocerebellar tract

The spinocerebellar tract (Fig. 4.7) deals with proprioceptive information and can be divided into two parts:

- The dorsal spinocerebellar tract is formed by the axons of cell bodies that lie in a column at the base of the dorsal horn (Clarke's column) running from T1 to L2. These cells receive information from muscle spindles and tendon organs (see Ch. 6). Below L2, the fibres ascend in the dorsal columns before they synapse with the cells in Clarke's column. The dorsal spinocerebellar tract conveys information about body movement, from the trunk and lower limb, to the cerebellum via the inferior cerebellar peduncle. The same kind of information from the upper limb is transferred via the external cuneate nucleus located laterally in the medulla. Information carried by dorsal spinocerebellar tract remains ipsilateral to the side of the body from which the fibres originate.
- The ventral spinocerebellar tract receives its input from cell bodies in lamina VII (the spinal interneuron layer). Most of the axons cross/decussate in their segment then travel up to the cerebellum via the superior cerebellar peduncle where most of the axons cross over again. This tract sends information primarily about inhibitory interneuron activity.

Spinocerebellar tract lesions

Friedreich's ataxia

This is an autosomal recessive disorder in which there is degeneration of many nerve tracts. The spinocerebellar tract is particulary disordered causing a wide-based gait (ataxia) and incoordination of the arms (dysdiadochokinesis and intentention tremor). Corticospinal tract and dorsal column degeneration also occur. The disorder begins in childhood and there is no cure. Surgery may provide symptomatic relief.

Descending tracts

Corticospinal tract

The corticospinal tract (sometimes called the pyramidal tract) is pimarily concerned with the control of skeletal muscle activity, particularly skilled voluntary movements in the distal parts of the limbs.

Two-thirds of pyramidal tract neurons originate from cell bodies in the motor cortex (Brodmann's areas 4 and 6; see Ch. 6). In the primary motor cortex, Betz cells give rise to the largest diameter corticospinal axons. The remaining third arise from the sensory cortices in the parietal lobes. Axons pass through the posterior third of internal capsule to the base of the cerebral peduncles. From here, the fibres descend through the pons to form a triangular fibre tract on the ventral surface of the medulla (hence the term pyramidal tract). The tract mostly decussates at the junction between medulla and spinal cord, after which they continue on the side contralateral to their origin in the motor cortex.

The corticospinal tract has two branches:

- 75–90% of fibres decussate to form the lateral corticospinal tract. This tract controls the precision movements of the limbs (innervating lateral motor neuron pools).
- 10–25% of pyramidal fibres remain uncrossed (ispilateral) forming the ventral corticospinal tract. They do, however, decussate near to their termination. This tract controls the less precise movements of the trunk (innervating medial motor neuron pools).

The fibres influencing motor neurons that innervate muscles in the head (e.g. extraocular muscles, tongue muscles and facial muscles, the bulbar muscles) run in the corticobulbar tracts to the appropriate cranial nerve nuclei. The somatotopic arrangement of the descending motor fibres from the cortex includes the head in the cerebral peduncles, but not at the level of decussation in the medulla.

The motor fibres carry signals for highly skilled voluntary movements. To achieve this:

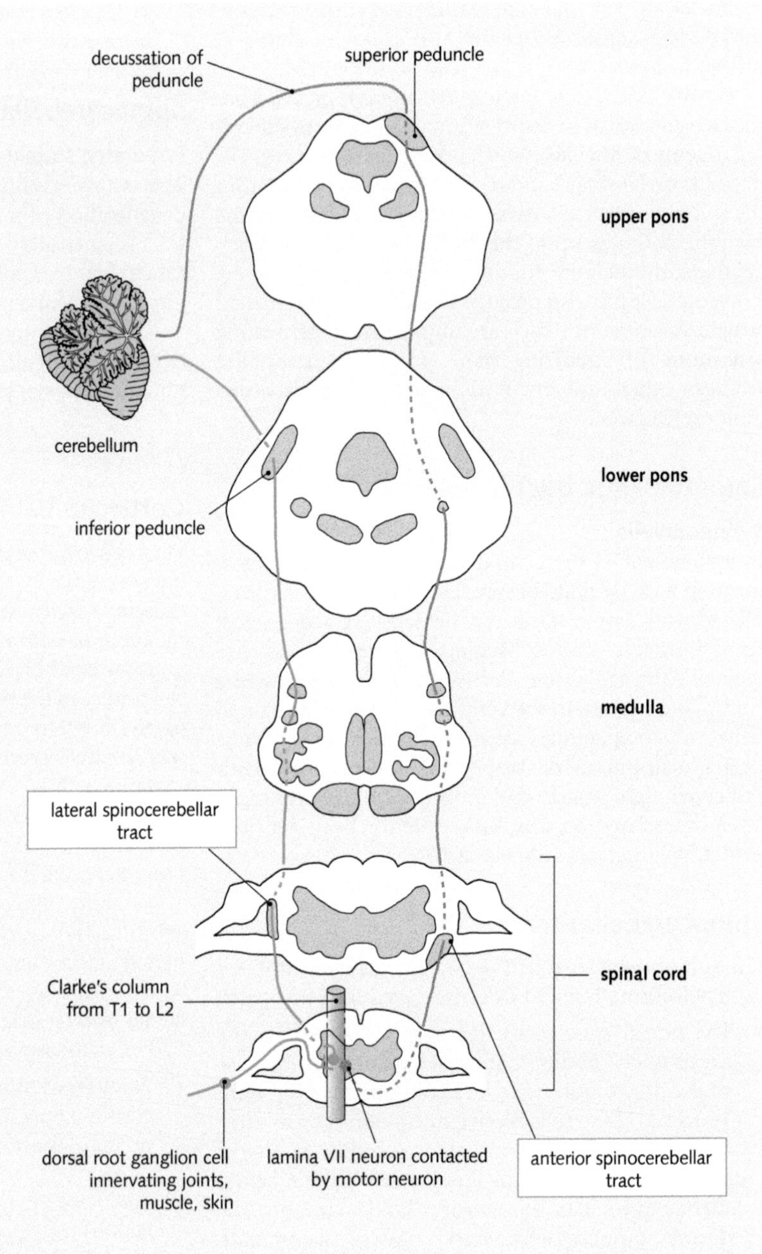

Fig. 4.7 The anterior and lateral spinocerebellar tracts.

- The tract needs to be highly somatotopic (see Ch. 6)
- The fibres must have few collaterals so that excitation from one fibre is communicated to the minimum number of spinal motor neurons (this allows a great deal of control over the execution of movement).

As well as motor axons, there are fibres that regulate spinal reflexes in the tract and feedback to the dorsal horn sensory circuits from the sensory cortex.

Upper and lower motor neuron lesions

Figure 4.8 demonstrates that there are two neurons involved in the descending corticospinal tract:

- An UMN that runs from the cortex to the ventral horn of the spinal cord
- A LMN that runs from the ventral horn to the skeletal muscle.

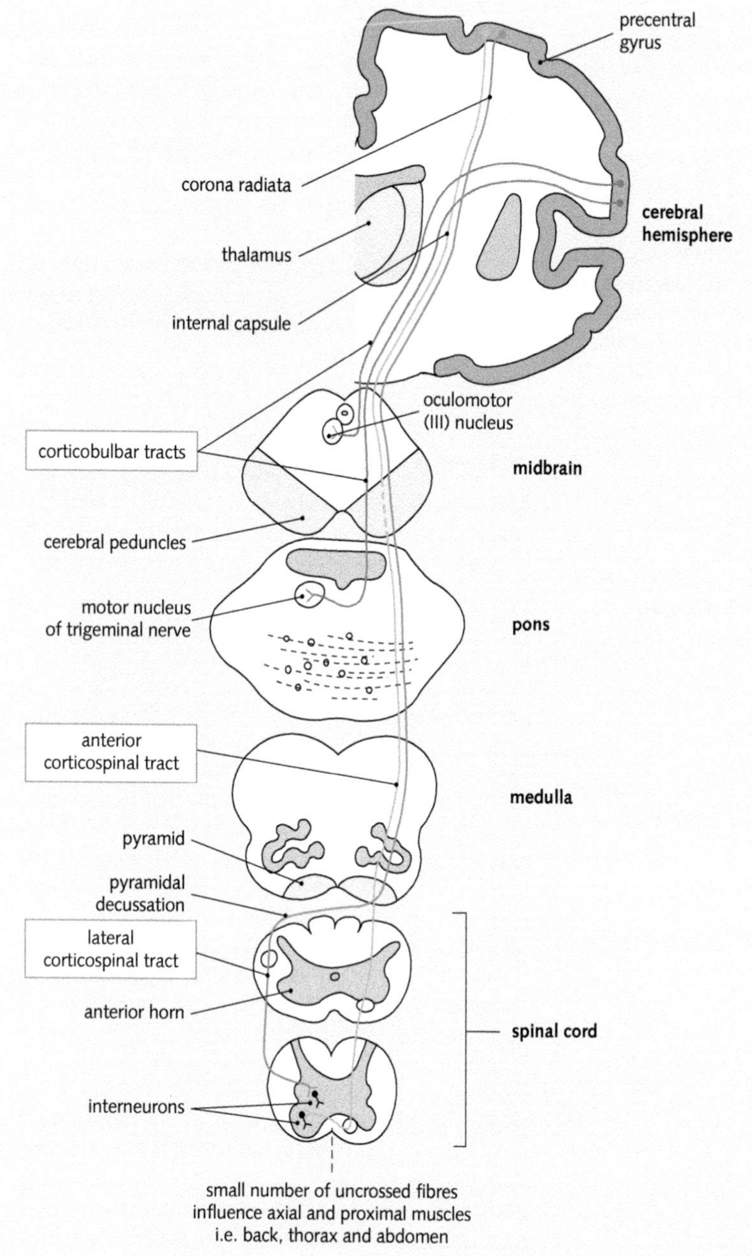

Fig. 4.8 The corticospinal and corticobulbar tracts. Note the decussation in the spinal cord.

Damage to the motor cortex leads to an absence of volitional movement but experimental evidence from cutting just the pyramidal tract in the medulla of monkeys results in very little motor deficit.

In humans, damage to the motor cortex and premotor areas after a cerebrovascular accident (or stroke) in the middle cerebral artery territory leads to a set of symptoms and signs affecting some of the contralateral muscles in the limbs and face. Because upper (i.e. cortical) motor neurons are involved, the effect is termed an 'UMN lesion', although other cells are involved too.

Voluntary paresis (weakness) is caused by loss of corticospinal input (i.e. a loss of UMN input). The symptoms and signs are:

- Weakness involving extensors of the upper limb and flexors of the lower limb

- Spasticity or abnormal distribution in muscle tone which affects flexors more than extensors (this may be caused by disruption of extrapyramidal systems)
- Stronger deep reflexes, e.g. knee jerk (hyperreflexia)
- Loss of superficial reflexes (e.g. abdominal, cremasteric)
- Positive Babinski's sign – extensor plantar response to stroking the lateral part of the sole from heel to toe
- Clonus – elicited by rapidly dorsiflexing the foot (≤ 3 rhythmic downward beats of the foot are normal).

The effects of an UMN lesion are typically seen on the side of the body contralateral to the lesion, because of the decussation of the corticospinal tract in the pyramids of the medulla (the left motor cortex, because of the decussation of fibres, controls the right side of the body). If there is localized damage to the motor cortex or pyramidal tract, all the input to an area will be affected due to homuncular and somatotopic organization.

Damage to the spinal motor neurons (or the LMNs), either in the cord or along their pathway to the site of innervation of the muscle, produces a different set of symptoms and signs, referred to as a LMN lesion:

- Weakness caused by loss of nervous innervation (flaccid paralysis)
- Atrophy as a result of disuse (this is a late sign)
- Fasciculations (wriggling movements of the muscle) caused by increased sensitivity at receptor level to any acetylcholine that is released from intact terminals
- Absent reflexes caused by loss of reflex output
- Plantars remain flexor.

The clinical differences between UMN and LMN lesions are summarized in Figure 4.9.

Fig. 4.9 Upper motor neuron (UMN) vs. lower motor neuron (LMN) lesions-clinical differences

	UMN	LMN
Inspection	Little wasting	Wasting ± fasciculation
Tone	Increased (spasticity)	Reduced
Power	Reduced (pyramidal distribution, i.e. weakness of extensors of upper limb and flexors of lower limb)	Reduced (distribution corresponds to muscles supplied by involved cord segment)
Reflexes	Brisk (hyperreflexia)	Reduced or absent
Plantars	Upgoing ± clonus	Downgoing

Lesions of the spinal cord

Damage to different parts of the spinal cord produce distictive clinical syndromes. Focal lesions of the cord and nerve roots result in clinical manifestations in two ways; lesions can either destroy function at the level of the lesion or disrupt ascending sensory and descending motor tracts. Figure 4.10 illustrates how damage to the cord at different levels can produce different degrees of deficit in both motor and sensory function. Lesions in the VPL nucleus in the thalamus and somatosensory cortex lead to deficits similar to those caused by dorsal column lesions, but on the contralateral side of the body.

HINTS AND TIPS

After transection of the spinal cord, there may be an initial period where no reflexes can be elicited below the level of the lesion (when you would expect exaggerated reflexes). This coincides with a period of 'spinal shock', which may persist for several weeks.

Peripheral nerves

The peripheral nervous system constitutes the link by which the CNS (brain and spinal cord) communicates with peripheral structures in the body. It consists of all the nerve trunks and branches that lie outwith the CNS, i.e. the cranial and spinal nerves. Peripheral nerves may be myelinated (by Schwann cells) or unmyelinated and consist of varying numbers of nerve fibre bundles (which may be either afferent or efferent with respect to the CNS). Fibres are ensheathed by three layers of connective tissue; the endoneurium, perineurium and epineurium, which are continuous with the pia, arachnoid and dura mater respectively.

Spinal nerves innervating the upper and lower limbs coalesce to form the brachial and lumbar plexuses respectively. Here, the nerve fibres are redistributed to form named peripheral nerves (Fig. 4.11). The area of skin that is supplied by a particular spinal nerve is known as a dermatome. The group of muscles innervated by a spinal nerve is known as a myotome. Figure 4.12 shows the dermatome map of the body.

Peripheral nerve pathology

Peripheral nerve trauma, degeneration and regeneration

Trauma to a nerve causes weakness or numbness in the area supplied by that nerve, although sensory nerve injuries tend to cause symptoms and signs in an area smaller than that which the nerve supplies owing to overlap in sensory territories. Trauma may partially or completely disrupt the nerve's function. When a

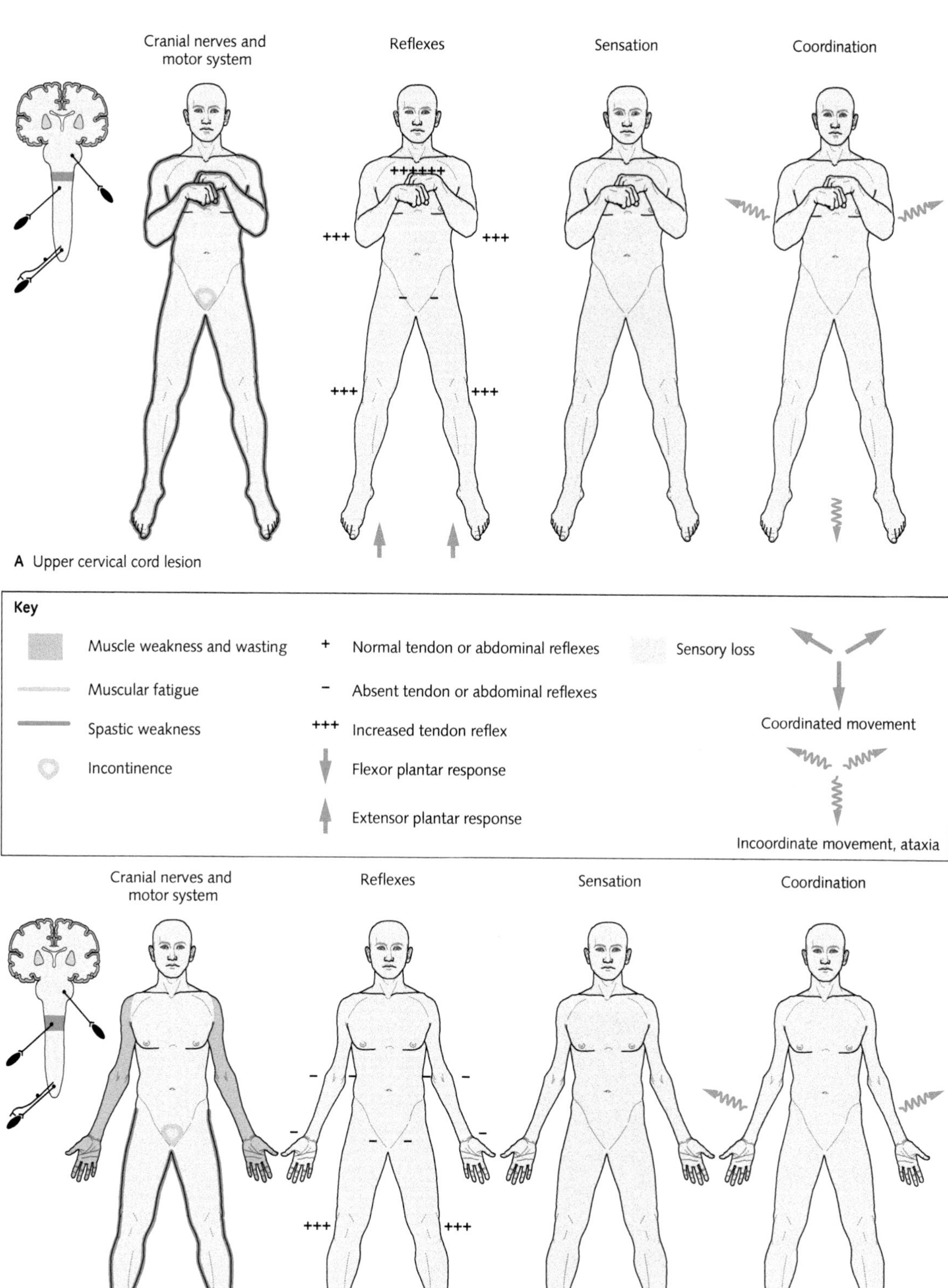

Fig. 4.10 Effects of spinal cord lesions in different areas. The area of lesion is shaded.

Continued

peripheral nerve is transected or seriously damaged, the part of the nerve distal to the transection dies and undergoes degeneration. This process is known as anterograde or Wallerian degeneration. The proximal neuron may survive and undergo regeneration. The further from the cell body that transection occurs, the more likely the cell body is to survive. Axons regrow at a rate of 1.0–1.5 mm/day and may eventually lead to reinnervation of the original structure and recovery of function. Types of nerve injury are given in Figure 4.13.

The main factors influencing restoration of neuronal function after trauma are:

- Integrity of the axon
- Integrity of the basal lamina
- Length of time needed for regrowth to the site of innervation (i.e. distal muscles may atrophy

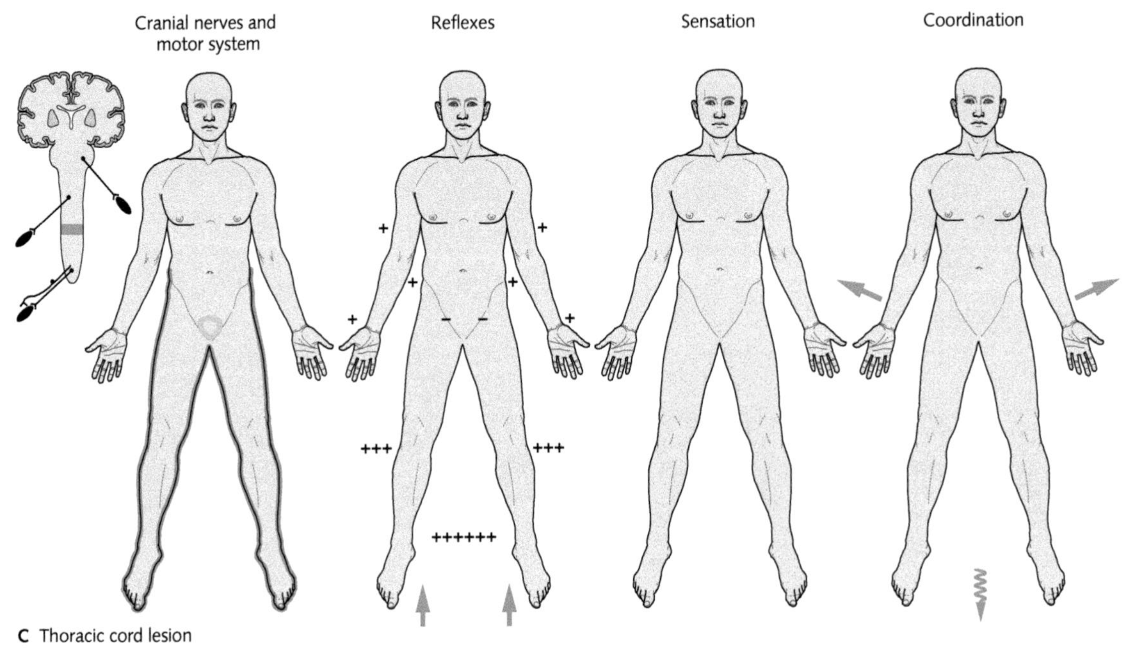

C Thoracic cord lesion

Cranial nerves and motor system
Reflexes
Sensation
Coordination
+
–

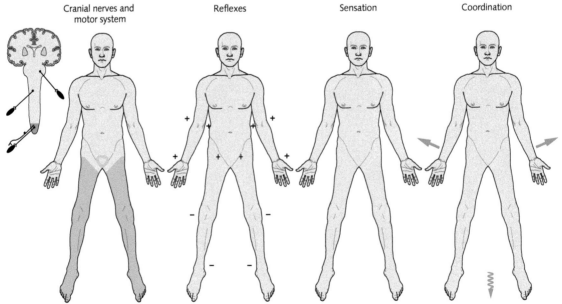

D Lumbar cord lesion

Figure 4.10—cont'd

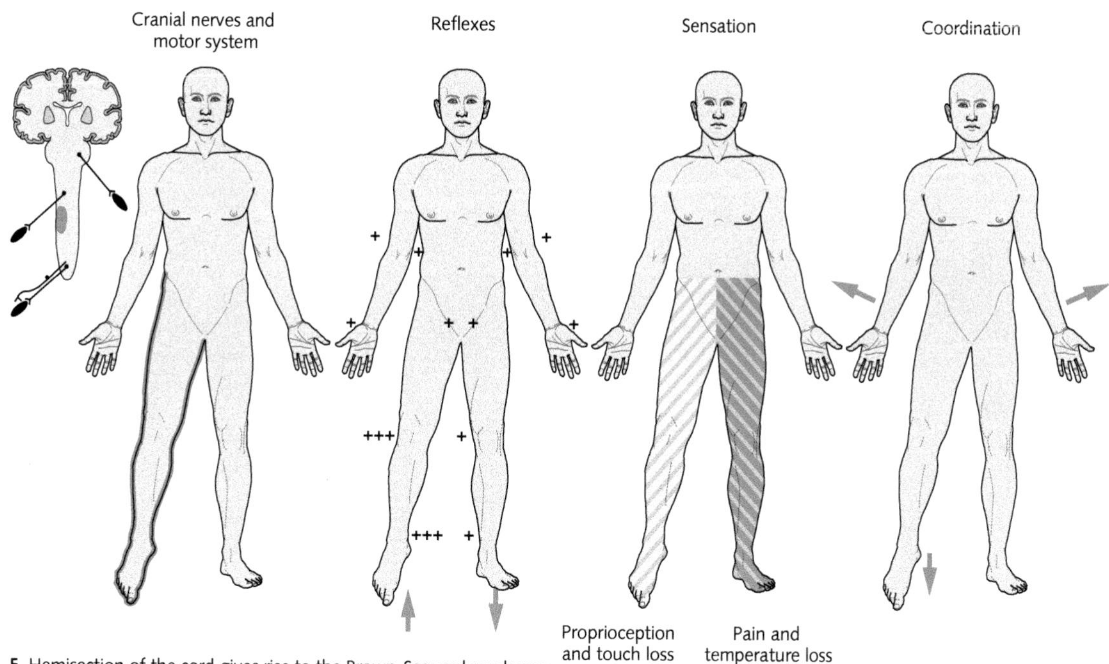

E Hemisection of the cord gives rise to the Brown-Sequard syndrome

Figure 4.10—cont'd

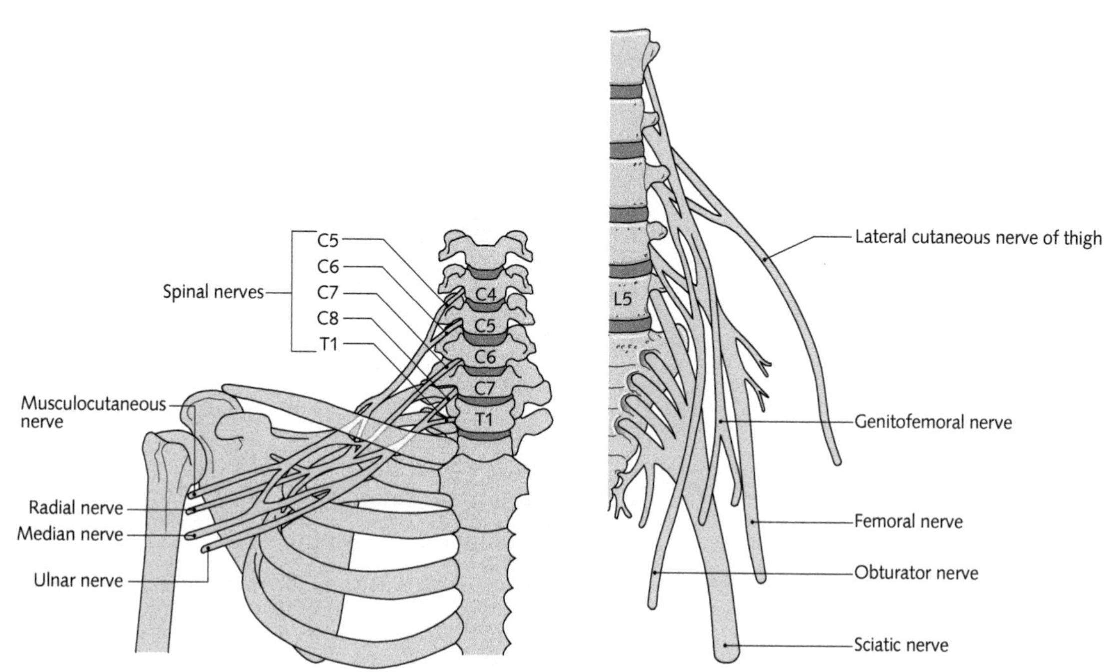

Fig. 4.11 The brachial and lumbosacral plexuses.

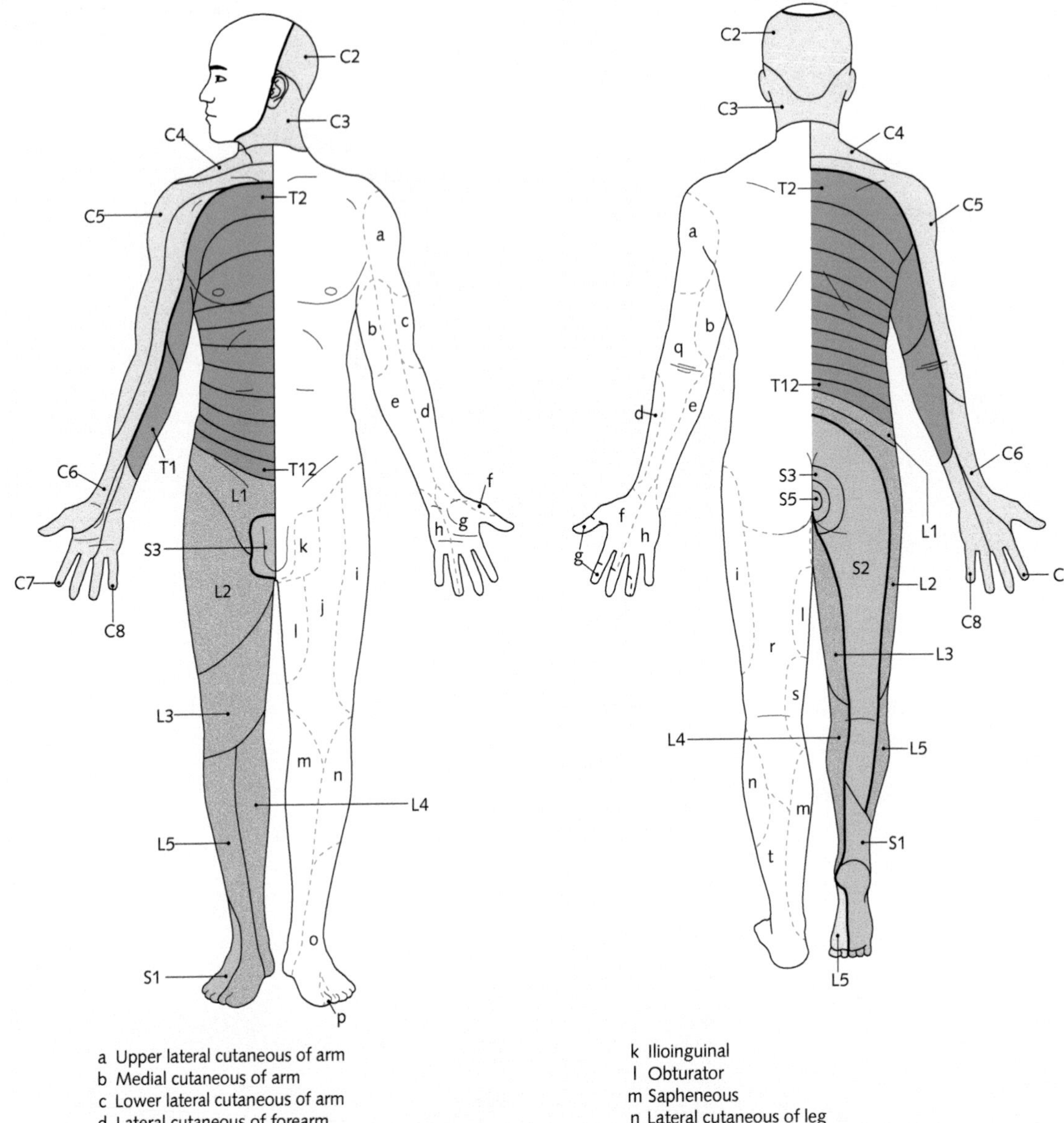

a Upper lateral cutaneous of arm
b Medial cutaneous of arm
c Lower lateral cutaneous of arm
d Lateral cutaneous of forearm
e Medial cutaneous of forearm
f Radial
g Median
h Ulnar
i Lateral cutaneous of thigh
j Medial and intermediate cutaneous of leg

k Ilioinguinal
l Obturator
m Sapheneous
n Lateral cutaneous of leg
o Superficial peroneal (musculocutaneous)
p Deep peroneal
q Posterior cutaneous of forearm
r Posterior cutaneous of thigh
s Medial cutaneous of thigh
t Sural

Fig. 4.12 Dermatome map.

Fig. 4.13 Types of nerve injury, their effects and potential for recovery

Injury	Extent	Effect
Neurapraxia	Transient block. No structural damage. Usually compression of nerve is the cause	No degeneration of nerve fibres. Temporary disruption to nerve function which recovers fully
Axonotmesis	Rupture of nerve fibres within intact sheath. Prolonged pressure or crushing is a cause	Wallerian degeneration. Nerves regrow within sheath. Effects on function may be severe but complete recovery is usual
Neurotmesis	Complete section of a nerve	Wallerian degeneration. Paralysis/sensory loss is complete. Regeneration may be slow and incomplete

Fig. 4.14 Effects of peripheral nerve injury				
	Compression	**Crush**	**Severed nerve**	**Severed limb**
Axon	Intact	Discontinuous	Discontinuous	Discontinuous
Basal lamina	Intact	Discontinuous	Discontinuous	Discontinuous
Regrowth possibilities	No regrowth needed, full remyelination within a few weeks	Trophic factors released by distal part of axon, and proximal axon (still attached to cell body) regrows at 1 mm/day	Trophic factors released by distal part of axon, but can grow into wrong basal lamina, previously occupied by nerve with different function	No distal part of axon present; nerve forms a neuroma
Restoration of function	Complete	Dependent on length of axonal growth needed for reinnervation	Four possibilities: (a) Grows into original basal lamina (b) Grows into basal lamina of same modality – altered function (c) Grows into basal lamina of different modality – no function (d) Forms neuroma – no function	No function; disturbed sensation and chronic/ transient pain

completely before a nerve sectioned far away grows and reaches them).

The effects of different types of peripheral nerve injury are outlined in Figure 4.14.

Peripheral sensorimotor neuropathies

Peripheral sensorimotor neuropathies are characterized by a 'glove and stocking' distribution of sensory loss, weakness and wasting especially of distal muscles and distal areflexia. Causes include:

- Systemic disease, e.g. diabetes mellitus
- Vascular disease
- Hereditary motor and sensory neuropathies (HMSNs) – Charcot–Marie–Tooth is the best described phenotype characterized by peroneal muscle atrophy, leading to an inverted champagne bottle appearance
- Infection
- Paraneoplastic syndromes.

There are two distinct pathological types of peripheral neuropathy; demyelinating neuropathies damage Schwann cells and myelin sheaths whereas axonal neuropathies cause axonal degeneration.

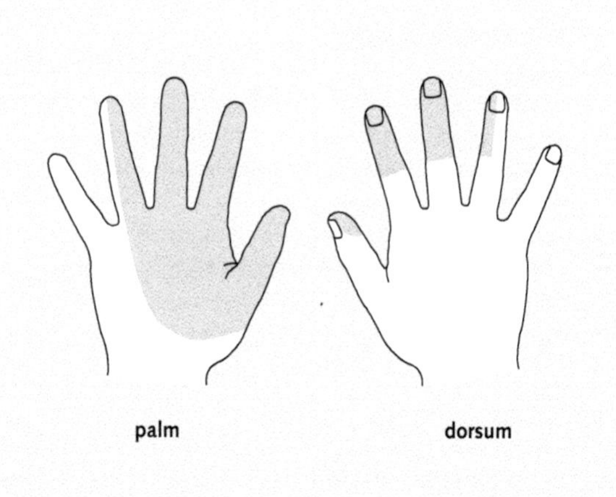

Fig. 4.15 Approximate area of sensory loss in a median nerve lesion.

Compression and entrapment neuropathies

Peripheral nerves are vulnerable to extrinsic compression and entrapment by either normal or diseased anatomical structures surrounding them.

Carpal tunnel syndrome

Carpal tunnel syndrome is common, especially in women. It is caused by pressure on the median nerve as it passes deep to the flexor retinaculum at the wrist. Initial symptoms are pain and tingling in the median nerve territory (most commonly the index and middle fingers), characteristically at night, causing the patient to shake the hand over the side of the bed for relief. Sometimes the pain shoots up the arm from the wrist. Signs may be absent initially. With time, median nerve innervated muscles, especially abductor pollicis brevis, may become weak and wasted and sensory signs may be found (Fig. 4.15).

Tinel's sign (tapping over the wrist) and Phalen's test (flexing the wrist for a minute) may reproduce symptoms, but a good history is the key to diagnosis. Predisposing factors for carpal tunnel syndrome are listed in Figure 4.16. The diagnosis may be confirmed with nerve conduction studies. The main differential diagnosis

Fig. 4.16 Predisposing factors for carpal tunnel syndrome
Arthritis of the wrist (usually rheumatoid)
Obesity
Pregnancy
Hypothyroidism and acromegaly
Repetitive wrist movements (washing floors, vibrating tools)
Hereditary neuropathy with liability to pressure palsies (HNPP)
Diabetes mellitus
Myeloma
But it is usually idiopathic

includes a C6 root lesion or a more central sensory abnormality.

Treatment may be non-surgical (wrist splints in slight extension, or local steroid injection) or surgical (division of the flexor retinaculum allowing decompression).

'Saturday night' palsy

'Saturday night' palsy is caused by compression of the radial nerve, especially if an arm is draped over a chair for some hours. It may also occur with fractures of the humerus (as the radial nerve runs in the spiral groove). Wrist drop and weakness of finger and thumb extension occur. There is a limited amount of sensory loss over the base of the thumb. There may be some weakness of triceps and brachioradialis and the triceps reflex may be impaired. It is important to examine finger abduction and adduction and abductor pollicis brevis. Patients generally recover spontaneously in a few months.

Ulnar nerve compression

This usually occurs at the elbow (in the groove of the medial epicondyle), particularly during general anaesthesia, with the use of crutches, and secondary to previous elbow injury. It can also occur in the cubital tunnel (the fibrous band between the heads of flexor carpi ulnaris). Symptoms include pain and paraesthesiae along the medial aspect of the forearm and numbness in the little and ring fingers, similar to that experienced when hitting your 'funny bone'. There may be wasting and weakness of ulnar-innervated small hand muscles, especially the first dorsal interosseous muscle. If the branch to flexor digitorum profundus is affected (in lesions above the cubital tunnel) there will also be weakness of flexion of the distal interphalangeal joint. The main complaint of patients is that they cannot grip objects.

Treatment involves avoiding unnecessary trauma to the nerve (no leaning on the elbows) and sometimes surgery.

Sciatica

Sciatica is a term used to describe symptoms within the distribution of the sciatic nerve. It is associated with lower back pathology, including prolapsed intervertebral discs. Prolapsed discs are most common at the L5/ S1 level and typically produce pain over the lateral aspect of the thigh and behind the knee, numbness of the lateral aspect of the foot, and weakness of ankle flexion. In severe cases surgical intervention may be required.

Common peroneal nerve neuropathy

The common peroneal nerve runs around the head of the fibula and can be injured by external pressure (e.g. from casts or trauma). Presentation is often with foot drop and sometimes with wasting of tibialis anterior producing weakened foot dorsiflexion, toe extension and foot eversion. Sensory function is usually preserved. Treatment is similar to the ulnar nerve.

Meralgia paraesthetica

This is a syndrome of tingling, pain/burning and numbness on the anterolateral surface of the thigh caused by compression of the lateral cutaneous nerve of the thigh under the lateral end of the inguinal ligament. It is more common in the obese, in pregnancy and with very tight trousers.

Treatment, other than weight reduction and reconsideration of wardrobe, is unnecessary.

Cervical spondylosis

Cervical spondylosis is a degenerative condition of the vertebral column and intervertebral discs, which is uncommon in patients aged under 50 years. It may cause compressive injuries of cervical roots as they pass through their foramina. The roots of C5, C6 and C7 are commonly affected. The symptoms are shown in Figure 4.17.

Fig. 4.17 Nerve roots commonly damaged in cervical spondylosis

Nerve root	Sensory supply	Motor supply	Reflexes
C5	Lateral arm and forearm	Shoulder abduction, elbow flexion	Biceps and supinator
C6	Lateral arm and lateral hand	Elbow flexion	
C7	Middle finger	Elbow extension, finger flexion and extension	Triceps (with C8)

Somatosensation and the perception of pain 5

Objectives

In this chapter you will learn about:

- The receptor mechanisms involved in somatosensation.
- The location and homuncular organization of the primary sensory cortex.
- The peripheral and central mechanisms of nociception and their regulation.
- The concept of referred pain.
- The differences between analgesia and antinociception.
- The mechanism of action of the main analgesics in clinical use.
- The features of chronic pain.
- The psychological aspects of pain.

SENSATION

Sensation is a remarkably important part of life. People who lose sensation may become unable to perform simple tasks such as undoing buttons and manipulating coins. In severe forms of sensory disturbance (such as the neuropathy that occurs with diabetes and leprosy) patients may sustain severe injuries partly because they cannot feel the pain.

There are four sensory modalities – touch, thermal sensation, pain and proprioception. In this chapter we will not look at proprioception, which is covered in Chapter 6.

There are individual receptors for submodalities within these groups. For example, the body can differentiate between light touch and pressure, between hot and cold and between mechanical and thermal pains.

In humans, no matter how a receptor is activated (electrically or electromagnetically), the subjective sensation reported is always that of its modality. Modality-specific channels convey information specific to one modality from the skin to the sensory receiving area.

RECEPTORS

Receptors are formed by peripheral terminations of axons of dorsal root ganglion cells. Receptors in the skin may be free nerve endings, or associated with different connective-tissue structures (e.g. Pacinian corpuscles, Merkel's discs).

The receptor membrane depolarizes in response to its modality stimulus, causing a generator potential. If sufficient, this causes the axon to depolarize to its threshold level and produce an action potential. Because the axon recovers after its refractory period, a long-lasting generator potential will cause the axon to fire a train of impulses whose frequency will be proportional to the magnitude of the generator potential. Essentially, all stimuli are encoded as analogue signals and the sensory systems function as analogue-digital 'translators'. To accommodate the wide range of sensory experience, different unimodal receptors have different thresholds, and the generator potential has a logarithmic relation between stimulus intensity, frequency of firing and ultimately perceived sensation.

Receptors can be divided into slowly adapting and rapidly adapting types. These two categories work in harmony to send different information about the same stimulus. The different signalling depends either on the linkage of the receptor to its incident energy or on a property called adaptation (i.e. a decline in receptor responsiveness even though the stimulus is still present). As a general rule, slowly adapting receptors signal the magnitude or location of a stimulus, whereas rapidly adapting receptors signal its rate of change and duration.

Figure 5.1 shows different fibre types for different modalities and their conduction speeds and axonal diameters.

Cutaneous mechanoreceptors

Mechanoreceptors are classified as either type I or type II (according to their location and receptor field) and as either slowly or rapidly adapting. Type I mechanoreceptors (e.g. Meissner's corpuscles and Merkel's discs) lie superficially at the boundary of the epidermis and dermis and have small, well-defined receptor fields. These receptors are more concerned with form and texture perception and their density varies across the body surface,

Fig. 5.1 Features of different sensory afferent fibres

Class	Modality	Axonal diameter (μm)	Conduction speed (m/s)	Pattern of termination in Rexed's laminae
Myelinated				
Aα	Proprioceptors from muscles, tendons	20	120	III, IV, V
Aβ	Mechanoreceptors from skin	10	60	III, IV, V
Aδ	Nociceptor, cold thermoreceptor	2.5	15	I, II, V
Unmyelinated				
C	Nociceptor, heat thermoreceptor	<1	<1	I, II

being greatest in the tongue, lips and fingertips and least in the trunk. Type II mechanoreceptors (e.g. Ruffini's corpuscles and Pacinian corpuscles) are positioned deep in the dermis and have large, poorly defined receptor fields. Pacinian corpuscles sense vibration whereas Ruffini corpuscles detect stretch.

Cutaneous thermoreceptors

Thermoreceptors are slowly adapting and are poor indicators of absolute temperature. Cold receptors increase their discharge frequency in response to decreasing temperature whereas warm receptors increase their discharge frequency in response to increasing temperature.

HIGHER PATHWAYS OF SOMATOSENSATION AND THE SENSORY CORTEX

The axons of somatosensory receptors enter the spinal cord via the dorsal root ganglion, with the fibres signalling modalities of touch travelling in the dorsal column pathway, and the fibres signalling thermal and pain information travelling in the spinothalamic tract (along with some information about crude touch). The region of skin innervated by a dorsal root is called a dermatome. The dorsal column pathway and spinothalamic tract are discussed in detail in Chapter 4.

The site of the sensory cortex and its organization are shown in Figure 5.2. The homunculus is disproportionately arranged with respect to body surface area, with more of the cortex responsible for processing information from areas used for exploration. Areas of greatest organized receptor density have the biggest representation in the sensory cortex.

The sensory cortex has a homunculus for each modality (i.e. a map for touch, another for pressure, etc., all lying next to each other). Within each homunculus, there is a columnar organization from the cortical surface to the corpus callosum. Within each column, the cells have similar receptive fields and modality. The layers in the column send and receive fibres from different areas of the cortex and thalamus. This is shown in Figure 5.3.

Nociception

Nociception is the sensory process detecting overt or impending tissue damage. Pain is the perception of irritating, sore, stinging, throbbing or painful sensations arising from the body. The way the body perceives pain not only depends on nociceptor input but also on other pathways giving information about, for example, emotional components. Pain is an 'experience' rather than a simple sensation.

Nociceptors are mechanical or polymodal. Mechanical nociceptors consist of a bare nerve ending at the end of one of 5–20 branches of an Aδ axon. They are concerned with the perception of well-localized, sharp pricking pain. Polymodal receptors (attached to C fibre afferents) are sensitive to temperature in excess of 46°C, skin puncture and several chemicals released by tissue injury (e.g. bradykinin, histamine, K^+, H^+). The pain resulting from polymodal nociceptor stimulation arrives last, after a mechanical injury, because C fibre conduction is so slow. Damage to tissue results in release of bradykinin and prostaglandin E_2. These substances reduce the threshold of nociceptors to mechanical and thermal stimuli such that the injury site becomes more sensitive to painful stimuli. Hyperalgesia is the phenomenon of increased sensitivity of damaged areas to painful stimuli:

- Primary hyperalgesia occurs within the damaged area
- Secondary hyperalgesia occurs in undamaged tissues surrounding this area.

Nociceptor afferent nerves release not only the excitatory transmitter glutamate (as do all sensory afferent nerves), but also the co-transmitter substance-P.

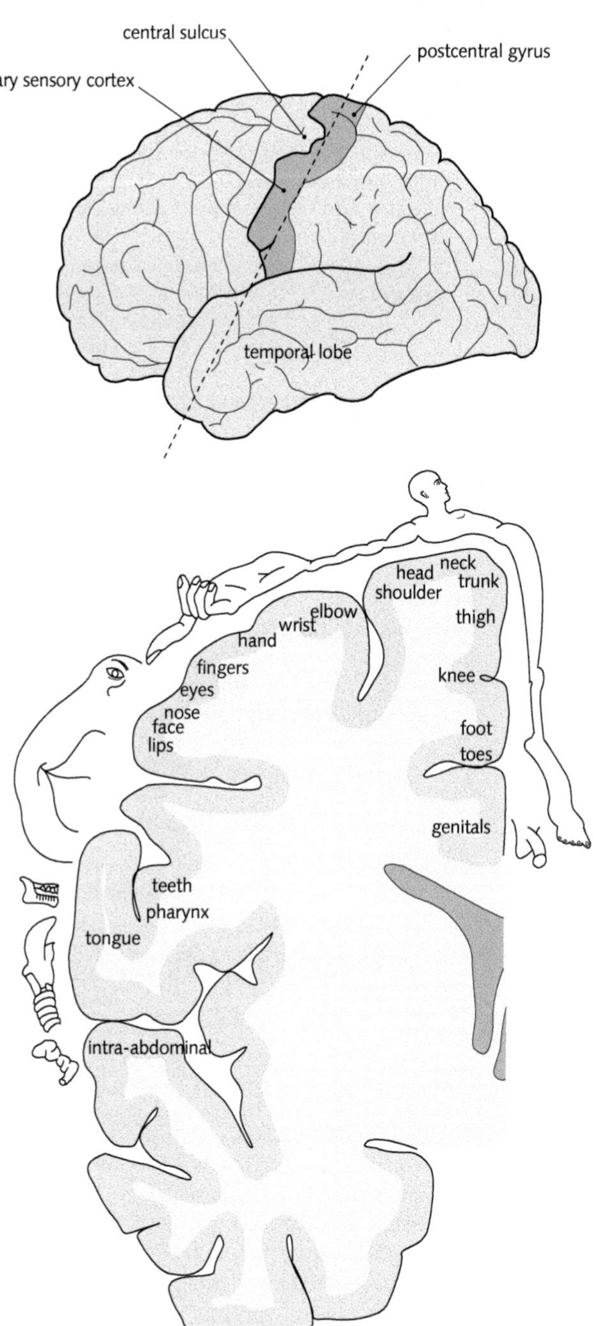

Fig. 5.2 Homuncular organization and location of primary sensory cortex (S1).

This causes a very long-lasting excitatory postsynaptic potential and helps sustain the effect of noxious stimuli.

Although nociceptors do not show adaptation (i.e. they fire continuously to tissue damage), pain sensation may come and go and pain may be felt in the absence of nociceptor discharge. In common with pain, itch is also mediated by Aδ and C fibres. People born without a sense of pain show no sense of itch, but itch is unaltered by opiate drugs.

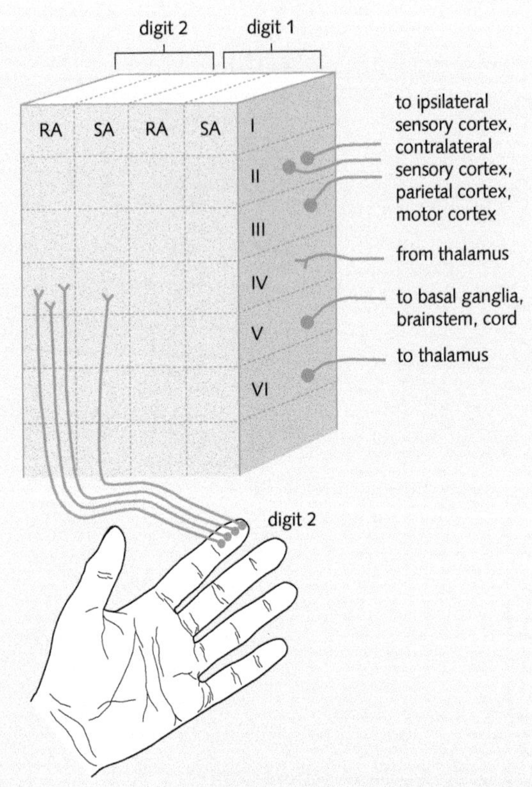

Fig. 5.3 Columnar organization of primary sensory cortex RA, rapidly adapting; SA, slowly adapting.

Processing of nociceptive afferent nerves begins in the circuits in the dorsal horn and a certain amount of descending control is exercised over the firing of spinothalamic cells in lamina I. Pain information is then transmitted to the cortex in the spinothalamic tract (see Ch. 4). Whether the cortex is the ultimate site of pain sensation is a matter for debate. Certainly, patients who are awake during neurosurgery do not report pain sensations when electrodes are passed through areas of the cortex. When these areas are stimulated, patients may report tingling or thermal sensation, but not pain. In addition, positron emission tomography illustrates activity in S1 and S2 in response to painful thermal stimulation. However, ablation of significant areas of somatosensory cortex has no measurable effect on perception of pain. It is likely then that the conscious sensation of pain has a large subcortical component, whereas the emotional response to pain is processed in the cingulate cortex.

Referred pain

Frequently, activation of nociceptors in the viscera results in pain felt at the body surface (referred pain). Nociceptor fibres from the viscera and from cutaneous structures can converge on a common dorsal horn cell. Therefore, the central nervous system cannot determine whether the source of the signal is superficial or deep, but it is programmed such that all pain is interpreted as coming from the surface. For example:

- Pain of myocardial infarction is classically felt centrally just behind the sternum, radiating down the left arm and up the root of the neck into the jaw.
- Inflammation affecting the diaphragm is felt in the tip of the shoulder (phrenic nerve root values C3–C5).

THE REGULATION OF PAIN

Peripheral regulation

Pain can be regulated by sensory input. Stimulation of large diameter (Aα and Aβ) low-threshold mechanoreceptors causes inhibition of spinothalamic cell discharge via the gate control theory. This mechanism accounts for the reduced pain sensation felt by rubbing a wounded area, by transcutaneous electrical nerve stimulation (TENS) and by acupuncture.

HINTS AND TIPS

Transcutaneous electrical nerve stimulation (TENS) can be used to activate large-diameter fibres to decrease the sensation of pain. This is particularly useful in chronic pain states (e.g. lower back pain) and increasingly is being used as non-invasive pain relief for women in labour.

Central regulation

In some situations stress, strong emotion or stoic determination can suppress the sensation of pain. Regions in the CNS that have been implicated in pain suppression are illustrated in Figure 5.4. Electrical stimulation of the periaqueductal grey matter in the midbrain causes profound analgesia. This area receives information from higher structures processing emotional states and projects to the midline reticular and raphe nuclei. Subsequent projections to the dorsal horns of the spinal cord depress the activity of nociceptive neurons. Two other parts of the reticular formation (the nucleus reticularis paragigantocellularis and the locus coeruleus) are also implicated in modulating nociceptive neuronal activity in the dorsal horns.

Opiates are thought to produce their anti-nociceptive action by activating these central regulating structures. Some of these regions contain endogenous opioid

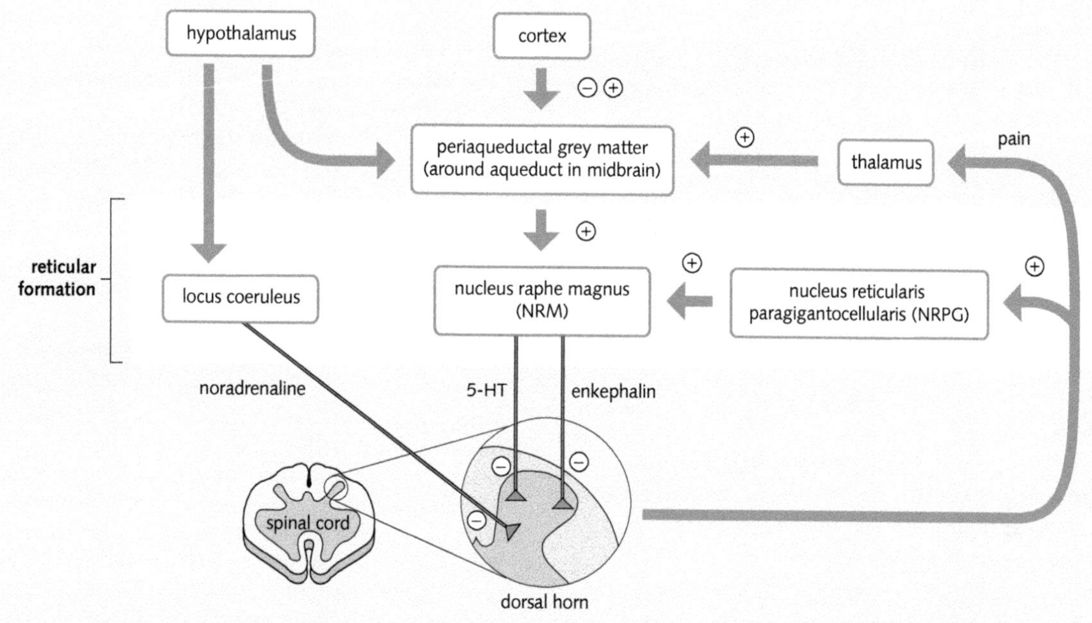

Fig. 5.4 Central regulation of pain.

peptides, although pain modulation also involves 5-hydroxytryptamine (5-HT) from the raphe nuclei and noradrenaline (norepinephrine) from the locus coeruleus. There are three classes of endogenous opioid peptides (Fig. 5.5).

There are three major classes of opioid receptor:

- μ (mu)
- δ (delta)
- κ (kappa).

Morphine is a potent μ agonist and naloxone is an antagonist. Endogenous enkephalins are active at both μ and δ receptors. Both receptor types are found in the periaqueductal grey matter and in laminae I and II of the dorsal horn.

Note that all of these receptors are found throughout the CNS, suggesting that they are involved in processes other than pain perception. This accounts for some of the other effects of opiates, such as euphoria and hallucinations.

ANALGESIA

Analgesia is relief from the psychological state of pain and is an important humanitarian undertaking. Antinociception is simply the blockage of nociceptive inputs. The main analgesics in clinical use are:

- Opioid analgesics acting on the endogenous system of pain control
- Non-steroidal anti-inflammatory drugs, which reduce the production of inflammatory mediators that sensitize nociceptors to bradykinin and 5-HT
- Simple analgesics (e.g. paracetamol)
- Local anaesthetics, which block action potential conduction along axons
- Miscellaneous drugs, e.g. sumatriptan (a 5-HT_{1D} agonist) in migraine; carbamazepine (antiepileptic) in trigeminal neuralgia; tricyclic antidepressants (amitriptyline) and GABA analogues (gabapentin) in some types of chronic neuropathic pain.

Fig. 5.5 Characteristics of the three classes of opioid peptides

Parent peptide	Opioid peptide	Amino acid sequence	Location
Proenkephalin	Enkephalins	Leu^5, Met^5, and longer sequences	Spinal cord, brainstem
Prodynorphin	Dynorphins	All contain Leu^5 within longer sequences	Spinal cord, brainstem
Pro-opiomelanocortin	β endorphin	Met^5 in 31 amino acid sequences	Hypothalamus

HINTS AND TIPS

Placebo (Latin for 'I shall please') can be a very effective analgesic, such that postoperative pain relief can be achieved simply by injection of sterile saline. Naloxone (an opioid receptor antagonist) can obstruct the analgesic effect of placebo just as it antagonizes the effect of true opiate analgesics. The belief that treatment will work is apparently enough to activate the endogenous pain relief systems of the brain.

HINTS AND TIPS

The World Health Organization analgesic ladder provides a useful structure with which to consider the management of acute pain. Initially, peripherally acting drugs such as aspirin, paracetamol, or NSAIDs are given. If pain control is not sufficient, the second stage is to introduce weak opioids such as codeine together with appropriate agents to minimize side-effects. If effective control is not achieved by this change the final step is to introduce a strong opioid drug such as morphine.

Opioids

Opioid drugs mimic endogenous opioids by binding to μ, δ and κ opioid receptors in the dorsal horn, periaqueductal matter and midline raphe nuclei. There are two classes of opioids:

- Opiates, which include morphine and analogues that are structurally similar to morphine and usually synthesized from it (e.g. diamorphine, codeine)
- Synthetic derivatives structurally unrelated to morphine (e.g. pethidine, fentanyl).

Opioids block pain information from being transmitted in the spinothalamic tract (anti-nociceptive action), but they also act in the brain to reduce the unpleasantness of the pain state (analgesic action):

- The weaker opioids (such as codeine) are widely used in over-the-counter pain preparations, and often in conjunction with a simple analgesic in prescription medications (e.g. co-codamol is codeine and paracetamol).
- Stronger opioids (such as morphine and pethidine) are used in postoperative pain and sometimes in severe chronic pain (such as cancer pain).
- Either fentanyl or morphine is commonly used as part of general anaesthesia.

The main effect of opioids is on the μ receptor, causing:

- Analgesia and anti-nociception
- Euphoria and drowsiness – depending on the circumstances of administration
- Respiratory depression – reducing the sensitivity of the brainstem to $PaCO_2$
- Miosis – pupillary constriction caused by stimulation of parasympathetic component of cranial nerve III
- Nausea – stimulation of the chemoreceptor trigger zone in the brainstem which sends signals to the vomiting centre
- Constipation – increased tone and reduced motility of gastrointestinal tract.

There are problems with repeated administration of opioids:

- Tolerance – a gradual reduction in effect over repeated administration of the same amount of drug. Doses of morphine, therefore, need to be increased over time to produce the same degree of pain relief, but this causes a greater degree of constipation.
- Dependence – this can be physical (where a withdrawal syndrome of physical symptoms and signs like influenza occurs when the drug is not administered) or psychological (where compulsive drug-seeking behaviour develops). Often, it is a combination of both.

The most common drug of misuse in this class is diamorphine (otherwise known as heroin). However, many patients taking legitimately prescribed opioids can also develop these side-effects and may be at risk from overdose.

Opioid overdose presents with:

- Coma
- Respiratory depression
- Pin-point pupils (there is no tolerance to pupillary constriction even in the hardened addict).

Treatment is with intravenous μ antagonists, such as naloxone (rapidly acting and short duration of action) or naltrexone (longer to act but longer duration of action). Note that antagonists may stimulate an acute withdrawal state and supportive therapy alone (e.g. ventilation) may be appropriate in some cases of opioid overdose.

HINTS AND TIPS

Naloxone is widely used in an emergency setting to treat opioid overdose, but its duration of action is much shorter than most opioids which are misused. Therefore, it is important to carry on monitoring the patient to look for signs of relapse.

Figure 5.6 summarizes the main opioids along with their pharmacological properties and clinical uses.

Fig. 5.6 Opioid drugs and their pharmacology

μ-Agonist	Bioavailability and administration	Metabolism	Potency and length of action	Clinical use	Notes
Morphine	Poor availability when given orally due to high rate of first-pass metabolism. Intravenous administration gives reliable dosing	Active metabolite morphine-6-glucuronide	$t_{1/2}$ 3 h	Acute and chronic pain	Cannot be given in labour as fetal liver cannot conjugate
Diamorphine (heroin)	More lipid soluble. Given orally or by intramuscular, intravenous or subcutaneous injection	Partly to morphine	Very potent, rapid onset, $t_{1/2}$ 2 h	Acute and chronic pain	
Codeine	High oral bioavailability	To other opioids including morphine	One-sixth potency of morphine	Mild pain, headache, dental pain	Potent antitussive, low side effect profile
Pethidine	High lipid solubility. Given orally and by intramuscular injection	Metabolite norpethidine interacts with MAOIs	One-tenth potency of morphine	Acute pain, labour	Does not cause miosis
Fentanyl	High lipid solubility. Given intravenously epidurally, transdermally		Very potent, short acting	Intraoperative pain	Intraoperative analgesia
Buprenorphine	Increased first-pass metabolism. Given sublingually, intrathecally		$t_{1/2}$ 12 h, slow onset	Acute and chronic pain	Partial agonist and difficult to reverse effects in overdose
Methadone	Given orally or by injection		$t_{1/2}$ >24 h, very slow onset	Maintenance of drug addicts	Does not produce euphoria

Note: MAOI, monoamine oxidase inhibitors – a type of antidepressant

Non-steroidal anti-inflammatory drugs

Non-steroidal anti-inflammatory drugs (NSAIDs) relieve pain by reducing the sensitization of nociceptors that occurs in inflammation. This is primarily achieved through inhibition of cyclo-oxygenase (COX), which impairs the ultimate transformation of arachidonic acid to prostaglandins, prostacyclins and thromboxanes (prostaglandins PGE_1 and PGE_2 lower the threshold of polymodal nociceptors to stimulation by the inflammatory mediators bradykinin and 5-HT). NSAIDs are also anti-inflammatory and antipyretic (decrease fever). There are two isoforms of the COX enzyme, COX-1 and COX-2:

- COX-1 is variably expressed in most tissues and might be described as a 'housekeeping' enzyme, regulating normal cellular processes (e.g. vascular homeostasis, gastric cytoprotection, platelet aggregation, kidney function).
- COX-2 is expressed constitutively in brain, kidney, bone and probably also in the female reproductive system. It is inducible and expression in other sites is increased during states of inflammation. Importantly, increased expression of COX-2 mRNA and protein has been noted in patients with hypertension, heart failure and diabetic nephropathy.

The desirable analgesic effect of NSAIDs is thought to be due to COX-2 inhibition. Certain side-effects of NSAIDs result from (COX-1-related) interference with the physiological role of prostaglandins in the regulation of blood flow. For example, interfering with blood flow in the gastric mucosa reduces bicarbonate production. Gastric acid can then attack the mucosal surface causing ulceration and potentially fatal gastrointestinal tract bleeding. This leads to the introduction of selective COX-2 inhibitors (e.g. rofecoxib) which have the presumed advantage of decreasing gastrointestinal toxicity compared with non-selective NSAIDs. However, an

Fig. 5.7 Uses and side-effects of non-steroidal anti-inflammatory drugs (NSAIDs)

Drug	Uses and side effects of NSAIDs
Aspirin	For mild pain; causes gastrointestinal upset, haemorrhage, salicylism (tinnitus, dizziness, nausea), Reye's syndrome in children (postviral encephalopathy and liver disorder)
Ibuprofen	Inflammatory joint disease, dental pain; much milder side-effect profile
Mefenamic acid	Moderately effective – especially for menstrual cramps; may cause gastrointestinal tract upset and diarrhoea

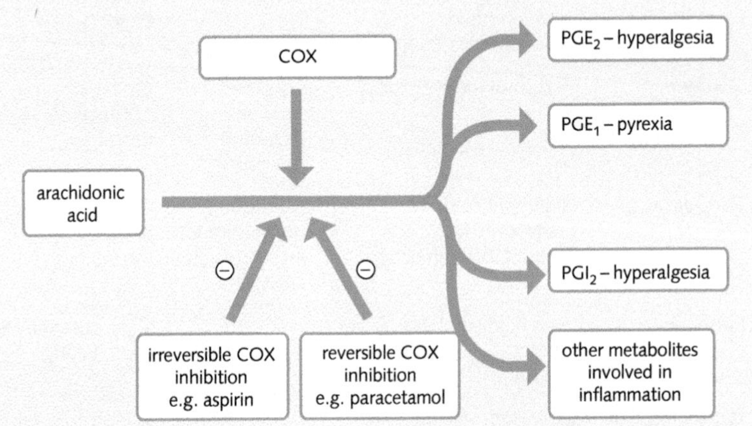

Fig. 5.8 Mechanism of action of non-steroidal anti-inflammatory drugs. COX, cyclo-oxygenase.

increased risk of cardiovascular disease has now been attributed to some selective COX-2 inhibitors. Figure 5.7 lists three NSAIDs commonly used in clinical practice with their effects and side-effects. Figure 5.8 shows the key mechanism of action of NSAIDs.

Local anaesthetic agents

Local anaesthetic agents block the ability of axons to conduct action potentials by blocking Na^+ channels in the axonal membrane. The blocking site on the Na^+ channel is on its intracellular portion. Local anaesthetics are weak bases that can exist, depending on their pK_a (the dissociation constant, calculated by the Henderson–Hasselbalch equation), in either a hydrophilic state, when bound to H^+, or in hydrophobic state without H^+:

- In the hydrophobic state, they can pass straight through the lipid membrane to gain access to the blocking site, whether the channel is closed or open.
- In the hydrophilic state, they can enter only through the open mouth of the Na^+ channel, and, therefore, need to wait until the channel opens to gain access to the blocking site. The hydrophilic route of the drug leads to 'use-dependent' block – the block of channels increases as more channels open.

Figure 5.9 shows both hydrophilic (XH^+) and hydrophobic (X) blocking of a Na^+ channel.

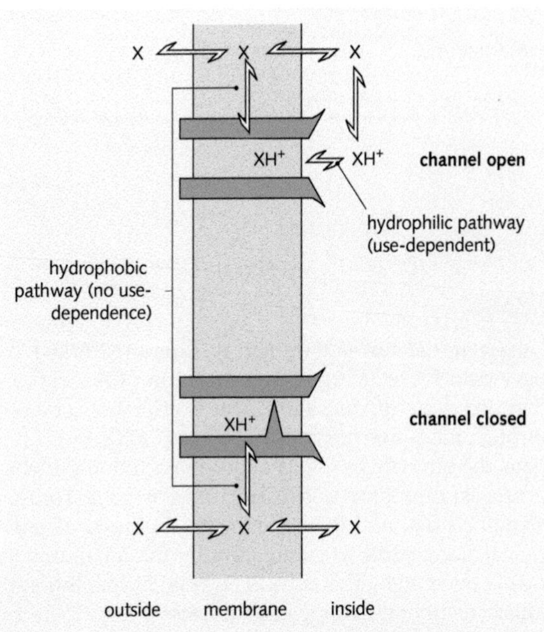

Fig. 5.9 Mechanism of action of local anaesthetics. Local anaesthetic agents (X) interact with ion channels. They can do this in an ionized (hydrophilic form-XH+), which passes through the open channel. This leads to use-dependent block. Alternatively, the uncharged species (X) can gain direct access to the membrane from the outside.

HINTS AND TIPS

To increase the effect of a given amount of local anaesthetic agent, a vasoconstrictor (e.g. adrenaline (epinephrine)) can be given with the local anaesthetic to reduce the rate at which the local anaesthetic is washed out of the tissue being anaesthetized. This is contraindicated when the tissue being anaesthetized relies on end arteries for supply (e.g. digital arteries in fingers and toes in a ring block) because ischaemic necrosis will result.

At low concentrations of local anaesthetic agents only small-diameter myelinated and unmyelinated fibres are affected. This means that administration of local anaesthetic agents can be used to produce a differential nerve block affecting only Aδ and C fibres. This reduces pain and temperature transmission, leaving proprioception, fine touch and motor functions intact.

The common local anaesthetic agents in use are summarized in Figure 5.10.

CHRONIC PAIN

Pain that continues when the causative stimulus is no longer present is chronic pain. Characteristic features include:

- Hyperalgesia – increased sensitivity to painful stimuli
- Allodynia – pain caused by innocuous stimuli such as light touch
- Spontaneous pain spasms – pain felt in the absence of any stimulation.

The chronic pain state is caused by a hyperactive acute pain pathway. Increased responsiveness of nociceptors is caused by sensitization by inflammatory mediators such as bradykinin, prostaglandins and nerve growth factor.

Increased excitability of neurons in the dorsal horn and thalamus is due to increases in synaptic transmission that occur after prolonged stimulation. This means that high nociceptor firing frequencies will set up a state of hyperexcitability in dorsal horn neurons. The process that facilitates this increase in synaptic effect is thought to involve the NMDA (*N*-methyl-D-aspartate) receptor, as NMDA antagonists can block the initiation of hyperexcitability.

Neurological disease can affect the pain pathway and produce neuropathic pain, a form of (often chronic) pain caused by damaged sensory neurons. Often α-adrenergic receptors are expressed on the neurons and, as a result, sympathetic activity can cause severe pain.

PSYCHOLOGICAL ASPECTS OF PAIN

Pain is a subjective experience influenced by emotional and social cues. It is essential to treat psychological conditions that exacerbate pain (e.g. depression, anxiety) and especially important to appreciate that fear magnifies pain. Chronic pain that is resistant to any drug therapy may respond to psychological treatments such as cognitive behavioural therapy.

Fig. 5.10 Local anaesthetic agents

Drug	Use	Side effects
Lidocaine	Nerve-block anaesthesia, e.g. dentistry; spinal anaesthesia – injection into subarachnoid space for surgery to lower trunk and legs	Spinal procedure affects many nerve roots – hypotension and bradycardia caused by sympathetic block, urinary retention caused by block of pelvic autonomic fibres
Bupivacaine	Epidural anaesthesia to block spinal roots for pain of labour	Less than for spinal as injection into epidural space minimizes diffusion to other nerve roots
Prilocaine	Intravenous regional anaesthesia (IVRA), e.g. Bier's block	Risk of local anaesthetic toxicity with IVRA. Early signs of systemic toxicity include tingling of the lips and tinnitus and later dysrhythmias and convulsions Methaemoglobinaemia

Motor control 6

Objectives

In this chapter you will learn about:

- Definitions of movement.
- Motor units and the control of muscle.
- Molecular basis of muscle contraction.
- Motor neuropathies, myopathies and disorders of the neuromuscular junction.
- Proprioception.
- Hierarchical control of movement.
- Planning and execution of movement.
- Control of posture.

MOVEMENT CONTROL

Types of movement

There are three basic types of movement:

- Reflex responses (e.g. the gag reflex) – stereotyped, involuntary responses graded to the eliciting stimulus
- Rhythmic motor patterns (e.g. walking) – sequences of stereotyped repetitive responses which are largely automatic, but require voluntary control to start and stop
- Voluntary movements – these are goal-directed movements, usually learnt and improved with practice.

Movements may also be categorized according to their speed: slow or ramp movements are controlled by sensory feedback; very fast or ballistic movements are not.

Muscle contraction is used to produce stabilization of the body (to provide the correct posture against gravity), as well as to produce movement. If the external force is smaller than that produced by the muscle, then movement occurs and an isotonic contraction is produced. When the external force is greater than that produced by the muscles an isometric contraction is produced. Force is generated but there is no movement.

Importance of sensation

Sensory information can be used in a feedback or feedforward control system.

In feedback control, the nervous system generates a movement and sensory information from that movement is used to obtain an error signal. This is the difference between the desired position and the current position. Our sense of proprioception gives us information about the position of our bodies (joints and muscles) and the movements of muscle groups. These sensations are transferred to the brain in both the dorsal column tract and the spinocerebellar tract. Patients who have lost their sense of proprioception due to a large-fibre sensory neuropathy do not know where their limbs are in space unless they can see them.

In feedforward control, sensory information is used to derive advance information and direct the movement towards a predicted position (e.g. picking up a drink).

Motor units and the recruitment of muscle fibres

Upper motor neurons

Upper motor neurons (UMNs) are outlined in Chapter 4 and travel to the ventral horn of the spinal cord via the pyramidal tract.

Lower motor neurons

Lower motor neurons (LMNs) innervate the skeletal muscle fibres, the cell bodies of which arise in the ventral horn of the spinal cord (see Ch. 4) and contain both sensory and motor fibres. Two types of LMN exist:

- Alpha motor neurons (AMNs): these large-diameter LMNs are responsible for the production of force by skeletal muscle.
- Gamma motor neurons (GMNs): these small-diameter LMNs cause contraction of spindle muscle fibres (see below).

One AMN and all of the muscle fibres it innervates make up the elementary component of motor control: the motor unit. The innervation ratio of a motor unit is the number of muscle fibres that a single motor

Fig. 6.1 Properties of motor neurons and functions, histology and biochemistry of muscle fibres

Motor unit	Properties of motor neuron	Functional properties of muscle fibres	Histology and biochemistry of muscle fibres
Slow fatigue-resistant (red; type II)	Constant low-frequency firing rate (10–20 Hz) with steady-state depolarization; smaller cell body, smaller diameter axon with slower conductance velocity	Longer contraction and relaxation times, lower force (10% of fast fatigable), very resistant to fatigue	Many mitochondria, high levels of oxidative enzymes (succinic dehydrogenase), high levels of myoglobulin
Fast fatigue-resistant (white; type I)	Intermediate firing rate response to steady-state depolarization; intermediate cell body size, axon diameter and conduction speed	Slightly slower than fast fatigable contraction and relaxation times, twice the force of slow units, very resistant to fatigue	Many mitochondria, high levels of glycolytic enzymes and oxidative, high levels of myosin ATPase
Fast fatigable (white; type 2)	Progressive drop in firing rate with steady-state depolarization; associated with high frequency bursts (30–60 Hz)	Fast contraction and relaxation times, high force during tetanus, fatigue after repeated stimulation	Few mitochondria, high levels of glycolytic enzymes (phosphorylase), high levels of myosin ATPase

neuron innervates. A high innervation ratio means that one motor neuron controls many fibres – such a motor unit produces coarse strong movements (e.g. the motor units in gastrocnemius have a ratio of 1:2000). A low innervation ratio means that only a few fibres are controlled by a motor neuron – such a neuron produces fine, well-controlled movement (e.g. the motor units in the extraocular muscles have a ratio of 1:10).

Motor units differ in their properties owing to the variation in the type of AMN innervating the muscle fibres (Fig. 6.1). Two functional types of motor unit can be distinguished by their histochemical features:

- Fast twitch (pale; type I) muscle, involved in quick phasic movements such as running and walking. This class is further divided into fast fatigue-resistant and fast fatigable categories
- Slow tonic (dark red; type II) muscle, involved in slow sustained contractions, such as those involved in the maintenance of posture.

A muscle fibre adopts the contractile properties of the nerve innervating it. If, for instance, a fast motor nerve were to be replaced by a slow motor unit the 'fast fibre' will change to a 'slow fibre'. This change is believed to be induced by the change in firing properties of the overlying nerves (see Fig. 6.1). All muscles have a variable number of each type of motor unit, as seen by staining techniques that pick up enzyme quantities (e.g. myosin ATPase). For example, postural muscles have many slow, dark red fibres, whereas extraocular muscles have mainly fast, pale fibres.

Recruitment

Recruitment describes the order in which types of motor units are activated when making any movement, whether it is reflex or voluntary. Most muscles have a range of motor unit sizes such that motor units with low innervation ratios will be recruited first and the largest last. This is why we have much more fine control when operating under light loads when compared with heavy loads.

Molecular mechanism of motor contraction

AMNs communicate with muscle fibres by means of synaptic transmission with the neurotransmitter acetylcholine (ACh) across a specialized synapse called the neuromuscular junction (NMJ). Presynaptic action potentials release ACh which induce the depolarization (and hence excitation) of the postsynaptic muscle fibre that, if large enough, triggers a postsynaptic action potential to sweep through the muscle fibre, initiating muscular contraction. If a series of high-frequency presynaptic activations occur at the same time (i.e. temporally summate) they can cause enough synaptic activity to trigger muscle contraction. Thus, rate of firing of motor units is an important way that the central nervous system (CNS) grades the amount of muscle contraction needed.

Figure 6.2 demonstrates the microscopic structure of a muscle fibre. A muscle fibre is made up of a number of cylindrical structures called myofibrils, which contract in response to an action potential that sweeps down the sarcolemma (which ensheaths the myofibrils). Myofibrils themselves are surrounded by the sarcoplasmic reticulum, an extensive intracellular sac which stores Ca^{2+} ions.

Action potentials that sweep down through the sarcolemma gain access to the sarcoplasmic reticulum by a network of T tubules, which are continuous with the sarcolemma. Where the T tubules and sarcoplasmic reticulum contact each other, a specialized coupling system exists between the two membranes. A voltage-sensitive protein in the T tubule membrane is linked

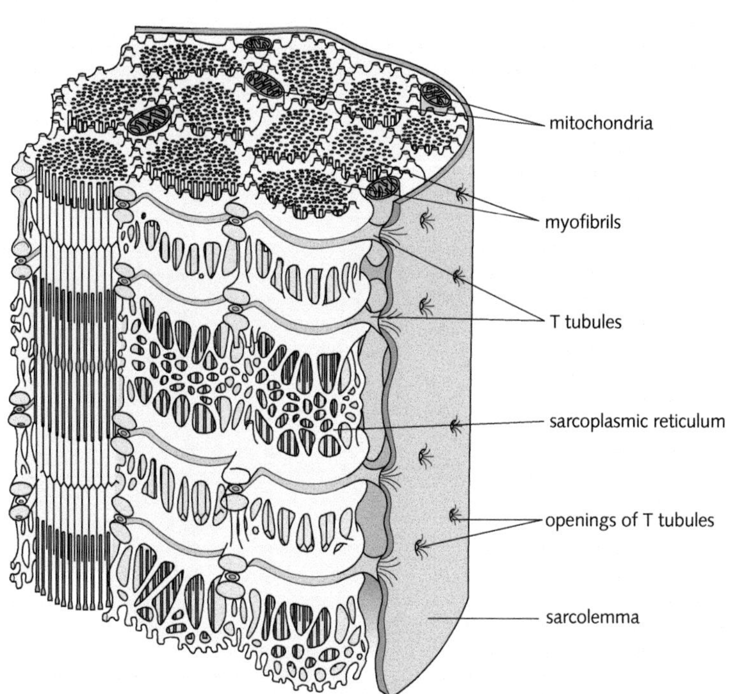

Fig. 6.2 Internal structure of a muscle fibre.

to a Ca^{2+} channel protein that lies in the sarcoplasmic reticulum. When action potentials arrive in the T tubule membrane it causes a conformational change in the voltage-sensitive membrane protein 'unblocking' the channel allowing Ca^{2+} flow out of the sarcoplasmic reticulum and into the myofibril cytosol. This process provides the Ca^{2+} needed for myofibril contraction.

Myofibrils are divided by a series of discs called Z lines. Anchored into the Z lines is a series of bristles called thin filaments and interdigitating between the thin filaments is another series of fibres called thick filaments. A segment consisting of two Z lines and the myofibril in between is known as a sarcomere. Muscle contraction occurs when thin filaments slide along the thick filaments, bringing the adjacent Z lines towards each other and shortening the sarcomere.

The major protein of the thick filament (myosin) binds to the major protein of the thin filament (actin). Movement occurs when a conformational change occurs in myosin such that the head rotates or 'nods' causing the thick filament to 'pull' the thin filament downwards towards the centre of the sarcolemma. If further contraction is needed then the myosin head can disengage, 'uncock' itself and repeat the process, much like a ratchet (Fig. 6.3). At rest myosin cannot interact with actin because the myosin attachment sites on the actin molecules are covered by the protein troponin. Contraction occurs when Ca^{2+} binds to troponin, exposing the myosin binding sites. Contraction can only occur as long as both Ca^{2+} and ATP are available.

Relaxation occurs when Ca^{2+} is removed by the sarcoplasmic reticulum. Reuptake of Ca^{2+} is driven by an active Ca^{2+} pump which requires ATP.

RESPONSES OF MOTOR UNITS IN DAMAGE AND DISEASE

Diseases affecting the different parts of the motor unit disrupt their normal function, as shown by changes in the pattern of motor unit arrangement, the size of muscle fibres and electrical recordings from muscle when active and at rest (electromyogram) (Figure 6.4).

Repeated activation of muscle fibres causes depletion of intracellular ATP stores, meaning that the muscle produces less force. However, the fibres remain in a state of some contraction for some time because relaxation is also an active process requiring ATP. This slow relaxation time has the effect of decreasing the force available to sustained contraction, but not that of single twitches (in early fatigue).

In myasthenia gravis, muscles (particularly those of the eyelid, neck and shoulders) are particularly fatigable. This is caused by a defect in the neuromuscular

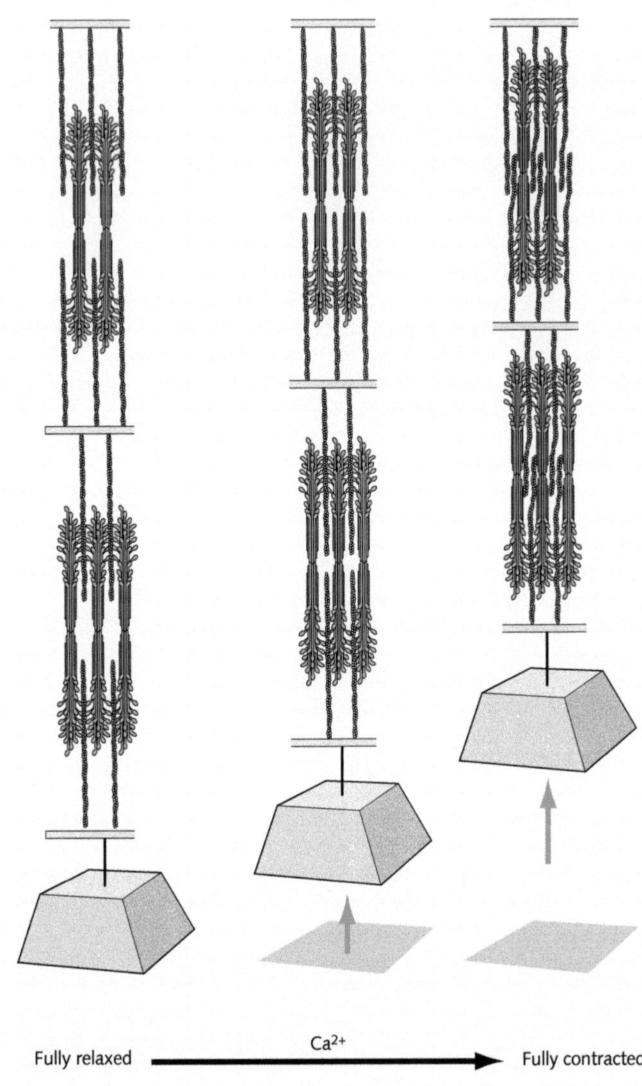

Fig. 6.3 Interaction between myosin and actin to effect sarcolemma contraction.

junction where there are autoantibodies to the acetylcholine receptor that prevent the depolarization of postsynaptic muscle fibre. The more activity there is, the more receptors become blocked hence the fatigability. This fatigue can be overcome temporarily by the use of acetylcholinesterase inhibitors, which is the basis of the diagnostic Tensilon' test.

Tetany occurs where hypocalcaemia or alkalosis reduce the threshold for action potential generation and neurons fire spontaneously, characteristically producing a spasm of the hands with the fingers and thumbs adducted and hand flexed at the metacarpophalangeal joints. It should not be confused with tetanus, which is a disease caused by a toxin from a soil-dwelling bacterium. The symptoms of tetanus include muscle contractions and 'lock-jaw' – it may be fatal if not swiftly treated.

Reflex action and muscle tone

Clinical relevance

Neurological examination of patients' limbs includes testing stretch reflexes. Tapping the patella tendon and observing the results indicates whether the spinal cord segments L2 and L3 are intact, excluding peripheral nerve damage. It can also indicate if the spinal motor neurons are receiving

Fig. 6.4 Diseases affecting the motor neuron cell body, peripheral axon and muscle fibres – clinical features and electromyographic (EMG) changes

Part of motor unit affected	Typical clinical features	Example	Effect on muscle fibres	EMG changes
Motor neuron cell body	Weakness, atrophy affecting distal muscles more than proximal, fasciculation (lower motor neuron lesion signs although hyper-reflexia is seen in amyotrophic lateral sclerosis (ALS))	Amyotrophic lateral sclerosis (motor neuron disease)	Atrophy and disappearance of groups of muscle fibres, with other fibres innervated by new collaterals from remaining motor neurons; this produces 'fibre clumping' where areas of muscle contain fibres of only one type (fibre type is determined by motor neuron type – response to disease results in collaterals of one motor neuron innervating many nearby fibres)	Spontaneous activity at rest (fibrillation), discrete pattern of potentials during voluntary contraction as fewer motor units active, potentials are larger as motor units innervate more fibres than usual; no change in axon conduction velocity
Motor neuron axon	Chronically – weakness, atrophy distally, loss of tendon reflexes, sensory symptoms (loss, paraesthesia) as all types of peripheral nerve are affected	Guillain–Barré syndrome		Fibrillation, discrete large potentials; demyelinating neuropathies (Guillain–Barré syndrome) result in reduced axon conduction velocity
Muscle fibre	Weakness initially affecting walking and lifting, proximal larger muscles involved more than distal ones	Duchenne's muscular dystrophy	No change in spread of type of motor unit; dead fibres and regenerating fibres are present; inflammatory cells and fat sometimes present	No spontaneous activity at rest, shorter smaller potentials as there are fewer remaining fibres in each motor unit; the overall pattern is still smooth as there is no reduction in the number of motor units firing

an abnormal drive from higher centres. In upper motor neuron lesions, there is a loss of descending inhibition, causing an increase in drive and therefore brisk reflexes.

Passive movement of a limb provides the examiner with information about the tone of the muscles in the limb; the greater the tone, the more resistance to movement.

Definitions

'Reflex action' is an automatic motor response (simple or highly coordinated) that is elicited by a stimulus. The stretch reflex (such as that elicited on tapping the patellar tendon) is simple because the stretch detector (the muscle spindle) makes a monosynaptic connection with the output spinal motor neuron. Other reflexes have neurons between the sensory input and the motor output (interneurons) and can produce more complex responses. The magnitude of the reflex can be influenced by higher centres.

'Muscle tone' is the resting tension in muscle. It is produced by tonic firing of spinal motor neurons and their firing frequency is set by various inputs from stretch receptors and from higher centres through the corticospinal, vestibulospinal, cerebellospinal and rubrospinal tracts.

HINTS AND TIPS

A stretch reflex can be 'reinforced' by performing Valsalva's manoeuvre or pulling the hands outwards against each other (Jandrassik's manouevre). This is useful in patients in whom reflexes are hard to elicit.

In parkinsonism, there is 'rigidity' where all muscles have increased tone but there is no change in the strength of the reflexes. Thus, there is no alteration in the reflex circuit but there is an alteration in the direct corticospinal input.

A stroke may cause cell death in the motor cortex due to haemorrhage or ischaemia. This leads to 'spasticity' on the contralateral side, where tone is increased more in limb flexors than extensors, and this is known as a pyramidal distribution of weakness. Stretch reflexes elicit stronger responses, and this may produce stretch-induced rhythmic involuntary muscle contractions known as clonus. Reduced cortical input to the reflex circuit frees it from inhibition and its activity is increased, both at rest and when appropriately stimulated.

Proprioceptors and reflexes

Muscle spindles

Spindles consist of specialized muscle fibres enclosed in a connective tissue capsule (these fibres are called 'intrafusal'; skeletal muscle fibres involved in active contraction are 'extrafusal'). The middle third of the capsule is swollen (Fig. 6.5) and is in contact with group Ia sensory neurons which wrap around the muscle fibres. Only the ends of these fibres can contract.

Discharge of the Ia sensory neurons is related to the length of the spindle; as the muscle is stretched the discharge rate of the neurons increases and when the muscle is shortened (and, therefore, goes slack) the discharge rate goes down. The stretching of the middle third of the intrafusal fibre leads to the depolarization of the Ia axon endings due to the opening of mechanosensitive ion channels.

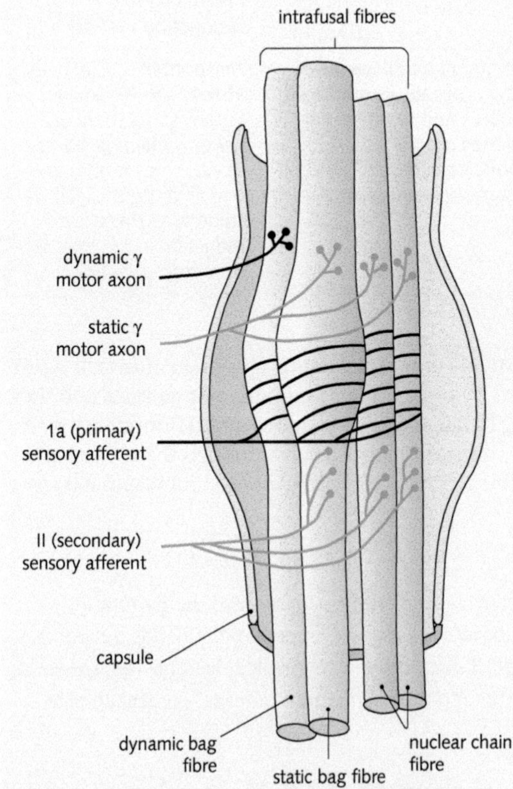

Fig. 6.5 Innervation and contents of a muscle spindle. Ia afferents are large, myelinated, fast fibres which are rapidly adapting. II afferents are small, myelinated, slower fibres which are slowly adapting.

The Ia efferents have an excitatory synapse in the spinal cords with AMNs. Following this through, stretching of the muscle spindle causes Ia neurons to fire, causing the excitation of AMNs. AMN stimulation causes skeletal muscle to contract shortening the muscle (and spindle), closing the mechanosensitive ion channels in the Ia sensory neuron.

The Ia fibres can be said to convey information to the CNS concerning muscle length.

Gamma motor neurons

GMNs innervate the contractile portions at the two ends of the intrafusal muscle fibres. Their function is to cause the contraction of the two poles of the intrafusal fibre when the extrafusal fibres contract. This happens so that when the extrafusal fibres contract the spindle does not become slack, reducing feedback from the Ia sensory neurons and, therefore, providing no information about muscle length.

Golgi tendon organs

Golgi tendon organs are found at the junction between muscle and tendon and are innervated by group Ib sensory axons. They are composed of a network of collagen fibres inside a connective tissue capsule with the sensory axon winding around the collagen.

The firing rate of the Ib afferent fibre increases when the tendon organ is stretched, with greater outputs for active contraction rather than passive stretching of the muscle. The Ib axons branch extensively in the spinal cord and synapse on several interneurons in the ventral horn. Some of these interneurons make inhibitory synapses with AMNs that innervate the same muscle the Ib axon originates from. As the muscle contracts the tension through the Golgi tendon organs increases, causing increased inhibition on the AMNs, which ultimately reduces AMN firing patterns and therefore reduces muscle contraction.

Proprioception from the joints

Various proprioceptive axons lie within the fibrous joint capsule and ligaments that surround joints. These axons are mechanosensitive and can respond to changes in the angle, direction and velocity of movement within a joint. It is likely these axons are most active during movement, but are 'quiet' when the joint is at rest. It seems that information from joint receptors is combined with information from muscle spindles, Golgi tendon organs and probably skin receptors to estimate joint angle and position in space.

Examples of reflexes

Basic pattern

The stretch reflex is elicited when a muscle is suddenly lengthened and a reflex contraction is produced (e.g. tapping the patellar tendon causing a reflex contraction of the quadriceps). Homonymous motor neurons (those supplying the same muscle) and synergist motor neurons (supplying a muscle with the same action) receive an excitatory input from the spindle (Ia) afferent. The spindle afferent also inhibits antagonistic muscles via Ia inhibitory interneurons in the spinal cord.

Tendon organs form part of a reflex circuit that inhibits homonymous and synergistic neurons, termed the inverse myotatic reflex. The pathways for these reflexes are shown in Figure 6.6.

HINTS AND TIPS

Understanding the basic spinal reflex arc is a common exam question. Make sure that you are able to talk through the arc in a couple of sentences.

Blink reflex

The blink reflex protects the cornea from foreign bodies (Fig. 6.7).

Gag reflex

This reflex protects the alimentary tract and upper airway from foreign bodies (Fig. 6.8).

Flexion withdrawal reflex

The flexion withdrawal reflex is a more complicated motor act that protects limbs against potentially noxious stimuli detected by cutaneous structures. The flexors of the affected limb contract and the extensors are relaxed. This withdraws the limb away from the noxious stimulus.

At the same time, a crossed extensor reflex is elicited in the contralateral limb where the extensors are contracted and the flexors relaxed. This provides postural support during the withdrawal of the stimulated limb.

Figure 6.9 shows the polysynaptic pathways in the spinal cord with extensor and flexor action of stimulated and non-stimulated limbs.

Plantar reflex

The plantar reflex is elicited when the plantar surface of the foot is stroked from heel to toe, causing reflex plantar flexion of the toes in normal individuals. However, in infants (whose corticospinal tract is not yet fully myelinated) and in patients with damage to the motor cortex or corticospinal tract (an upper motor neuron lesion), dorsiflexion of the toes is elicited. This is known as positive Babinski's sign.

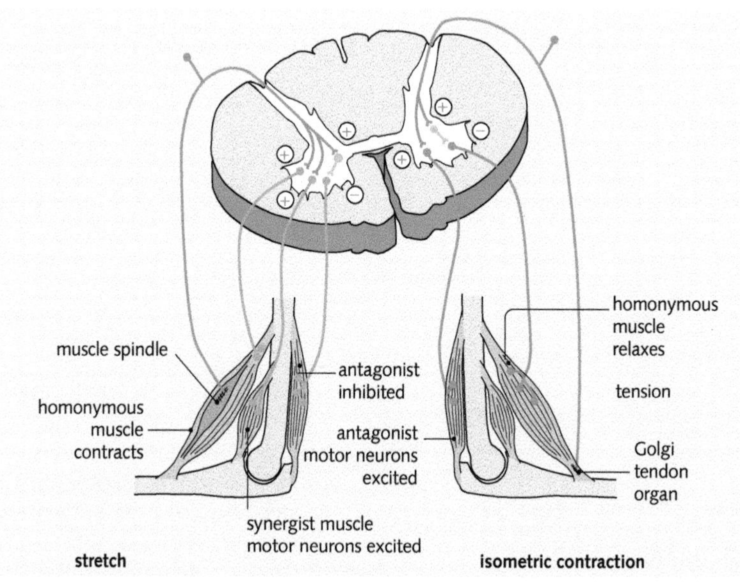

Fig. 6.6 Muscle spindle and Golgi tendon organ reflexes. Muscle spindles detect the rate of change and absolute muscle length during movement. Golgi tendon organs provide information on tension, and are particularly useful in exploratory movements as they have the protective effect of decreasing muscle force when resistance is met. They are modulated by higher centres to allow their response properties to be modified.

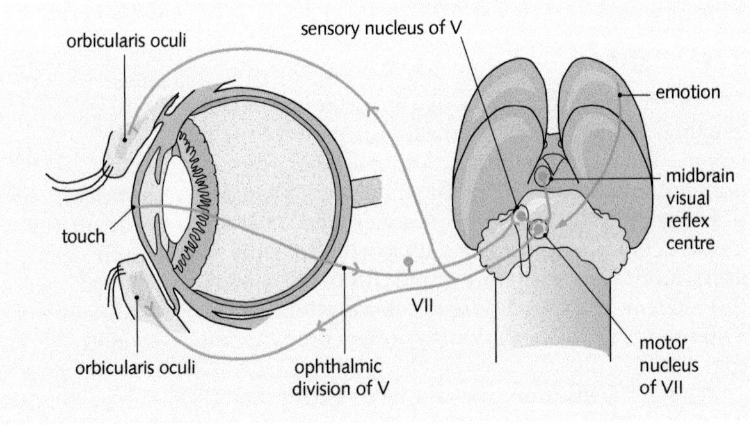

Fig. 6.7 Corneal (blink) reflex. Primary afferent fibres running in the opthalmic division of the trigeminal nerve (V) sense the stimulus on the cornea. Efferent fibres carried by the facial nerve (VII) initiate the motor respone.

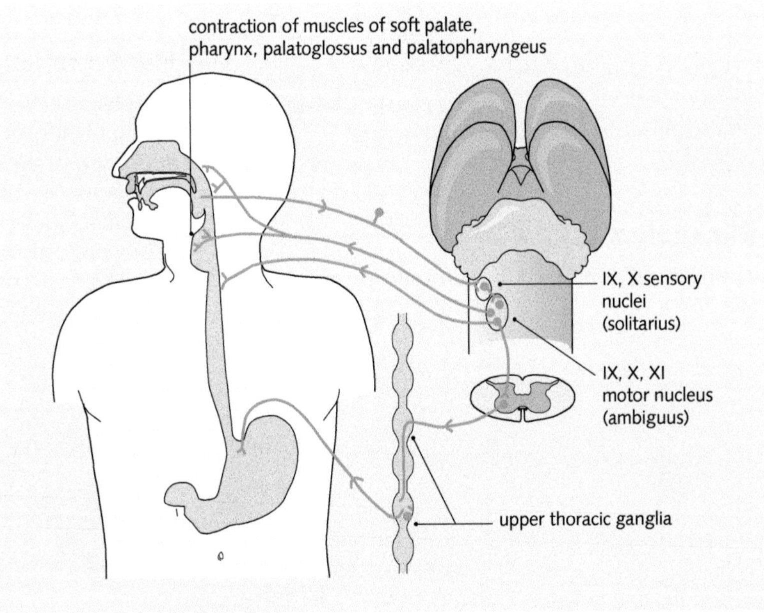

Fig. 6.8 Gag reflex consists of a combination of skeletal muscle action (e.g. muscles of pharynx) and smooth muscle action (e.g. contraction of stomach).

PATHOLOGY OF MOTOR UNITS

Anterior horn cell disorders

Motor neuron disease

The annual incidence of motor neuron disease is approximately 2–3 per 100 000. It usually presents between the ages of 50 and 70 years. Three major types are recognized:

- Amyotrophic lateral sclerosis – the classic form of motor neuron disease. This is a combination of upper and lower motor neuron limb and also, possibly, bulbar weakness
- Progressive muscular atrophy – a lower motor neuron limb weakness
- Primary lateral sclerosis – a predominantly upper motor neuron problem which may progress to include lower motor symptoms.

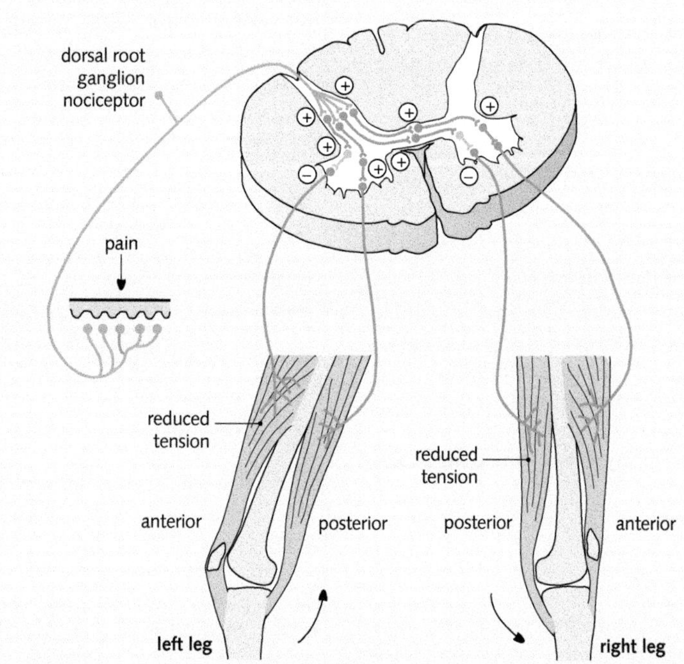

Fig. 6.9 The flexion withdrawal reflex showing withdrawal to pain on the left side, with a crossed extensor reflex in the right leg. Primary afferent fibres activate interneurons within the spinal grey matter, which in turn excite alpha motor neurons innervating the limb flexor muscles. The crossed extensor reflex is mediated by axon collaterals which cross the midline of the cord and excite alpha motor neurons innervating contralateral limb extensor muscles.

These syndromes represent a continuum, and patients progress from one syndrome to the other. Sensory symptoms and signs are absent. Treatment is aimed at maintaining a reasonable quality of life for as long as possible using a multidisciplinary approach. Prognosis is extremely poor and the survival is approximately 2–3 years.

Spinal muscular atrophy

SMA is a group of hereditary conditions characterized by progressive lower motor neuron degeneration. Features include hypotonia, proximal weakness and wasting. There are four main types:

- Acute infantile SMA (Werdnig–Hoffmann disease) – presents at birth or shortly after, death occurs by age 3 years
- Chronic infantile SMA – presents at 6 months, death occurs by 10 years
- Juvenile onset SMA (Kugelberg–Welander disease) – presents at approximately 10 years, death occurs around 35 years
- Peroneal/scapuloperoneal SMA – adult onset, survival is roughly normal.

Guillain–Barré syndrome

This is a clinical syndrome caused by an acute peripheral neuropathy, affecting motor more than sensory nerves, and in most cases follows infection. The incidence is approximately 1:50 000. Following the illness, 20% of patients remain so disabled that they are unable to work after a year and 5% die. By definition, the illness progresses for less than 4 weeks. Approximately 70% of the patients recall a preceding diarrhoeal illness or upper respiratory tract infection a few days or weeks before neurological signs develop. These are most commonly *Campylobacter* (30% of cases) or cytomegalovirus (10% of cases) infections. There is also an association with Epstein–Barr and herpes zoster viruses.

In most cases, there is inflammation and demyelination, hence the alternative name 'acute inflammatory demyelinating polyradiculopathy' (AIDP). In approximately 5% of cases, the same clinical picture (i.e. syndrome) may be produced by an acute motor or acute motor and sensory axonal neuropathy (AMAN and AMSAN), where the brunt of the injury falls on the axons primarily and the potential for spontaneous recovery may be less.

The clinical features are:

- Development of symptoms over days or weeks
- Bilateral flaccid weakness (and later wasting) of proximal and distal limb muscles
- Loss of tendon reflexes
- Progression of weakness in some cases to affect the respiratory and bulbar (speech and swallowing) muscles
- Burning pains and numbness, but often without sensory signs.

Important complications include:

- Respiratory failure and associated respiratory infections. Management includes measuring vital capacity (VC). VC less than 1 L requires ventilation
- Variable autonomic involvement producing cardiac arrhythmias, hypo- or hypertension
- Pressure sores and prophylaxis against deep vein thrombosis
- Anxiety and depression.

Investigations

In AIDP, in particular, nerve conduction studies show prolonged distal motor latencies in the upper and lower limbs. Slowing of conduction velocities is a late sign and may not be seen at all. Action potentials are often reduced.

Cerebrospinal fluid protein is usually raised (up to 50 g/L (5 g/dL)), but the cell count is normal.

The Miller–Fisher syndrome is a variant of Guillain–Barré syndrome with:

- An eye movement disorder caused by cranial nerve III, IV or VI palsy
- Cerebellar ataxia
- Areflexia.

Management

Management involves avoidance of complications, by regular measurement of the vital capacity (deterioration may be rapid; the patient may require ventilation only hours after symptoms begin), constant electrocardiogram recording and careful nursing. Patients may require long stays in intensive care, with 25% requiring respiratory support. Plasma exchange and intravenous immunoglobulin are equally effective at hastening recovery. Pain may be a prominent feature – good physiotherapy and non-steroidal anti-inflammatory drugs are helpful.

The disease ultimately is self-limiting, with remyelination of axons within a matter of weeks.

Peripheral nerve disorders

Peripheral nerve pathology is discussed in Chapter 4.

Myopathies

Myopathy is a term embracing all forms of primary skeletal muscle disorders (Fig. 6.10). Myopathies may be due to dystrophies, a group of inherited myopathies in which progressive degenerative changes occur in muscle fibres, inflammatory conditions, neurogenic damage, or metabolic and drug-related causes.

Duchenne's muscular dystrophy

Duchenne's muscular dystrophy (DMD) is relatively common, with an incidence of 1:3500. It is an X-linked condition which is caused in most cases by a mutation in the dystrophin gene, resulting in reduced levels or absence of dystrophin, a protein that links the sarcolemma with actin molecules (see Ch. 15). Becker muscular dystrophy (BMD) is caused by mutations in the same gene, but these result in a truncated rather than an absent/non-functional protein, and thus is a milder disease.

In affected cases, there is progressive proximal muscle weakness presenting between the ages of 3 and 6 years and pseudohypertrophy of the calf muscles (pseudohypertrophy because the 'enlargement' is due to the wasting of the thigh muscles, making the calves look bigger). The

Fig. 6.10 Classification of muscle/neuromuscular junction

Type of disorder	Examples
Muscular dystrophy	Duchenne's, Becker's, facioscapulohumeral, limb-girdle, myotonic dystrophy
Inflammatory myopathy	Polymyositis, dermatomyositis, inclusion body myositis, infective myositis, polymyalgia rheumatica
Metabolic myopathy	McArdles's disease, mitochondrial disorders, periodic paralyses
Endocrine myopathy	Thyroid disease, Cushing's disease
Drug-induced myopathy	Clofibrate, D-penicillamine, steroids, alcohol
Disorders of neuromuscular transmission	Myasthenia gravis, Lambert–Eaton myasthenic syndrome, stiff-man syndrome

weakness eventually spreads to involve both limbs. Most are wheelchair bound by 12 years and die by 25 years due to respiratory or cardiac complications.

Investigations include muscle creatine kinase (elevated) and muscle biopsy (no fibres staining for dystrophin).

BMD follows a similar but milder course.

Other muscular dystrophies include the limb-girdle muscular dystrophy (LGMD) group and facioscapulohumeral muscular dystrophy.

Inflammatory myopathies

Polymyositis is an acquired inflammatory myopathy, which affects women more commonly than men. The incidence of this together with dermatomyositis is approximately 1:100 000. It is a disorder of acute or subacute onset, with fever, muscle pain and tenderness, and weakness of proximal limb, trunk, neck, pharyngeal and oesophageal muscles. This may be so severe as to require ventilation. Pathologically, infiltration of $CD8^+$ T cells occurs in association with necrosis of muscle fibres. The primary cause is unknown. Investigations include creatine kinase (elevated), myopathic changes on electromyography (EMG) and biopsy showing inflammatory changes. Treatment is with corticosteroids and immunosuppression (e.g. azathioprine). Creatine kinase can be used as a marker of disease and, therefore, a marker of response to treatment.

Dermatomyositis pathologically shows B cell and $CD4^+$ T cell infiltration of the vessels and is associated with photosensitivity, a 'heliotrope' rash around the eyes and a linear red rash over the knuckles and proximal phalanges (Gottren's papules). In adults, but not in children, it may be associated with underlying malignancy (in 40% of those aged over 40 years).

Both conditions respond to steroids.

Disorders of the neuromuscular junction

Myasthenia gravis

The prevalence of myasthenia gravis is approximately 1:20 000. Women are affected twice as frequently as men. The condition is characterized by fatigable weakness of periocular, facial, neck, bulbar and proximal muscles (i.e. it worsens with exercise, and usually gets worse as the day goes on (diurnal)).

Myasthenia gravis is associated with acetylcholine-receptor antibodies at the neuromuscular junction preventing the entry of calcium into the postsynaptic cell and subsequent muscle depolarization. Both immunological and genetic factors appear to be important in its pathogenesis.

The condition is associated with lymphoid hyperplasia and tumours of the thymus. Weakness may respond to surgical thymic removal, especially in young patients with a short history. Otherwise, treatment is with immunosuppression and with anti-cholinesterases (pyridostigmine or neostigmine).

Lambert–Eaton myasthenic syndrome

This is characterized by weakness that is initially lessened with exercise. It is a rare disorder that is more common in men. It is caused by destruction of presynaptic voltage-gated calcium channels at the neuromuscular junction by autoimmune antibodies, causing a reduction in the amount of acetylcholine released (calcium is crucial to vesicle transmission). The antibodies originate de novo or in association with carcinoma of lung, breast, prostate, stomach or lymphoma. Clearly this will reduce the amount of acetylcholine arriving at the postsynaptic cell and therefore reduce the amount of muscle contraction. Treatment is with guanidine or 3,4-diaminopyridine. Immunosuppression and plasmapheresis may help.

HINTS AND TIPS

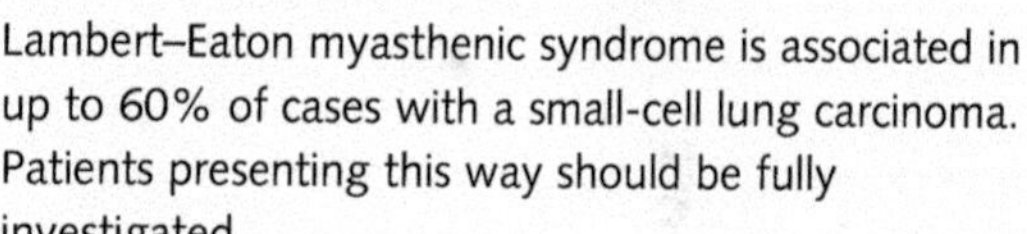

Lambert–Eaton myasthenic syndrome is associated in up to 60% of cases with a small-cell lung carcinoma. Patients presenting this way should be fully investigated.

MOTOR PROGRAMMES AND VOLUNTARY MOVEMENT

Definitions

Motor programme: a sequence of nerve impulses that, when sent to a group of muscles, will execute a movement. In essence, the brain 'remembers' its output to the muscles that cause a desirable movement. The same motor programme can be scaled and timed differently and sent to different muscle groups, for example, it is possible to hold a pen and write with either hand (with different levels of success!).

Motor strategy: a set of motor programmes that have been selected and sequenced to achieve a recognized goal.

Playing a slice shot in tennis is a motor strategy which is reliant upon the motor programmes that constitute the movement. Motor programmes include how the arm holds the racket, how the legs perform the correct footwork and how the truncal muscles work to produce the correct swing.

Development of motor programmes

Motor programme development is best known to anyone trying to learn their sport. Think of trying to learn how to kick a football or hit a tennis shot or take a rowing stroke. It is a lengthy process of trial and error, where one must monitor every movement to 'remember' what they did when the movement was 'right', and then repeat that process (practise) until the movement becomes 'automatic' thus developing the pattern of muscle activity changes.

Now to apply the science: initially, discontinuous movement occurs where the muscles work to achieve the task (agonists) by moving the limb nearer and nearer towards the 'target' (kicking the ball with swing or hitting a topspin shot), judging the end-point with feedback. This is self-monitoring of the trial and error 'phase'. This gives a slow, clumsy and unsmooth movement.

Faster, continuous movement then develops, with a single agonist burst stopped by an antagonist, then smaller adjustments guided by feedback made with agonist muscles. This is smoother movement, which gets closer to the target in a shorter time. This is where you know the movement you need to achieve the 'target' (see above) and practise the movement to make it become 'automatic'.

Eventually, the movement becomes ballistic, with a single agonist burst to move the limb towards the target and a single antagonist burst to stop the limb moving so it comes to rest at the target. The movement is learnt and committed to memory! You can now reliably and consistently perform the movement whenever you choose.

HIERARCHY OF MOVEMENT CONTROL

There are three levels of the central motor system, with the forebrain at the top and the spinal cord at the bottom:

- High – involved with the strategy or what is to be achieved by the movement according to recognized demands and how the movement will be carried out. Structures for this level include the frontal lobes and limbic system and basal ganglia.
- Middle – the tactics or the sequence of muscle movements in time and space required to achieve the goal. This includes the selection of appropriate known motor programmes. Structures that carry out this level include the motor cortex and cerebellum.
- Low – execution or the activation of motor neuron and interneuron pools that generate the movement. This level also adjusts posture if necessary. Structures involved in this level are the brain stem and spinal cord.

Planning of movement

Control of voluntary movement is a process that involves practically the whole neocortex. To move we need to know where our body is in space, where we intend our body to go and the selection of a plan to get us there, which must be issued to execute the plan. This plan must, however, be held in memory for an appropriate length of time (so we do not forget what we are trying to do). Before movement is initiated the brain needs information concerning whereabouts in space it is. This is overcome with a 'mental' body image generated by somatosensory, proprioceptive and visual inputs to the posterior parietal cortex. Two regions which are of paramount importance to the whole process are area 5 (receives inputs from the primary somatosensory cortical areas 1, 2 and 3) and area 7 (receives information from higher order visual cortical areas).

The parietal lobes are heavily interconnected with areas in the anterior frontal lobe (the prefrontal areas), areas that are important for abstract thought, decision making and anticipating the consequences of action. Together the prefrontal and parietal lobes are the highest level of the motor control hierarchy and both send axons that converge on cortical area 6. Area 6 is split into two sections, a lateral premotor area (or PMA) and a medial supplementary area (or SMA).

Premotor and supplementary motor areas

The premotor (PMA) and supplementary motor areas (SMA) play similar roles in the planning and execution of movement, but on different groups of muscles. The SMA sends axons which innervate distal motor units (i.e. limb muscles) and the PMA primarily innervates proximal motor units (i.e. axial muscles).

What is the function of these area 6 cortices? Both the PMA and SMA lie at the junction where the signals for what actions are required (the prefrontal and parietal innervation) meet signals for how these actions will be executed (innervation from M1; see below). Positron emission tomography (PET) shows that when asked to plan but not execute a movement, area 6 showed increased metabolism along with the prefrontal cortex. If the region of the prefrontal area addresses what movement should be performed then area 6 addresses how that movement should be converted from intention into a plan of action of what movements will be needed.

Area 6 also receives a large subcortical input from the thalamus and is discussed below.

The motor cortex

Movement begins in area 4 (the primary motor cortex, M1), which lies anterior to the central sulcus on the precentral gyrus. M1 contains a somatotopic organization,

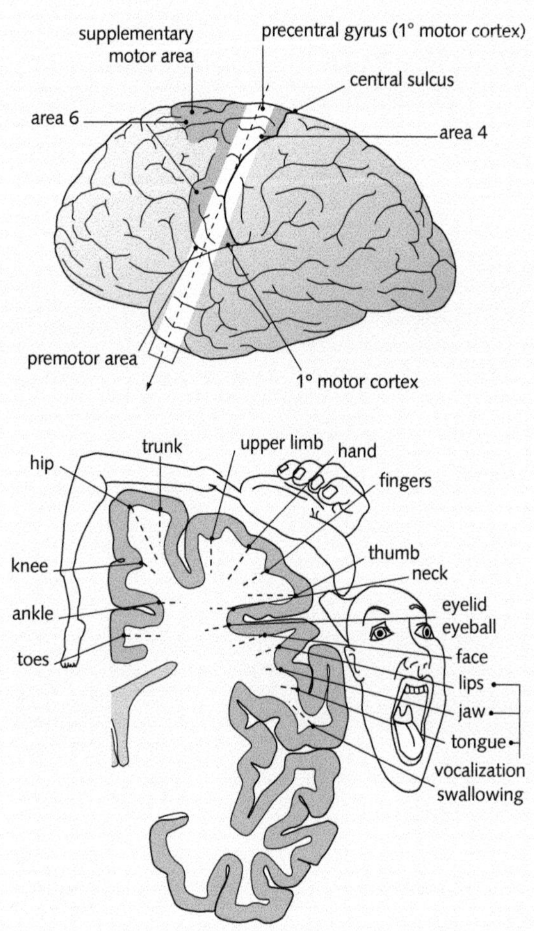

Fig. 6.11 Location and homuncular organization of the motor cortex.

similar to the somatosensory homunculus, which controls muscle movement (Fig. 6.11). Movement originates in cortical layer 5 of M1 in a population of pyramidal neurons called Betz cells, which receive synaptic input from other cortical areas and the thalamus. The thalamic input arises from a part of the ventrolateral nucleus that relays information from the cerebellum (which will become important later).

HINTS AND TIPS

In epilepsy, disordered neuronal firing during a fit can affect the motor cortex. This produces a wave of muscle activity, termed a 'jacksonian march', that moves over the body as the disruption of function spreads over the motor cortex. This partly led to theories of homuncular organization of the motor cortex.

HINTS AND TIPS

Dyspraxia is the inability to perform skilled actions despite intact basic motor and sensory abilities. Dyspraxia originates from problems with the planning and initiation of movement, which depends on the frontal and parietal lobes, so patients 'forget' how to perform previously learned movements.

THE BASAL GANGLIA AND THALAMUS

The major subcortical input to area 6 arises from a nucleus of the dorsal thalamus, the ventrolateral nucleus. The input to this nucleus arises from the basal ganglia, which lie deep within the telencephalon. The basal ganglia themselves receive input from several targets especially the prefrontal, frontal and parietal cortices. The function of basal ganglia, in any context, appears to be the voluntary selection and initiation of higher functions, so in this case the selection of willed movements.

Anatomy

Chapter 1, Figure 1.13 shows the relation between the putamen, caudate nucleus and the elements of the basal ganglia. Figure 6.12 shows the thalamus as a rugby ball-shaped collection of cell groups with thalami on either side joined by the interthalamic connexus.

The thalamus is organized around a Y-shaped collection of white matter called the 'internal medullary lamina'. This splits the thalamus into three sections – the anterior, lateral and medial sections. Each section is composed of several cell groups with particular inputs and functions, and there are also groups of cells inside the medullary lamina.

In general, sensory systems project from their receptors along peripheral sensory nerves and then, via a relay in the thalamus, to the 'primary' sensory cortex for that sensory modality (e.g. V1 for vision or S1 for sensation). The thalamus acts as a gateway to the cortex for sensory information and its output to the cortex can be modified, such as by the brainstem reticular activating system. The thalamus can, therefore, exert considerable influence on cortical processing.

Connections and circuits of the basal ganglia

Caudate and putamen

The caudate and putamen contain identical cell types and together they form the main cortical target input to the basal ganglia: the corpus striatum (or simply the striatum).

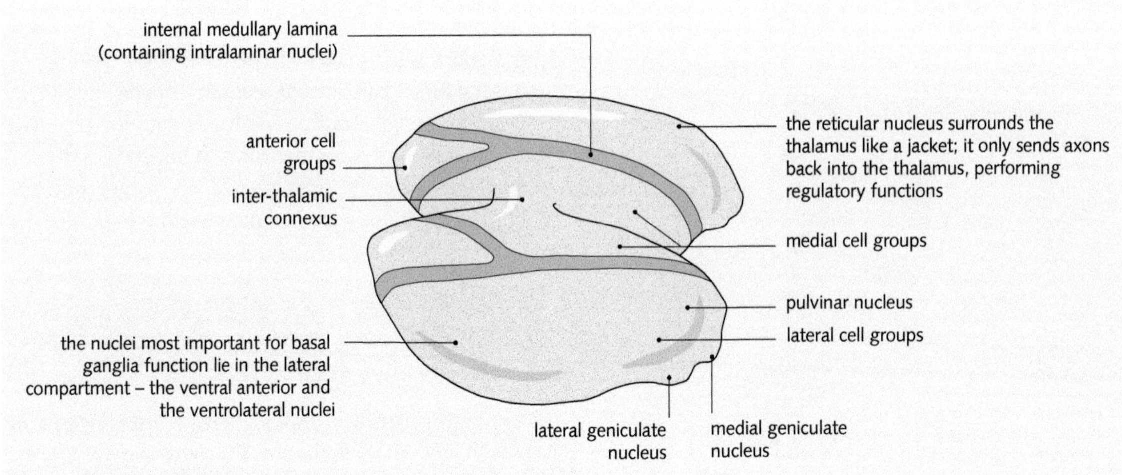

Fig. 6.12 The thalamus.

The striatum receives somatotopic information from motor, sensory, association and limbic areas as well as the intralaminar nuclei of the thalamus.

The corticostriate projection is topographically and functionally organized so that the putamen is chiefly concerned with motor control and the caudate with eye movements and cognition.

Globus pallidus

The globus pallidus is the output source to the thalamus. The globus pallidus can be divided into internal (GPi) and external (GPe) segments lying lateral to the internal capsule and medial to the putamen. The GPi is the major output nuclei of the basal ganglia projecting to the ventrolateral and ventral anterior nuclei of the thalamus. The connection from the striatum to the GPi and thence to the thalamus is known as the direct pathway (Fig. 6.13).

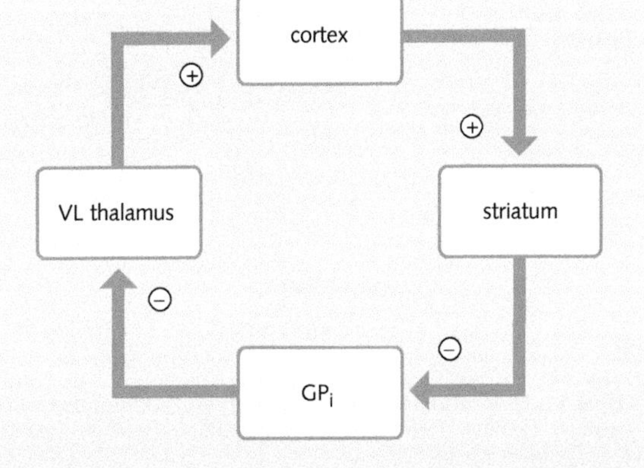

Fig. 6.13 The direct corticostriatal loop. When the striatum inhibits the internal globus pallidus (GPi), it reduces the ability of the GPi to inhibit the thalamus. This effectively encourages the thalamus to fire, and thus stimulates the cortex (supplementary motor area) (VL, ventrolateral).

Subthalamic nucleus

The subthalamic nucleus lies below the thalamus at its junction with the midbrain and communicates bidirectionally with the GPe. There is also an excitatory output to the GPi, therefore establishing a second loop of information through the basal ganglia travelling via the subthalamic pathway: the indirect pathway (Fig. 6.14).

Substantia nigra

The substantia nigra lies in the midbrain and is divided into a ventral pale part, the pars reticulata, which projects to the ventrolateral and ventral anterior thalamic nuclei and the superior colliculus, and a dorsal pigmented part, the pars compacta, which projects to the caudate and putamen. These use dopamine for the transmission of information.

The substantia nigra helps to facilitate the role of the direct pathway by activating cells in the putamen, which in turn releases the ventrolateral nucleus from the inhibitory influence of the globus pallidus.

Re-entrant processing loops

In Figures 6.13 and 6.14 it is possible to see that the direct and indirect pathways have opposing roles in the production of movement; the direct pathway facilitates movement and the indirect pathway inhibits it.

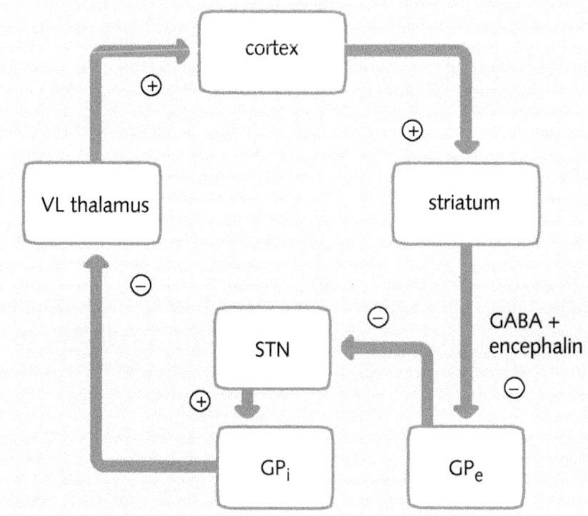

Fig. 6.14 The indirect loop. Striatal output inhibits the GPe, reducing the inhibition of the subthalamic nucleus. The GPi is then excited, and in turn inhibits output from the VL thalamus. The cortex therefore gets less stimulation (GABA, γ-aminobutyric acid; VL, ventrolateral; GPe, globus pallidus external segment; GPi, globus pallidus internal segment).

The easiest way to work through this is mathematically. The direct pathway consists of two inhibitory synapses (let us call them -1). When -1 is multiplied by itself we get $+1$ ($-1 \times -1 = +1$); therefore the facilitation of movement. The indirect pathway has three inhibitory synapses therefore $-1 \times -1 \times -1 = -1$. Thus the indirect pathway when activated inhibits movement.

The cellular interactions of the basal ganglia are shown in Figure 6.15.

Functions of the basal ganglia

The global role of the basal ganglia in any domain (e.g. movement or cognition) is thought to be selection. For instance it is used by the brain to select the movement that M1 wants and inhibit the ones it does not. Other roles include:

- To scale the output of the motor programme so that appropriate movements are made. This is particularly important in motor programmes with fine movement (e.g. hand writing) and also where similar repetitive movements are needed (e.g. in walking).

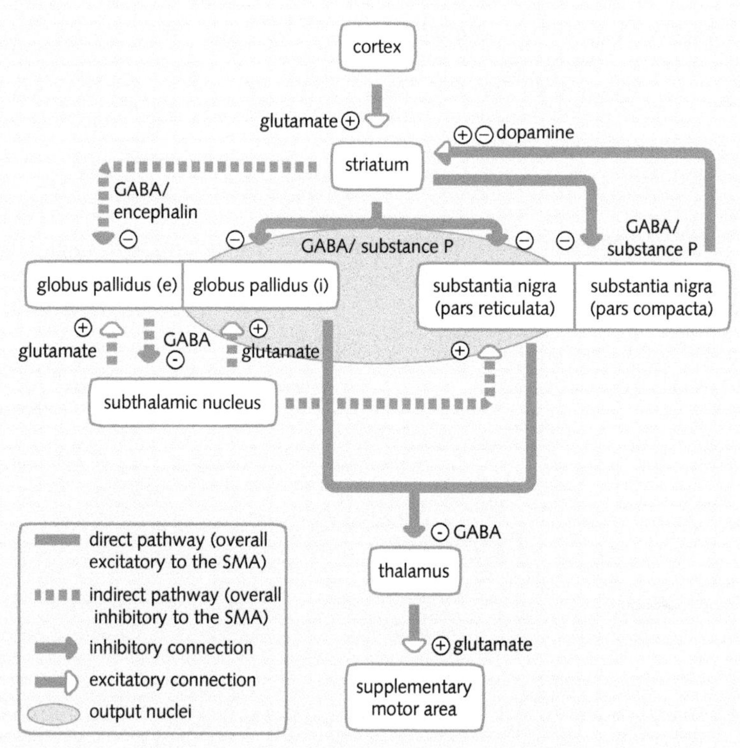

Fig. 6.15 Overview of the pathways through the basal ganglia with their neurotransmitters. Inhibitory signals from the output nuclei (GPi and substantia nigra (pars reticulata)) cause decreased output to the supplementary motor area (the direct and indirect pathways are considered in Figures 6.15 and 6.16, respectively) (GABA, γ-aminobutyric acid).

- To project to the frontal eye fields via the thalamus and have a role in the control of saccadic eye movements.
- A circuit with the prefrontal and other association cortices which may have a role in memory relating to body orientation.
- Connects with the orbitofrontal cortex which may indicate a role in the 'selection' of behaviour.

Whereas the basal ganglia loops participate in the activation of motor programmes it is important to note that they only modulate descending output to the spinal cord. Therefore lesions to the basal ganglia produce extrapyramidal signs (e.g. tremors, rigidity and slowness of movement). This is in contrast with pyramidal signs seen with damage to the descending pyramidal tracts.

THE CEREBELLUM

Movement requires a detailed sequence of muscle contraction each timed with great precision. This control is carried out by the cerebellum.

Anatomy

The cerebellum is divided into four functional areas – the flocculonodular lobe, the vermis and the intermediate and lateral parts of the cerebellar hemispheres. The visible (dorsal) part of the cerebellum is a thin sheet of cortex repeatedly folded and is characterized by a series of ridges which run transversely across the surface of the cerebellum.

There are three functional units:

- The flocculonodular lobe (vestibulocerebellum) involved in the control of posture and eye movements.
- The vermis with the intermediate part of the hemisphere or paravermis (together known as the spinocerebellum), involved in the control of both postural and distal muscles.
- The lateral part of the hemisphere (cerebrocerebellum) involved in coordination and planning of limb movements (in conjunction with the basal ganglia).

Figure 6.16 shows the divisions of the cerebellum, including the deep nuclei that integrate cerebellar cortical processing, forming an output that passes through the superior cerebellar peduncle. Figure 6.17 shows the folding of the cerebellar cortex into lobules and folia that give the cerebellum its furrowed appearance. Figures 6.18 and 6.19 show the inputs to and outputs from the cerebellum.

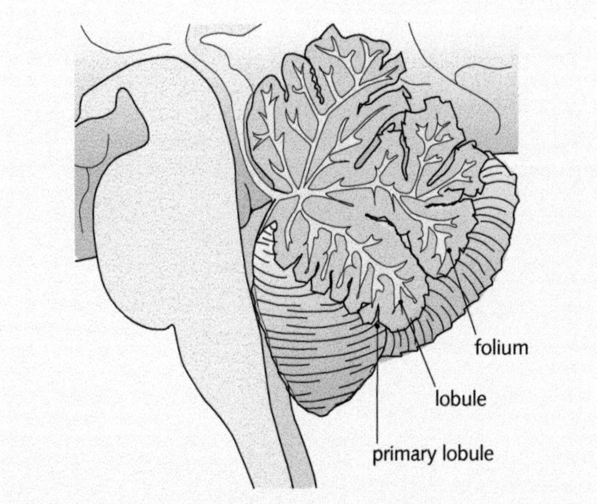

Fig. 6.17 Sagittal section through cerebellar cortex showing lobules and folia.

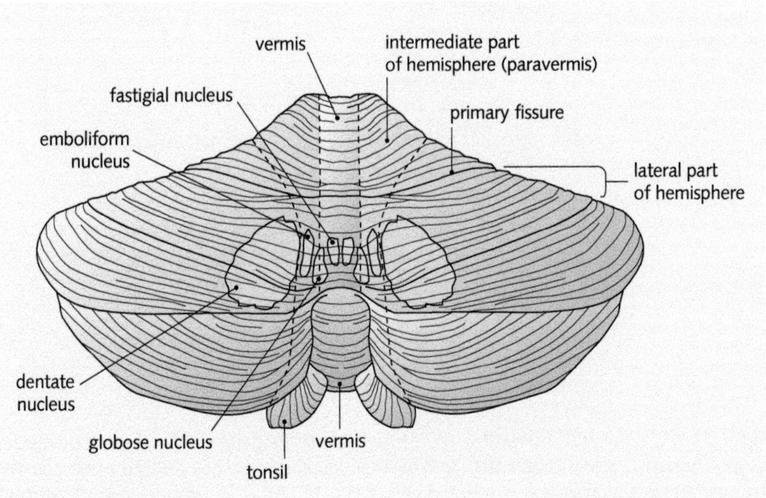

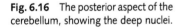

Fig. 6.16 The posterior aspect of the cerebellum, showing the deep nuclei.

Fig. 6.18 Inputs to the cerebellum

Input from	Tract	Peduncle	Termination	Processing
Spinal cord	Spinocerebellar (anterior)	Superior	Vermis	Control of axial muscles, muscle tone
Medulla (gracile, cuneate + trigeminal nuclei)	Spinocerebellar (posterior)	Inferior	Paravermis	Distal limb coordination, muscle tone
Midbrain	Tectocerebellar	Inferior	Vermis	Visual + auditory
Olivary nucleus	Olivocerebellar (via medulla)	Inferior	Paravermis	Sensory
Vestibular nucleus	Vestibulocerebellar (via medulla)	Inferior	Vermis + floccus	Balance
Cerebral cortex	Pontocerebellar (via pons)	Middle	Lateral hemispheres	Motor planning

Fig. 6.19 Cerebellar outputs

Region	Via deep nucleus	Termination	Function
Vermis	Fastigial	Motor cortex, reticular formation	Control of axial muscles as movement progresses
Paravermis	Interposed	Red nucleus – influencing fibres to thalamus and motor cortex, and those in rubrospinal tract	Control of distal muscles as movement progresses
Hemispheres	Dentate	Red nucleus and premotor cortex	Movement planning, timing and initiation
Flocculonodular lobe	Direct projection	Lateral vestibular nucleus	Control of balance and postural reflexes

The cerebellar cortex

The processing circuit in the cerebellar cortex, as shown in Figure 6.20, can be divided into input axons, processing interneurons and output neurons.

Mossy fibres from the spinocerebellar tract, the dorsal column nuclei and the pontocerebellar tract form the inputs, terminating on granule cells. Inputs from the inferior olivary nucleus in the brainstem (carrying information from the spino-olivary tract, brainstem and cortex) enter the circuit as parallel fibres and make many contacts on Purkinje cells. Climbing fibres from the spinal cord (via the inferior olive) also synapse with the Purkinje cells. Both parallel and climbing fibres also send inputs to the deep cerebellar nuclei.

The interneurons in the circuit have different functions:

- Granule cells, which receive most of the input to the cortex from the mossy fibres, send axons up towards the cortical surface, branching in parallel and making many contacts with other cell types in the cortical circuit.
- Golgi cells, after receiving excitation from granule cells, inhibit them in a feedback loop.
- Stellate and basket cells are also inhibitory and inhibit the output cell of the circuit – the Purkinje cell.

The inhibition produced by Golgi, stellate and basket cells helps to prevent submaximally stimulated Purkinje and granule cells from firing (reducing noise).

The output of the circuit is from the Purkinje cell which also receives input from climbing fibres. Purkinje cells make GABAergic (inhibitory) projections to the deep cerebellar nuclei which project to other parts of the CNS.

Functional units of the cerebellum

The vestibulocerebellum receives information from the vestibular nuclei (changes in head position relative to body position and gravity) and visual information from the lateral geniculate nuclei, superior colliculi and visual cortex. It projects to the vestibular nuclei, and thence to the oculomotor centres, and is involved in the control of axial muscles (balance) and the coordination of head and eye movements.

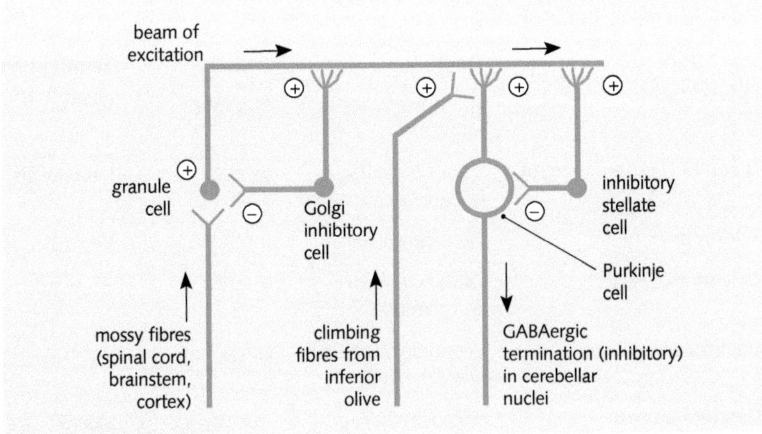

Fig. 6.20 The processing circuit in the cerebellar cortex.

The spinocerebellum receives its main input from the spinocerebellar tract and is concerned with the control of postural muscle tone (by setting GMN drive which affects alpha motor neuron activity through the reflex loop) and movement execution.

The vermis receives information from auditory, visual and vestibular systems, and sensory information from the proximal body. It projects to the ventromedial descending motor pathway and reticular formation.

The intermediate hemisphere receives sensory information from the distal body and projects through the red nucleus (via the superior olive) and thence to the descending rubrospinal tract. It also projects to the contralateral motor cortex (via the thalamus).

The cerebrocerebellum controls precision in rapid and dextrous movements, receiving information from cortical motor and sensory areas. It is inserted in a processing loop like the basal ganglia (motor cortex to pontine nuclei to cerebellar cortex to dentate nucleus to contralateral ventrolateral thalamic nucleus and red nucleus to motor cortex).

Error detection in cerebellar movement control

The Purkinje cells show an alteration in their firing pattern when errors in planned movement occur. This change consists of 'complex' spikes where, after the initial depolarization from the incoming Na^+, there is a smaller continued depolarization, a 'plateau' caused by incoming Ca^{2+}, and then further spikes superimposed on the plateau, again because of the opening of Ca^{2+} channels. This pattern of firing is produced by climbing fibre input and shows that the role of the olivocerebellar tract is in error detection.

When a new movement is performed, a large and long-lasting activation of Purkinje cells is seen. This corresponds to error correction signals being stored in motor memory at a special type of modifiable synapse capable of long-term depression. As the movement becomes more practised, fewer errors are made and the Purkinje activation decreases.

CONTROL OF LOCOMOTION

Locomotion requires a coordination of the systems controlling posture and the systems producing voluntary movements. This ensures that the body is supported in gravity and that the centre of gravity lies over the support base during propulsion.

A rhythm of muscle activity is needed as each limb takes its turn in supporting the body and moving it forwards. The circuits that generate this pattern of activity are in the spinal cord and can be activated by higher centres (e.g. the brainstem).

A network of interneurons in the spinal cord govern the activity of motor neurons; these are known as central pattern generators (CPGs). One CPG will activate flexor muscles, and another extensors, the two being mutually inhibitory. Renshaw cells in the spinal cord inhibit interneurons which are firing. Therefore activation of CPG-1 will cause its own inactivation (via Renshaw cells), which then removes the inhibition of CPG-2. This rhythmic switching may be modified by 1b afferent information from the Golgi tendon organs which prevent excessive tension in either muscle group.

So often an example is useful in tidying up new concepts. Consider Shane Warne bowling to Andrew Flintoff and hopefully the areas in controlling movement will become clear: Warne knows that he has had some success with his 'sliders' (the limbic system) so he decides to try the same with Flintoff (prefrontal cortex). His motor strategy (the slider delivery) is set and consists of several motor programmes (how to hold the ball, how to spin it, his run up). Warne's prefrontal region projects the 'plan' to the SMA and PMA so they can prepare M1 with a plan of how to carry out the slider delivery (the tactics of the delivery; the middle level of motor control hierarchy). The Betz cells of the M1 prepare to tell the descending spinal tracts which muscles to activate in a somatotopic way.

The motor circuit of the basal ganglia (via the ventrolateral thalamus) helps to 'select' the chosen delivery (the direct pathway) and 'select out' (via the indirect pathway) the other possible deliveries (e.g. topspin, the flipper). This circuit ends in PMA and SMA to help with 'planning' of the movement. The projection from the cerebellum (via the thalamus) to M1 helps coordinate the intended movement and the muscle movements required.

The selected and coordinated motor strategy is relayed to the muscles via the descending tracts of the spinal cord (the lowest level of the hierarchy). Upper motor neurons from M1 synapse with AMNs which instruct which muscles should contract and by how much. Warne's muscles are therefore able to carry out the movement. He carries out the delivery and the cerebellum helps to compare the intended movement with the actual movement.

The result of this motor planning sequence? Flintoff hits a six.

CLINICAL ASPECTS OF THE MOTOR CONTROL SYSTEM

Now that the 'how' of movement has been cleared up, the consequences of motor system pathology should be more easily understood.

Disorders involving basal ganglia function and their treatment

Parkinsonism

The signs resulting from low dopaminergic input from the substantia nigra (pars compacta) to the striatum (and, therefore, reduced facilitation of the direct pathway) are collectively called 'parkinsonism' and are due to the basal ganglia not processing motor programmes correctly. The signs are:

- Akinesia – poverty of movement, usually noticed first by lack of blinking and producing a characteristic expressionless face.
- Bradykinesia – when movement does occur it is very slow.
- Tremor at rest – characteristically in the hands, it is called a 'pill-rolling' tremor and has a frequency of 3–6 Hz.
- Rigidity – caused by an increased tone in skeletal muscle. When passive movement is attempted, the limbs move in a series of jerks as if catching on something. This is termed 'cog-wheel' rigidity.
- Micrographia – small handwriting results from inappropriate motor scaling.
- Shuffling gait– which increases in pace as walking distance increases, termed a 'festinating' gait.
- Abnormal postural reflexes producing a stooped, flexed posture.

Parkinson's disease

The commonest cause of parkinsonism is Parkinson's disease, an idiopathic condition where cells in the compact part of the substantia nigra which project to the striatum die, and so the dopaminergic input is lost. Other cell groups are also affected – the ventral tegmental area (dopamine to ventral striatum), locus coeruleus (noradrenaline (norepinephrine) projected diffusely in central nervous system) and the raphe nuclei (5-hydroxytryptamine projected diffusely in central nervous system).

The annual incidence is 1 in 5000, with a prevalence of about 1 per 500. Age of onset is generally approximately 50 years onwards, but 8% of patients develop symptoms before the age of 40 years. The cause remains unclear although genetic (particularly in early-onset Parkinson's) and environmental factors are likely to be important. The main pathological changes are:

- Loss of the pigmented cells in the substantia nigra, which results in severe striatal dopamine deficiency
- Atypical eosinophilic inclusion bodies, called 'Lewy' bodies.

Clinical features include:

- Bradykinesia (cardinal feature). Patients present with slowness of gait, difficulties in writing and using their hands, turning in bed and reduced facial expression
- Resting tremor classically of four or five cycles per second
- Rigidity of lead-pipe or (with superimposed tremor) cog-wheeling type
- Impaired postural control and loss of righting reflexes, causing flexed posture and falls in advanced cases
- Dementia in approximately 30% of cases
- Affective disorders are very common (particularly anxiety and depression).

Investigations

- The diagnosis is usually based on the clinical features and response to treatment.
- Imaging, autonomic function tests and sphincter electromyogram are occasionally needed to exclude other parkinsonian syndromes.

Treatment

- Anticholinergic and dopaminergic drugs are the main line of treatment (see below).
- Dopaminergic neuronal implantation is still a research procedure.
- Prognosis with treatment – life expectancy is now only slightly shorter than that of the general population.

Drug treatment of Parkinson's disease

Dopamine precursors

This approach bypasses the rate-limiting step of dopamine synthesis – tyrosine hydroxylase. L-dopa, the drug of choice for most Parkinson's disease patients, is metabolized by dopa decarboxylase to dopamine. Dopamine itself cannot be given because it has many peripheral effects, and does not cross the blood–brain barrier well.

Side effects of L-dopa include: nausea and vomiting caused by stimulation of D_2 receptors in the chemoreceptor trigger zone in the brainstem; reduction in gastric emptying due to effects on gastric dopamine receptors; dyskinesias – the striatum becomes very sensitive to its dopamine input and overdose of L-dopa can occur producing involuntary movements (dyskinesias), which can be very disabling; and psychiatric effects (psychosis, depression, acute confusional state) due to alteration of all dopaminergic pathways that influence cortical function (e.g. ventral tegmental area to limbic system nuclei).

Side effects can be treated with a peripherally acting dopamine antagonist, domperidone, counteracting gastric emptying and nausea.

To increase the proportion of L-dopa reaching the CNS, drugs need to be given to prevent L-dopa from being used by peripheral nervous structures, such as sympathetic nerve terminals. Carbidopa and benserazide are inhibitors of dopa decarboxylase that act only in the periphery, as they do not cross the blood–brain barrier, and are an essential addition to L-dopa therapy.

In long-term treatment ($>$ 5 years) deterioration is inevitable and akinesia recurs. Tolerance develops, meaning equivalent doses give shorter periods of relief and the response to L-dopa becomes unpredictable.

Antimuscarinics (e.g. trihexyphenidyl and benzatropine)

Combining the arrangement of striatal circuitry (Fig. 6.14) whereby dopamine facilitates striatal direct pathway output and acetylcholine antagonizes dopamine, acetylcholine antagonists can be given to increase dopaminergic transmission. They reduce tremor and rigidity but have little effect on bradykinesia. Side effects are drowsiness, confusion (which can exacerbate dementia in Parkinson's disease) and reduced parasympathetic function. Acetylcholine is not the only excitatory input and this therapy will not work for long.

Inhibitors of monoamine oxidase B

Inhibitors of monoamine oxidase B, such as selegiline, reduce the rate at which dopamine is degraded in nerve terminals and potentiates the effect of L-dopa. It is often reserved for severe disease when L-dopa is beginning to lose its efficacy.

Direct dopamine agonists

Direct dopamine agonists (e.g. bromocriptine) stimulate striatal receptors but do not mimic the normal conditions of dopamine release in the striatum. Side effects are similar to those of L-dopa – nausea and psychiatric disturbance. Again, they are reserved for severe disease.

Newer methods to treat Parkinson's disease include:

- Neurosurgery to ablate the hyperactive globus pallidus internal segment (pallidotomy)
- The placement of electrodes for deep brain stimulation in the globus pallidus internal segment and substantia nigra (pars reticulata), which depresses their function (via conduction block)
- Implantation of dopamine-rich material from fetal tissue (this remains a controversial and, as yet, unproven therapy).

The different mechanisms of action of the various agents used in Parkinson's disease are illustrated in Figure 6.21.

Other degenerative disorders which can produce parkinsonism:

- Progressive supranuclear palsy (Steel–Richardson–Olzewski syndrome) – characterized by more tone in the neck than the limbs and falls early on in the disease
- Multiple system atrophy

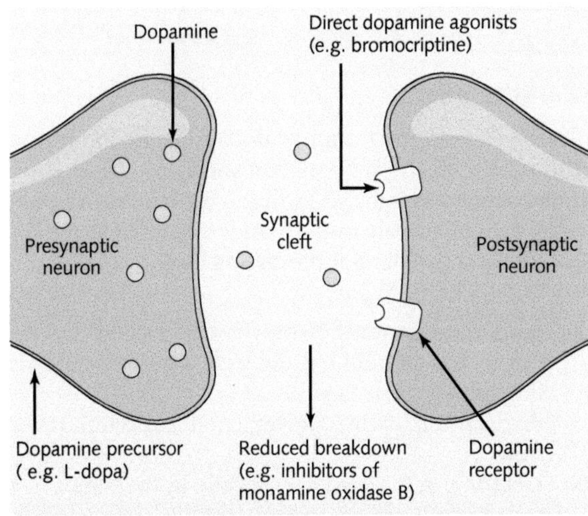

Fig. 6.21 Drugs used in the treatment of Parkinson's disease.

- Wilson's disease – a disorder of copper metabolism
- Diffuse Lewy body disease
- Diffuse cerebrovascular disease with abnormal gait.

Drug-induced parkinsonism

- Neuroleptic medication – taken for psychosis, which antagonizes the dopamine input to the striatum
- Neurotoxin ingestion – infamously by drug misusers taking a synthetic morphine analogue contaminated with MPTP (1-methyl-4-phenyl-1,2,3,6-tetrahydropyridine). This is metabolized by monoamine oxidase B to a compound MPP^+, which inhibits NADH dehydrogenase in dopaminergic terminals, reducing ATP production and promoting cell death.

Non-parkinsonian disorders

Huntington's disease

This autosomal dominant condition is caused by a trinucleotide repeat on chromosome 4 (Ch. 15). It typically presents in mid-life, but may show anticipation in subsequent generations. The symptoms are caused by selective cell death in the striatum of both acetylcholine and GABA-containing neurons. Hyperkinesia develops with squirming dance-like or 'choreic' movement. This is because initially GABAergic output cells projecting to the external globus pallidus die, releasing it from inhibition and resulting in greater inhibition at the next set of cells in the group – the subthalamic nucleus. Subthalamic lesions reduce the inhibitory tone from the GPi onto the ventrolateral thalamus thereby signalling to M1 that inappropriate movements are to be made (the direct pathway; Fig. 6.13). Subthalamic lesions by themselves produce contralateral involuntary movement). Cognitive functions also deteriorate as striatal cell death continues, affecting the processing loops with the frontal lobes.

Effects of cerebellar lesions

Cerebellar disease produces disorders in limbs ipsilateral to the lesion; volitional movements are still present, although defective.

Lesions can result from head injury, tumours, haemorrhage, ischaemia and Friedreich's ataxia. The white matter pathways carrying the connections can be damaged in multiple sclerosis.

Effects include the following:

- Disturbances of posture – wide-base standing position, ataxic gait, nystagmus in flocculonodular damage
- Disturbances of muscle tone (hypotonia) and axial and truncal control – in vermis and intermediate hemisphere damage
- Disturbances in control of precision movements – delays in starting and stopping movements, tremor increasing in severity through a movement, disorders in movement timing so that movements become decomposed into their components, and poor coordination of similarly acting muscle groups, making rapidly alternating movements very difficult (dysdiadochokinesis).

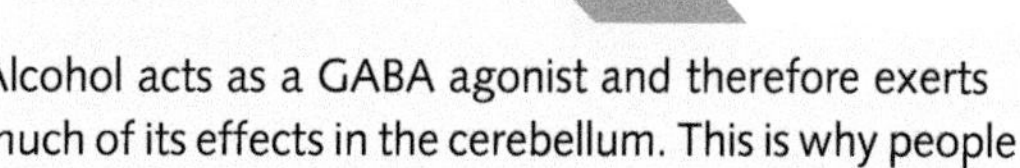

Alcohol acts as a GABA agonist and therefore exerts much of its effects in the cerebellum. This is why people become dysarthric and uncoordinated when drunk.

THE VESTIBULAR SYSTEM, POSTURE AND LOCOMOTION

Control of posture

Posture is the relative position of the trunk, head and limbs in space. To keep posture stable, the body's centre of gravity needs to be maintained in position over its support base.

Postural reflexes are required to correct changes caused by displacement of the centre of gravity (by either external forces or deliberate movement). Postural change is detected by musculoskeletal proprioceptors, the vestibular apparatus and the visual system.

Vestibular system

The components of the vestibular system can be seen in Figure 6.22. It is the vestibular system that is responsible for the detection of changes in head position, linear acceleration and angular acceleration. Output from the vestibular system is by efferents called Scarpa's ganglion which feed into the auditory (VIII) nerve that runs through to the auditory nucleus. The vestibular nuclei use this information together with afferent nerves from neck muscles and cervical vertebrae to determine if the head is moving alone or if the head and body are both moving. The nuclei influence antigravity and axial musculature via a direct projection into the spinal cord. The vestibular system also has outputs which affect eye movements.

Receptor system

The inner ear apparatus is contained within a number of interconnected membranous tunnels. These are cavities within the petrous temporal bone – the bony labyrinth – which contain fluid (perilymph). Within the bony labyrinth and bathed in perilymph is the

Fig. 6.22 The vestibular system.

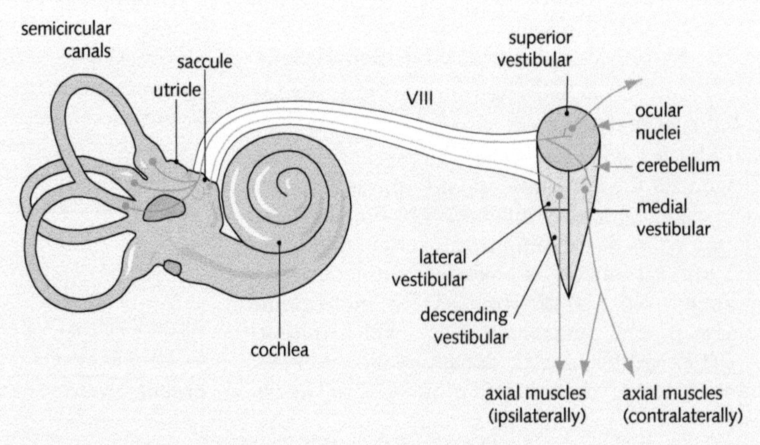

membranous labyrinth which is filled with endolymph. Perilymph closely resembles cerebrospinal fluid, but endolymph is much similar to intracellular fluid in terms of ion concentration.

Vestibular labyrinth

The vestibular labyrinth includes two types of structures with different functions:

- The otolith organs (Fig. 6.23), which detect the force of gravity and tilts of the head
- The semicircular canals (Fig. 6.24), which are sensitive to head movement and rotation.

The otolith organs are a pair of relatively large chambers, the saccule and utricle, which lie in the middle (the vestibule) of the inner ear, but have different functions:

- The saccular otoliths are orientated vertically and detect changes in linear acceleration in the vertical plane and changes in head position during lateral tilt.
- The utricular otoliths are orientated horizontally and detect changes in linear acceleration in the horizontal plane and changes in head position during flexion and extension of the neck.

Each otolith organ contains a sensory epithelium called a macula, which is vertically orientated in the saccule and horizontally orientated in the utricle, when the head is upright. The macula hair cells lie amongst a bed of supporting cells and project their cilia into a gelatinous cap. The gelatinous cap of the otoliths organs are encrusted by tiny crystals of calcium carbonate (otoliths literally means ear stones; see Figure 6.23). The otoliths have a higher density than the endolymph that

Fig. 6.23 Structure of the otolith organs.

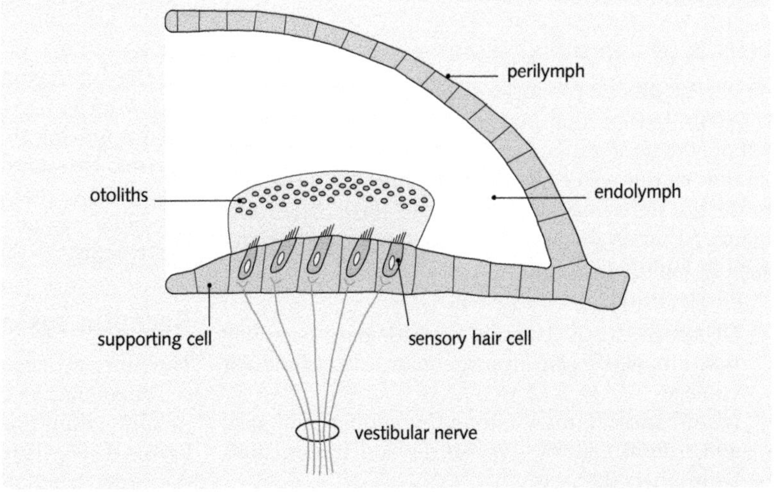

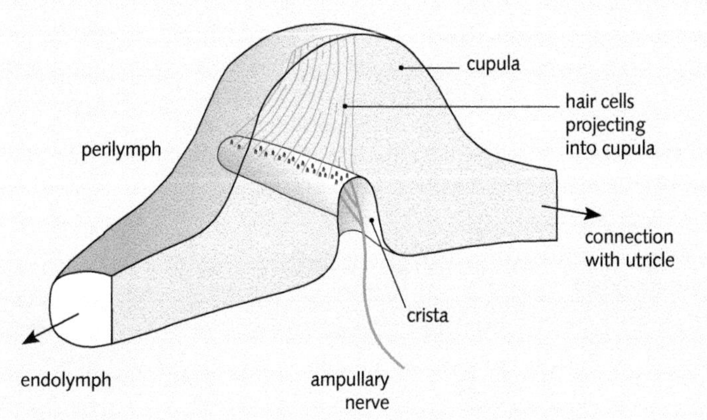

Fig. 6.24 Structure of ampullar crista.

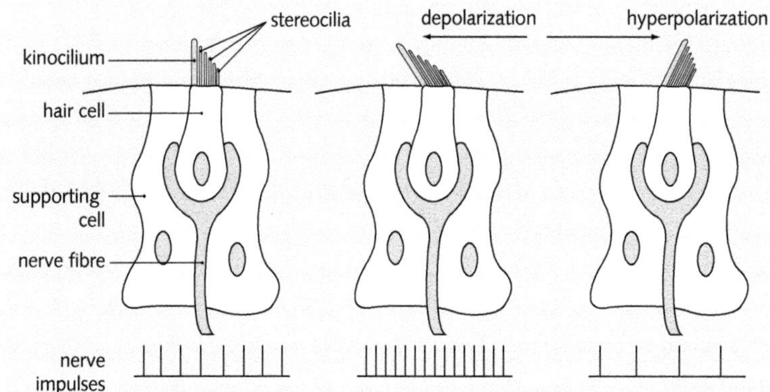

Fig. 6.25 Vestibular hair cells. Bending of the stereocilia towards the kinocilium causes ion channels to open and therefore depolarization of the cell. The opposite happens when the stereocilia are bent the other way.

surrounds them, such that when the angle of the head changes or when the head accelerates a force is exerted on the otoliths, which then exerts a force in the same direction on the gelatinous cap. This causes the hair cells to bend. Each hair cell contains one tall cilium, the movement of which is crucial to the detection of head movement (Fig. 6.25):

- The bending of the hairs towards the kinocilium results in a depolarizing (therefore excitatory) receptor potential, causing more neurotransmitter release.
- The bending of the hairs away from the kinocilium results in a hyperpolarizing (therefore inhibitory) receptor potential, reducing neurotransmitter release.

Membrane deformation produces alterations in the shape of cation channels, which causes the change in membrane potential (i.e. bending towards the kinocilium opens the cation channels permitting depolarization).

If the cells are perpendicular to their preferred direction of movement then they barely respond. Only tiny movements are needed for transmission to occur.

Semicircular canals

The semicircular canals detect turning movements of the head (e.g. nodding or shaking your head). The canals detect acceleration like the otolith organs; however, this acceleration is angular acceleration generated by sudden rotation movements.

The semicircular canals are arranged at right angles to each other and together they detect the angular acceleration in all three planes of three-dimensional space. Each canal has a swelling (ampulla) near its attachment to the utricle, which contains the hair cells projecting from a ridge (crista) again into a gelatinous substance (the cupula; see Figure 6.24). All the hair cells in the ampulla are orientated in the same direction, which means they all get excited or inhibited together.

HINTS AND TIPS

Disturbance of the vestibular system (such as might be caused by infection in the middle ear) may lead to a false sense of rotational movement (vertigo), nausea and eye movement problems. It is often caused by disruption to endolymph flow due to debris, and may be worse in particular positions.

Head movement is detected when the wall of the canal and cupula begin to spin. As they do the endolymph tends to stay behind because of inertia. The viscous endolymph exerts a force upon the cupula causing it to fill out, bowing the cupula. This movement bends the cilia which depending on the direction of the rotation either excites or inhibits the release of neurotransmitter from the hair cells onto the vestibular nerve (see Fig. 6.25).

Improving the quality of postural information

Hair cells show greatest alteration in membrane potentials when the stereocilia are moved in one direction. To detect different degrees of tilt and different degrees of flexion, the hair cells in the maculae are orientated in various planes so that they respond best to a particular head position.

The left and right saccules, utricles and semicircular canals are basically arranged in a mirror-image orientation. This means that that when a head movement excites hair cells on one side, it will tend to inhibit hair cells in the corresponding location on the other. In this way the vestibular nuclei can use this information to assess head position precisely.

Vestibular nuclei

The vestibular nuclei lie in the medulla, on the floor of the fourth ventricle and receive information from the hair cells through the vestibular nerve (VIII). The semicircular canals project to the superior and medial nuclei. The otolith organs project to the lateral nuclei.

The medial vestibulospinal tract projects bilaterally and the lateral vestibulospinal tract projects ipsilaterally. Both tracts influence antigravity, axial and limb extensor muscles. The vestibular nuclei also project to the thalamus, cerebellum, oculomotor nuclei and contralateral vestibular nuclei. These connections are important in maintaining eye position in the presence of head rotation.

Responses to external and self-generated disturbance

External disturbance alters the postural equilibrium. The vestibular system detects postural change and mediates postural adjustment. Together with the cerebellum, the vestibular system can adapt postural reflexes (e.g. responses on a moving platform; Fig. 6.26).

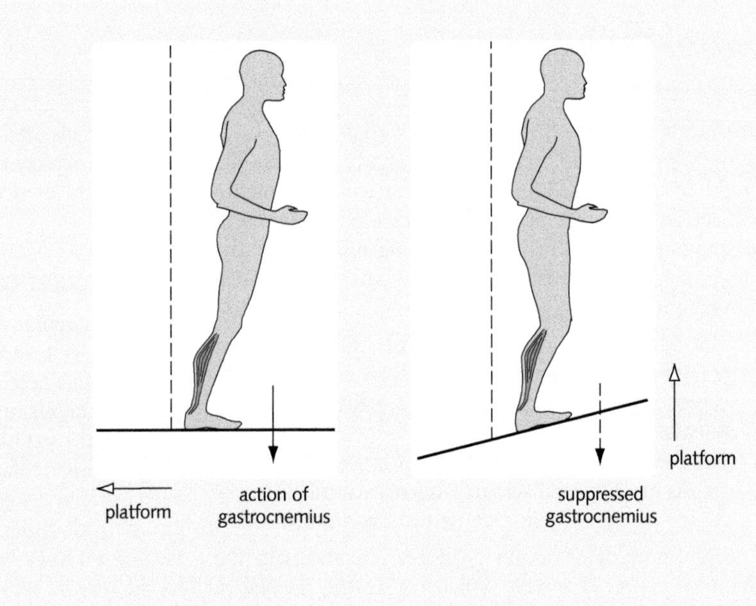

Fig. 6.26 Reflex responses to postural change can be altered.

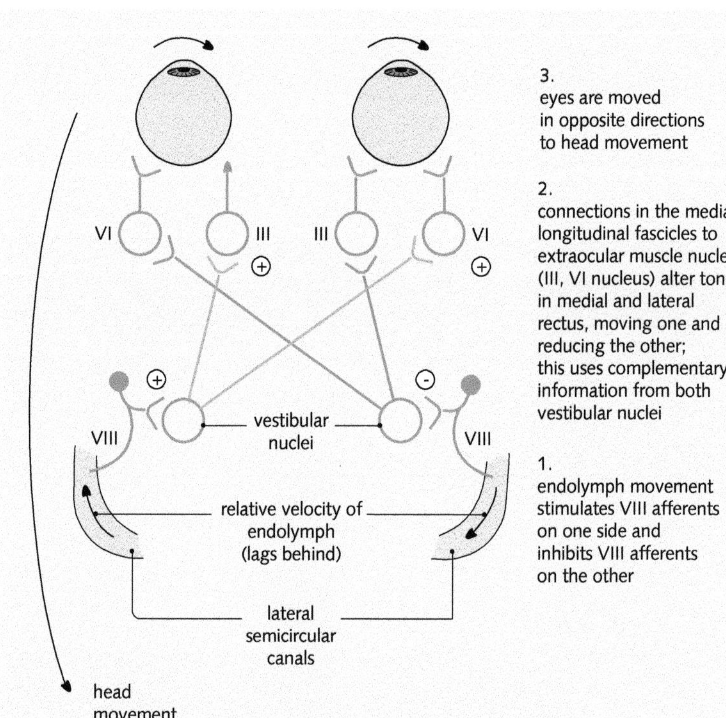
3.
eyes are moved
in opposite directions
to head movement
2.
connections in the medial
longitudinal fascicles to
extraocular muscle nuclei
(III, VI nucleus) alter tone
in medial and lateral
rectus, moving one and
reducing the other;
this uses complementary
information from both
vestibular nuclei
1.
endolymph movement
stimulates VIII afferents
on one side and
inhibits VIII afferents
on the other
VI
III
III
VI
VIII
VIII
vestibular
nuclei
relative velocity of
endolymph
(lags behind)
lateral
semicircular
canals
head
movement

Fig. 6.27 The horizontal vestibulo-ocular reflex.

Responses to self-generated disturbance show that the vestibular system has a feed-forward control mechanism. This is important for eye movements, as a change in head position will alter the image on the retina. To stabilize the retinal image, the vestibular system detects head movements and drives compensatory eye movements. The circuit for this is shown in Figure 6.27. The vestibulo-ocular reflex is an open loop reflex as it works without feedback. The cerebellum regulates the gain of the reflex (amount of eye movement to compensate for head movement). Eye movement control is discussed more fully in Chapter 8.

Vestibular and neck reflexes

The vestibular system mediates some of the neck reflexes (Fig. 6.28).

Fig. 6.28 The vestibular neck reflexes. Note that these are overcome by cortical control in normal situations

Reflex	Action
Vestibulocolic	Stabilizes the position of the head, e.g. if the body is tilted forwards, it returns the head to the vertical position. Synergistic with the cervicocolic reflex of the neck musculature
Vestibulospinal	Tilting the head forwards (e.g. when falling) causes extension of the upper limbs, and flexion of the lower limbs. This protects from the impact of the fall. Antagonistic with the cervicospinal reflexes

The autonomic nervous system

Objectives

In this chapter you will learn about:

- The anatomy and physiology of the sympathetic nervous system.
- The anatomy and physiology of the parasympathetic nervous system.
- Pharmacology and the autonomic nervous system.
- The enteric nervous system.
- Disorders of autonomic function.

INTRODUCTION

Along with the somatic motor system, the autonomic system constitutes the total neural output of the central nervous system. The autonomic nervous system controls involuntary internal processes such as digestion and the regulation of blood flow. It acts mainly on the heart, smooth muscle (such as that in blood vessel walls), metabolic processes and glandular structures. The autonomic nervous system has three branches:

- Sympathetic
- Parasympathetic
- Enteric.

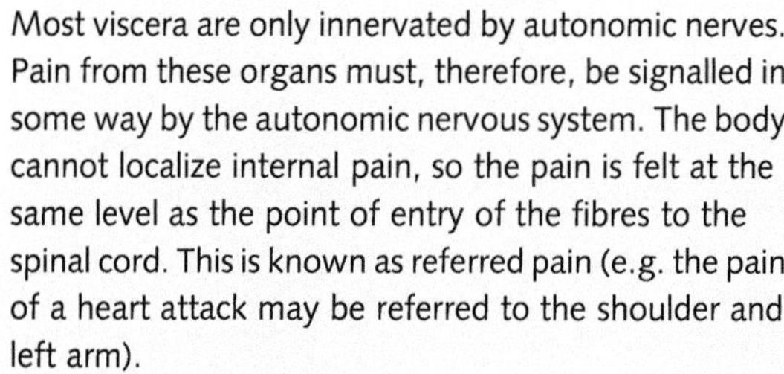

HINTS AND TIPS

Most viscera are only innervated by autonomic nerves. Pain from these organs must, therefore, be signalled in some way by the autonomic nervous system. The body cannot localize internal pain, so the pain is felt at the same level as the point of entry of the fibres to the spinal cord. This is known as referred pain (e.g. the pain of a heart attack may be referred to the shoulder and left arm).

The actions of the autonomic system are multiple, widespread and relatively slow, and unlike the somatic motor system, the autonomic nervous system balances the excitation and inhibition of targets to achieve widely coordinated and graded control. As such, the sympathetic and parasympathetic divisions are often thought of as mutually antagonistic. This is true in certain organ systems (such as the heart), but it is an oversimplification. Some parts of the body receive input from only one of the divisions, and in other areas (such as the salivary glands) their effects are similar. Their actions are coordinated and balanced by the hypothalamus and the nucleus of the solitary tract (NTS).

The autonomic nervous system innervates three types of tissue:

- Secretory glands (e.g. salivary, sweat, tear and mucus-producing glands)
- Smooth muscle (e.g. blood vessels to control blood pressure and flow; respiratory bronchi to meet oxygen demands of the body and to regulate digestive and urogenital function)
- Cardiac muscle (e.g. to control heart rate in response to homeostatic challenges).

Central control of the autonomic nervous system

Central control of the autonomic nervous system is controlled primarily by the hypothalamus. The hypothalamus receives many efferents from many different sensory modalities (i.e. water status and pain). In this way it is able to integrate information about the homeostatic status of the body and to adjust output accordingly. Output comes in the form of both neural and hormonal (via the pituitary gland) outputs. Neural output runs from the periventricular zone to the brainstem and spinal cord nuclei that contain the preganglionic neurons of the sympathetic and parasympathetic divisions.

The NTS (located in the medulla) also plays a role in autonomic control and communicates with the hypothalamus. The nucleus of the solitary tract integrates sensory information from the internal organs and helps to coordinate output to the autonomic brainstem nuclei.

STRUCTURE AND FUNCTION OF THE SYMPATHETIC NERVOUS SYSTEM

Physiological role of the sympathetic nervous system

The sympathetic system prepares the body for responses to stressful challenges, and causes a 'fight or flight' response, allowing sudden strenuous exercise and increased vigilance.

The sympathetic nervous system also helps control blood pressure, thermoregulation, gut function and urogenital function.

Structure of the sympathetic nervous system

There is a column of efferent cell bodies (intermediolateral column) in the lateral grey horn of the spinal cord, running from T1 to L2. These 'preganglionic' neurons have axons that travel through the ventral root of their segmental spinal nerve. They contact a chain of ganglia outside the central nervous system lying along the vertebral column (paravertebral ganglia) (Figs 7.1 and 7.2).

HINTS AND TIPS

The paravertebral ganglia are often referred to as the 'sympathetic chain'.

Each preganglionic neuron can influence many neurons in different ganglia by collaterals, coordinating the activation of ganglia at different spinal levels (Fig. 7.3). The postsynaptic cells in the ganglia are the 'postganglionic' neurons. Postganglionic axons are unmyelinated (therefore conduct more slowly) and pass into peripheral nerves to target sites. For the head and neck, they form a plexus around the carotid arteries and gain access to the interior of the skull travelling alongside the internal carotid artery.

Afferent fibres pass through the paravertebral ganglia without synapsing, reaching their cell bodies in the dorsal root ganglia.

Exceptions to the general pattern of sympathetic nervous system innervation

Some preganglionic fibres do not synapse in the paravertebral ganglia, but carry on to ganglia closer to their target organs via the splanchnic nerves. The coeliac, aorticorenal, superior mesenteric and inferior mesenteric ganglia contain cell bodies providing the sympathetic nervous system innervation to the gut, kidney, liver, pancreas and urogenital organs. Some preganglionic fibres continue to the adrenal medulla. Here, they are responsible for the glandular secretion of catecholamines from cells that are functionally similar to postgang lionic sympathetic neurons.

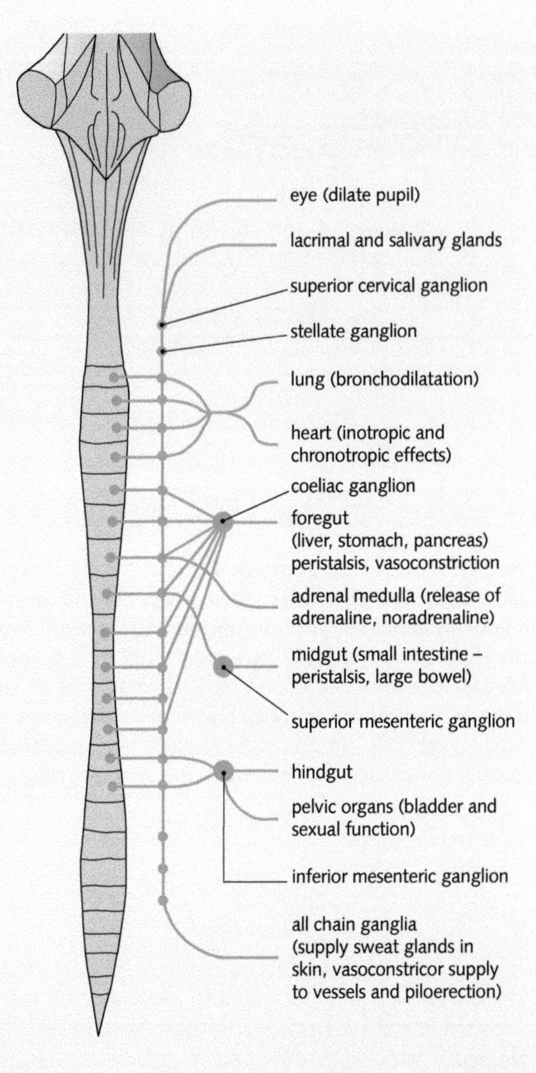

Fig. 7.1 Organization of the sympathetic nervous system.

Neurotransmission in the sympathetic nervous system

The transmitter released by preganglionic neurons at the ganglia (and also those synapsing in the adrenal medulla) is acetylcholine, which binds to postsynaptic nicotinic receptors. The nicotinic receptor is a cation

Fig. 7.2

Cord segment	Organ	Effect	Origin of postganglionic neuron
Th1–2	Eye Lacrimal gland Salivary gland	Pupillary dilatation, vasoconstriction	Superior cervical ganglion
Th1–4	Heart	Heart rate (chronotropic) Stroke volume (inotropic) Coronary artery dilatation	Superior, middle and inferior cervical and upper thoracic ganglia
Th1–4	Skin and muscles of the head and neck	Sweat, vasoconstriction and piloerection	Superior and middle cervical ganglia
Th2–7	Bronchi Lungs	Dilatation Vasodilatation	Inferior cervical and upper thoracic ganglia
Th3–6	Skin and muscles of upper extremity	Sweat, vasoconstriction and piloerection	Stellate and upper thoracic ganglia
Th6–10	Stomach Pancreas Small intestine, ascending and transverse large bowel	Decreased peristalsis and secretion Decreased secretion Vasoconstriction, decreased peristalsis and secretion	Coeliac ganglion Coeliac ganglion Coeliac and superior and inferior mesenteric ganglia
Th10–L2	Skin and muscles of lower extremity	Sweat, vasoconstriction and piloerection	Lower lumbar and upper sacral ganglia
Th11–L2	Descending large bowel and rectum Ureter and bladder	Decreased peristalsis and secretion Relaxes detrusor, contracts internal sphincter	Inferior mesenteric, hypogastric ganglia and pelvic plexus Hypogastric ganglion and pelvic plexus

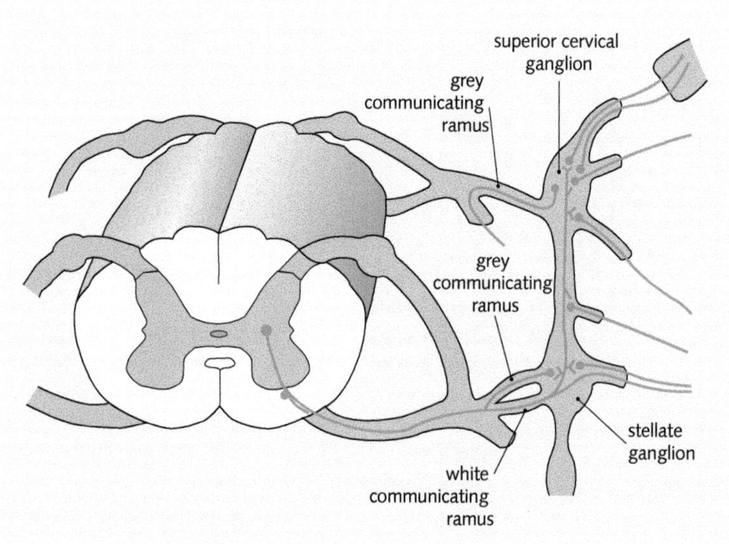

Fig. 7.3 Spinal cord efferents to the sympathetic chain.

Fig. 7.4 Adrenergic receptors: location, second messenger and function

Adrenergic receptor	Location	Second messenger	Function
α_1	Smooth muscle in blood vessels and bronchi, dilator pupillae	IP_3	Contraction
α_2	Smooth muscle in blood vessels, presynaptically on adrenergic synapses	Decreased cAMP	Contraction, reduced transmitter release
β_1	Heart muscle, presynaptically on adrenergic synapses	Increased cAMP	Increased heart rate and force of contraction, increased transmitter release
β_2	Smooth muscle in blood vessels and bronchi	Decreased cAMP	Relaxation

channel which, when opened, produces a fast excitatory postsynaptic potential. The transmitter released by postganglionic neurons (and, therefore, the neurotransmitter released to perform sympathetic function) is noradrenaline (norepinephrine), except in sweat glands where acetylcholine is released and binds to muscarinic receptors (which are slower metabotropic receptors).

Transmission occurs at specialized structures along the length of the postganglionic axon called varicosities, which synthesize, release, take up and metabolize noradrenaline. This process is called 'en passage' transmission, as the action potential does not end when noradrenaline is released but carries on to the next varicosity.

Cells of the adrenal medulla release noradrenaline and adrenaline (epinephrine) into the circulation from the adrenal medulla, permitting the sympathetic nervous system to have a general humoral action on adrenergic receptors in the body ('flight or flight' features).

The effect of noradrenaline release is dependent on the type of receptor that is present in the target organ (Fig. 7.4).

Other transmitters

Often, co-transmitters are released with the main transmitter in the sympathetic nervous system to give a longer-lasting and more subtle modulatory influence on postsynaptic activity (e.g. ATP is released along with noradrenaline at postganglionic sympathetic nerve endings).

Drugs acting on the sympathetic nervous system

The ganglia

Drugs affecting ganglionic transmission have no clinical use. They have complex actions because parasympathetic and sympathetic postganglionic neurons are influenced at the same time, often with opposing effects. Agonists at ganglionic acetylcholine receptors (e.g. nicotine) produce hypertension and tachycardia. Antagonists (e.g. hexamethonium) produce hypotension, but cannot be used as antihypertensive agents because of their side-effect profile.

HINTS AND TIPS

Although nicotine initially stimulates the ganglia, it causes a depolarization block in high concentrations. This causes hypotension and decreased gut motility.

Target organs

Noradrenergic transmission can be altered by interfering with noradrenaline synthesis, release or postsynaptic interaction with different receptor subtypes. Drugs used clinically are shown in Figure 7.5.

STRUCTURE AND FUNCTION OF THE PARASYMPATHETIC NERVOUS SYSTEM

Physiological role of the parasympathetic nervous system

The parasympathetic nervous system has many actions, which can be described as:

- Opposing some effects of the sympathetic nervous system (heart rate, gut motility and bronchiolar diameter)
- Controlling body functions under non-stressful conditions, working either alone or with the sympathetic nervous system (e.g. ciliary muscle for accommodation for near objects; gastrointestinal secretions; secretions of the nose, mouth and eye; micturition; defaecation; sexual function).

The functions of the parasympathetic system can be broadly summarized as 'rest and digest'.

Fig. 7.5 Drugs acting on the sympathetic nervous system

Drug	Action	Clinical use	Side-effects
Adrenaline	α, β agonist	Anaphylaxis, cardiac arrest	Hypertension, dysrhythmia
Salbutamol	β_2 agonist	Asthma	Tachycardia, dysrhythmia, tremor
Clonidine	partial α_2 agonist	Hypertension	Drowsiness, postural hypotension
Prazosin	α_1 antagonist	Hypertension	Hypotension, tachycardia, impotence
Atenolol	β_1 antagonist	Hypertension, acute coronary syndromes, tachyarrhythmias	Heart failure, fatigue, cold extremities, less bronchoconstriction than non-selective β antagonists

Structure of the parasympathetic nervous system

There are two clusters of preganglionic neurons at either end of the spinal cord (Fig. 7.6). The cranial parasympathetic nervous system outflow comes from several nuclei in the brainstem. Structures in the head are supplied by the ciliary, pterygopalatine, otic and submandibular ganglia which receive inputs from cranial nerves III, VII and IX. Organs in the thorax and abdomen receive their parasympathetic supply via the vagus (Xth) nerve, which forms diffusely distributed collections of postganglionic neurons in the walls of, or close to, the target organs. The sacral parasympathetic nervous system outflow comes from preganglionic neurons whose cell bodies lie in a column running from segment S2 to segment S4 of the spinal cord. Their axons leave the cord through the ventral root for a short distance and leave the spinal nerves as separate small pelvic nerves. The postganglionic neurons are found in the pelvic plexus located near the target organs.

Neurotransmission in the parasympathetic nervous system

As in the sympathetic nervous system, parasympathetic preganglionic neurons release acetylcholine onto ganglionic nicotinic receptors.

At target organs, postganglionic neurons release acetylcholine onto muscarinic receptors, which show subtype variation localized to different target organs (Fig. 7.7). Unlike the sympathetic nervous system, the acetylcholine released at the postganglionic neuron does not have widespread systemic effects.

Drugs acting on the parasympathetic nervous system

Therapeutic drugs that affect the function of the parasympathetic nervous system interact with the receptors on target organs (Fig. 7.8).

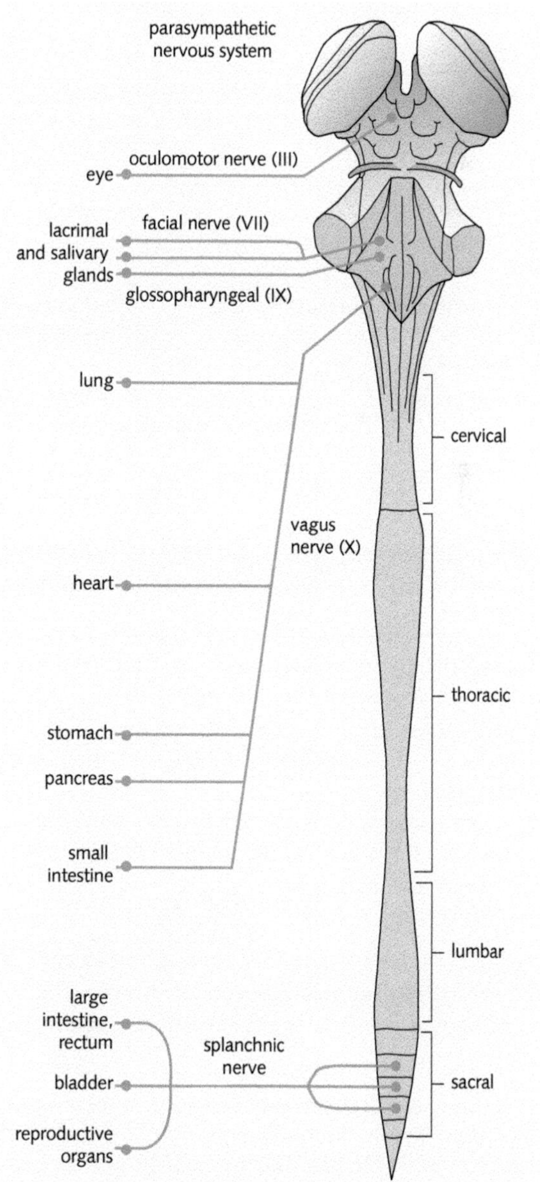

Fig. 7.6 Organization of the parasympathetic nervous system.

Fig. 7.7 Muscarinic receptors

Muscarinic subtype	Location	Function
M_1	Gastric parietal cells, enteric nervous system	Slow excitation of ganglia. Gastric acid secretion, gastrointestinal motility
M_2	Cardiac atrium	Vagal inhibition of heart. Decreased heart rate and force of contraction
M_3	Smooth muscle, glands	Secretion, contraction of smooth muscle, vascular relaxation

Fig. 7.8 Drugs acting on the parasympathetic nervous system

Drug	Action	Use	Side effects
Pilocarpine	Partial muscarinic agonist	Glaucoma (increased intraocular pressure), where increased constrictor pupillae action allows greater drainage of aqueous humour	Cardiac slowing, increased gastrointestinal tract activity causing abdominal pain
Atropine	Muscarinic antagonist	Cardiac arrest, sinus bradycardia after myocardial infarction	Dry mouth, dilated pupil, blurred vision, bronchodilatation, urinary retention
Ipratropium	Muscarinic antagonist	Asthma, causing bronchodilatation and inhibiting increases in mucous secretion	Inhaled and does not pass easily into the circulation, so few side effects
Dicyclomine	M_1 antagonist has direct relaxant effect on smooth muscle	Reduces spasmodic activity of gastrointestinal tract in irritable bowel syndrome	Less severe than atropine

THE ENTERIC NERVOUS SYSTEM

The enteric nervous system is a neural system embedded in the wall of the gastrointestinal tract, pancreas and gall bladder. It consists of two tubular systems:

- The submucosal (Meissner's) plexus which lies between the mucous membrane and the circular muscle layer
- The myenteric (Auerbach's) plexus which lies between the circular and longitudinal muscle layers.

HINTS AND TIPS

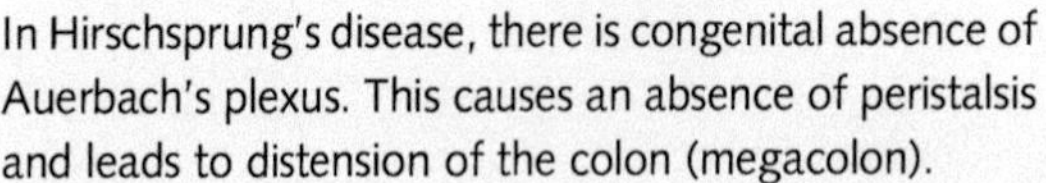

In Hirschsprung's disease, there is congenital absence of Auerbach's plexus. This causes an absence of peristalsis and leads to distension of the colon (megacolon).

Both systems contain both sensory and motor modalities. They have inputs from other parts of the autonomic nervous system but have intrinsic activity of their own:

- The sensory neurons monitor the mechanical state of the alimentary canal, the chemical status of the stomach and intestinal contents, and the hormonal levels in the portal blood vessels.
- The output motor neurons control gut motility and secretions, as well as the diameter of local blood vessels.

An enteric interneuronal circuit exists that uses information from the sensory enteric neurons to control the activity of the enteric motor neurons. The enteric nervous system to a large degree is autonomous; however, it does receive input from both the sympathetic and parasympathetic nervous systems. These connections permit supplementary control of the enteric nervous system and can, in certain situations (i.e. acute stress) overcome enteric control.

The parasympathetic and sympathetic nervous systems can override the enteric division.

DISORDERS OF THE AUTONOMIC NERVOUS SYSTEM

Loss of sympathetic innervation to the face causes Horner's syndrome. This is characterized by:

- Ptosis (drooping of the eyelid)

- Miosis (pupillary constriction)
- Anhidrosis (loss of sweating; more usual with central lesions)
- Enophthalmos (eyes appear withdrawn into the orbit).

The innervation may be interrupted anywhere along its course; the brainstem and cervical spinal cord are rare sites of 'central Horner's syndrome'. Classically, compression of the stellate ganglion may occur in the presence of a carcinoma in the apex of the lung (Pancoast's tumour). Injury can also happen as the sympathetic fibres gain access to the head wrapped around the internal carotid artery (e.g. after dissection of the artery). Surgical exploration of the neck may also cause lesions to sympathetic fibres.

HINTS AND TIPS

Sympathetic innervation of the eye differs from the parasympathetic innervation which arises from the oculomotor nerve. The sympathetic innervation travels up from the neck along the carotid artery into the orbit. Therefore, a widened pupil is a sign of a lesion of the oculomotor nerve and a narrow pupil may be associated with neck pathology.

HINTS AND TIPS

The sympathetic nervous system innervates a third of levator palpebrae superioris via Müller's muscle. It is this innervation that is lost in Horner's syndrome producing the partial ptosis seen.

As well as several other clinical patterns of neuropathy, diabetes mellitus can cause autonomic neuropathy. This may affect the genitourinary system (with impotence and bladder problems), sweating (e.g. during eating), the gastrointestinal tract (with gastricatony, nocturnal diarrhoea, constipation) and the cardiovascular system (especially with postural hypotension).

Section of the sympathetic trunk disrupts the control of structures controlled by that spinal level. Surgical section of sympathetic nerves in the cervicothoracic region has been used to treat Raynaud's syndrome (where vasoconstriction causes painfully cold hands) with little success. A poorly understood feature of peripheral sympathetic injury is 'reflex sympathetic dystrophy', which is chronic pain, accompanied by dry, shiny, red skin and poor wound healing. When this can be localized to a particular nerve root, it is called 'causalgia'.

The effects of disrupting parasympathetic innervation depend on the level of the lesion:

- A neurosyphilitic lesion in the oculomotor nerve causes loss of the pupillary light reflex, dilation of the pupil and preservation of the accommodation reflex (Argyll Robertson pupil).
- Controlled ablation of a highly selective part of the vagal innervation to the stomach may be used as a treatment for excessive gastric acid secretion.
- Damage to the parasympathetic components in the cauda equina causes loss of bladder control and sphincter dysfunction.

Phaeochromocytomas are tumours of the adrenal medulla that secrete vast quantities of catecholamines. This causes hypertension (which may be extremely severe, with headaches and even intracranial haemorrhage as presenting features). A combination of α and β adrenoceptor blockade is required until surgical removal is possible.

Vision 8

Objectives

In this chapter you will learn about:

- The macro- and microscopic anatomy of the eye.
- Retinal structure and function.
- Central visual pathways.
- Mechanisms of attention.
- Loss of vision.

THE EYE

The anatomy of the eye

Figure 8.1 illustrates the structures inside the eye.

The cornea is the transparent outer coat covering the pupil. It is continuous with the sclera (the white of the eye, which is continuous with the dura mater) and consists of five layers. From the exterior inwards they are:

- An epithelial layer of stratified squamous non-keratinizing cells richly innervated with sensory nerves from cranial nerve V and continuously bathed in tear fluid.
- The basement membrane and Bowman's membrane, which gives strength to the cornea.
- The corneal stroma, which occupies 90% of the thickness of the cornea. It consists of thin sheets of collagen fibrils that are oriented parallel to each other in the same sheet and at right angles to fibrils in sheets on either side. The spacing and arrangement of the fibrils gives the cornea its transparency. The stroma is avascular.
- The basal lamina (Descemet's membrane), which lines the inner surface of the stroma.
- The endothelial layer, which is a single layer of squamous cells, providing mechanisms for metabolic exchange between the aqueous humour and the cornea. It regulates the water content of the corneal stroma, preventing oedema and consequent opacity.

The iris is the part of the eye that regulates how much light enters the eye. It is a pigmented muscular structure that lies in front of the lens. The lens is seen in the central space in the iris (the pupil). It appears black as it is transparent. The lens consists of three parts:

- A capsule made of basement membrane, which is elastic and strongest at the insertion of the suspensory ligament around the perimeter of the lens.
- A layer of cuboidal cells (subcapsular epithelium), which lines the inside of the capsule on its anterior surface. Epithelial cells near the perimeter differentiate into lens fibres.
- Lens fibres, which are thin, flattened and devoid of organelles and nuclei. They become filled with proteins (crystallins) and extend towards the centre of the lens, producing a very dense central section.

The ciliary muscle contracts to alter the curvature of the lens and change its refractive power. This is the basis of accommodation.

With time the properties of the lens change. The elasticity of the lens becomes reduced and, therefore, the lens loses the ability to accommodate. Furthermore, transparency is lost either because of changes in the constituent proteins of the fibres or because of dehydration of the lens. Opacity in the lens is known as a cataract.

The shape of the eye is maintained by the tough sclera and an internal pressure (the intraocular pressure) exerted by the aqueous humour lying anterior to the lens. This is produced in the ciliary body and flows into the posterior chamber through the pupil and into the anterior chamber. It passes out through the trabecular meshwork (a network of tissue bands defining the edge of the anterior chamber) and via the canal of Schlemm into the episcleral veins. The normal intraocular pressure is 10–20 mmHg. If it exceeds 22 mmHg the condition of glaucoma is produced, in which compression of the blood supply to the optic nerve can result in blindness. Blockages in the trabecular meshwork (e.g. by drugs which dilate the pupil, thereby pushing the iris up against the lens) can cause sharp rises in intraocular pressure. Such drugs should obviously be avoided in this condition. Glaucoma is discussed later in this chapter.

The vitreous humour fills the posterior part of the eyeball. It is more viscous than the aqueous humour.

Fig. 8.1 Cross-section through the eye showing the main structures.

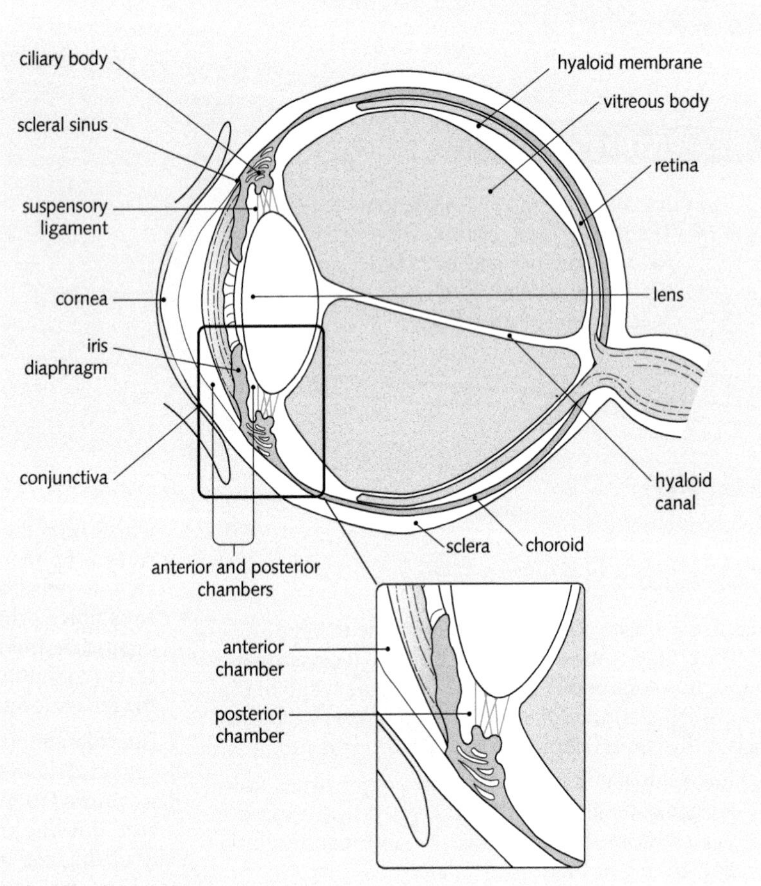

The eye is adapted for acute changes in visual information. The centre of a small circular region (macula lutea) in the sensory layer (retina), called the fovea, contains an extremely high density of photoreceptors (specifically for colour vision in good illumination). These receptors can be directed accurately and quickly to different areas of space by the extraocular muscles. The fovea lies 3 mm lateral to the optic disc (Fig. 8.2), and it differs from the rest of the retina because:

- Only cone (wavelength-specific) receptors are present at a very high density
- It has no overlying vascular network
- Overlying nerve cell bodies are displaced to allow maximal light access.

On examination with an ophthalmoscope, the pigmented epithelium underlying the macula shows through, giving it a darker appearance than the rest of the retina. The visual axis of the eye does not correspond to its geometrical axis and is displaced so that the visual axis runs through the fovea (Fig. 8.3).

HINTS AND TIPS

There are no photoreceptors overlying the origin of the optic nerve (optic disc). This area corresponds to the blind spot.

The optics of the eye

Light from a point of visual fixation is bent (refracted) so that a clearly focused image appears on the retina (Fig. 8.4). This occurs mainly at/within the cornea:

- Between the anterior chamber and the lens
- Between the lens and the vitreous body
- The lens for the visual system is a compound lens with interfaces of different refractive power (measured in dioptres, D). The total refractive power is 58.6 D, with most of the power (42 D) at the air-cornea interface.

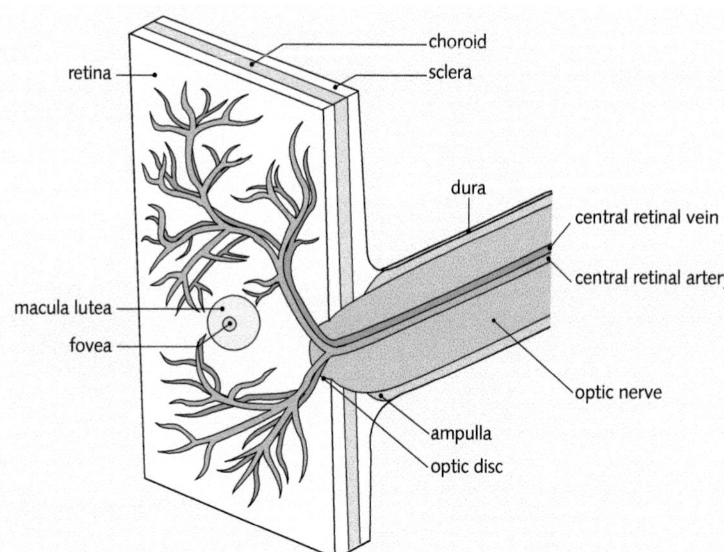

Fig. 8.2 Section of retina containing the fundus.

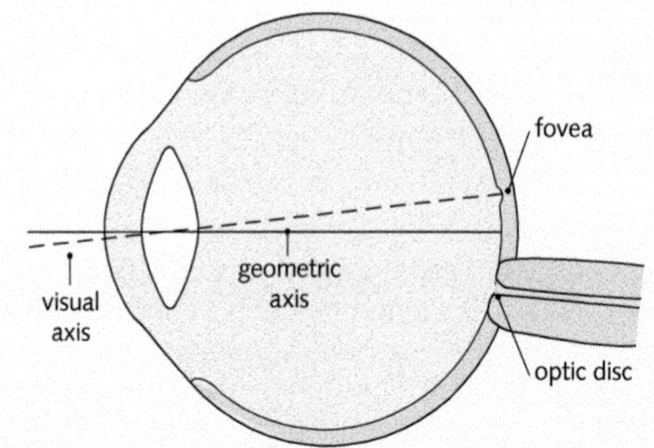

Fig. 8.3 Visual axis of the eye.

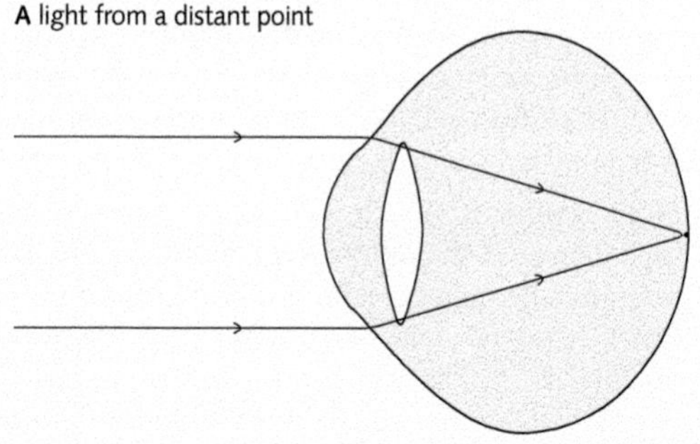

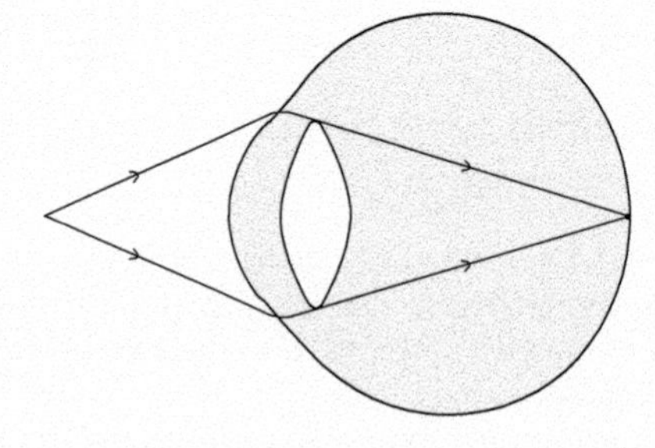

Fig. 8.4 To change from distant to near vision the refractive power of the lens has to increase by around 3.3 D. For near vision the lens becomes better by a process called accommodation.

Accommodation

The refractive power of the lens is changed by accommodation. When the ciliary muscle contracts, it moves downwards and forwards. This reduces the tension in the suspensory ligament and allows the elastic lens to become fatter and shorter. This has the effect of increasing the refractive power of the lens allowing light from near targets (which reaches the surface of the eye as divergent rays) to be focused by convergence onto the retina. The lens is an elastic structure in young people, but it gradually hardens with age and can no longer readily change shape. Near vision, therefore, becomes impaired with increasing age, a phenomenon called presbyopia or long-sightedness.

HINTS AND TIPS

The accommodation reflex demonstrates that when the eye is focused on a distant object the pupil is dilated. However, if the patient is asked to suddenly focus on an object close to their face, the pupil constricts. This is mediated by cranial nerves II (optic) and III (oculomotor).

Structure of the retina

The neural part of the retina detects light via photoreceptors, and it processes these light signals, eventually sending visual information to the thalamus and brainstem. The functions of the different neurons in the retina depend on their connections. All the neural elements are supported by a particular type of glial cell called Müller's cell.

There is a blood–retina barrier at the endothelium of the capillary network on the anterior surface of the retina from the central retinal artery, and at the endothelium of the capillary network in the choroid (the middle layer of the wall).

The photoreceptors are situated in the deepest layer of the retina (the outer nuclear layer; Fig. 8.5). This means that light has to travel through several cell layers before reaching the photoreceptors. This is particularly true in the peripheral areas of the retina.

Two different types of photoreceptor exist: rods and cones. These two cell types have different structures (Figs 8.6 and 8.7) but share the following features:

- Outer segments, which contact the pigmented epithelial layer of the retina and contain highly folded membrane structures with visual pigments
- Inner segment, which contains the nucleus and organelles
- A synaptic terminal (the most anterior structure) which synapses with the output cells – the bipolar cells.

Figure 8.8 compares the connections and functions of rods and cones.

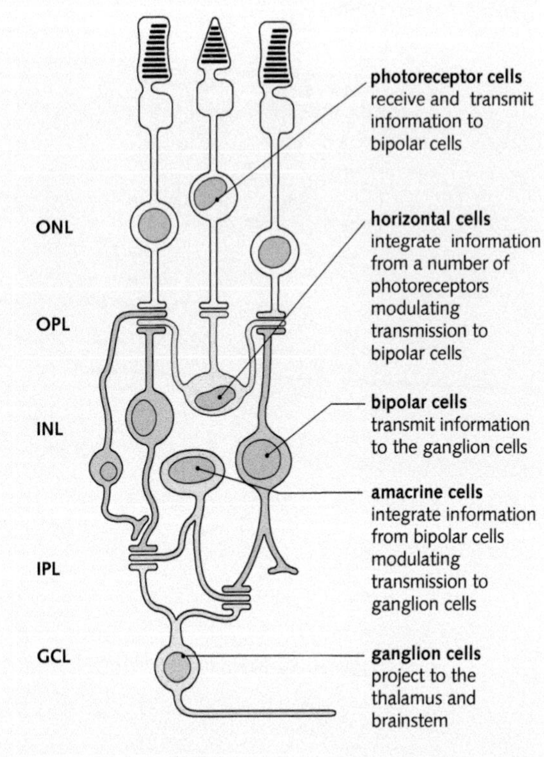

Fig. 8.5 Processing of visual information in the retinal layers. ONL, outer nuclear layer; OPL, outer plexiform layer; INL, inner nuclear layer; IPL, inner plexiform layer; GCL, ganglion cell layer.

Retinal function and image processing

Light is converted to electrical impulses and this information passes to the visual cortex for interpretation. This process begins with the photoreceptors. The photoreceptors contain receptor proteins (called opsins) and a prebound receptor agonist molecule (retinal; a derivative of vitamin A). Absorption of light causes retinal to undergo a conformational change, such that it can then 'activate' its receptor opsin. Opsin ('receptor') activation causes the stimulation of a G-protein 'receptor system' called transducin, which in turn activates an effector enzyme called phosphodiesterase (PDE). PDE, once activated, breaks down another intracellular second messenger called cyclic guanosine monophosphate (cGMP) (see Fig. 8.9). How then does this 'receptor system' translate, or more appropriately transduce, light into electrical activity?

Photoreceptor cells (both rod and cones) in darkness have a resting membrane potential of approximately −30 mV (remembering that the normal resting potential of a neuron is −65 mV) and thus can be described as depolarized. Remember the principle of synaptic transmission – when a presynaptic terminal is depolarized it releases neurotransmitter. Photoreceptor cells are no different; in darkness they continually release glutamate from their presynaptic terminal. This depolarization is caused by a steady influx of Na^+ through special membrane channels (known as 'the dark current'), which are stimulated to open by cGMP.

When light arrives at the photoreceptor it causes the conformational change in retinal, which activates its 'receptor' (opsin) and starts a cascade that ends in the cleavage of cGMP by PDE. Reduction in cGMP causes Na^+ channels to close reducing Na^+ flow

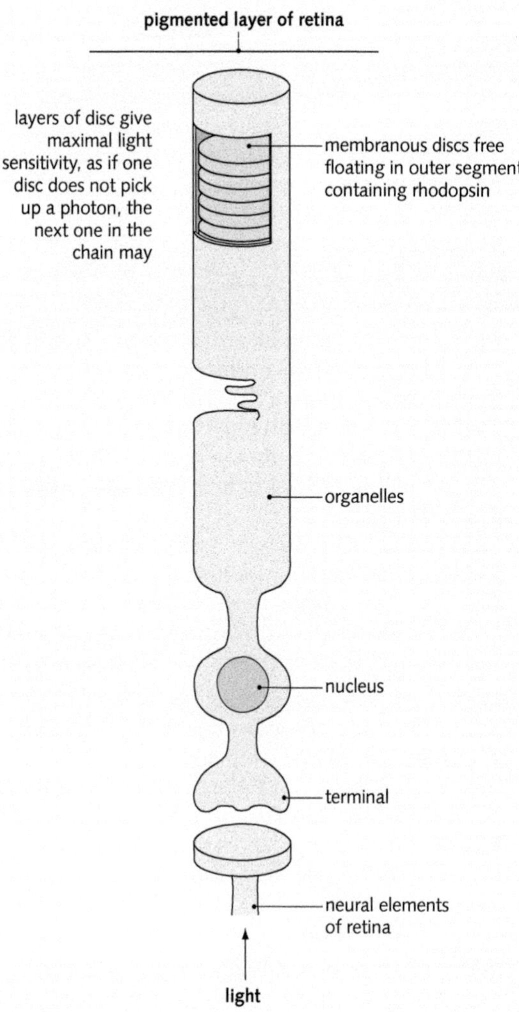
pigmented layer of retina
layers of disc give maximal light sensitivity, as if one disc does not pick up a photon, the next one in the chain may
membranous discs free floating in outer segment, containing rhodopsin
organelles
nucleus
terminal
neural elements of retina
light

Fig. 8.6 Structure of a rod.

facilitating the hyperpolarization of the cell, reducing glutamate transmission from the presynaptic terminal, thus 'silencing' the cell. In fact the stimulus that 'activates' photoreceptors is darkness; however, in

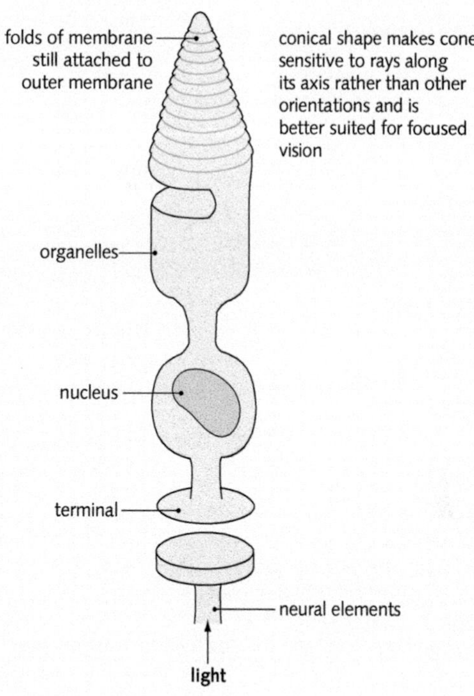
folds of membrane still attached to outer membrane
conical shape makes cone sensitive to rays along its axis rather than other orientations and is better suited for focused vision
organelles
nucleus
terminal
neural elements
light

Fig. 8.7 Structure of a cone.

neuroscience silence can mean as much as shouting. This is especially so when one considers the postsynaptic cell (see later).

The two photoreceptors (cones and rods) differ in their response to light (see Fig. 8.8):

- Rods are very sensitive to the level of light (scotopic vision), but prolonged illumination of the rods causes cGMP levels to fall to a point where they become saturated and can no longer respond to increasing amounts of light. They are mostly found in the periphery of the retina. Scotopic vision is mainly used at night when light levels are low.
- The photopigment in cone cells requires more energy to become fully activated; hence vision during

Fig. 8.8 Comparison of rods and cones

Receptor	Total number	Location	Connection to output cells	Function
Rod	120×10^6	Peripheral retina, around the fovea	Convergent pattern where many rods send information to a few output cells and this compresses information	Responding to dim light with low spatial resolution and mediating visual reflexes from stimuli in the peripheral field
Cone	6×10^6	Clustered in the fovea	No convergence; each cone projects to one bipolar cell, which projects to one output cell	Focused, highly detailed colour vision with high spatial resolution

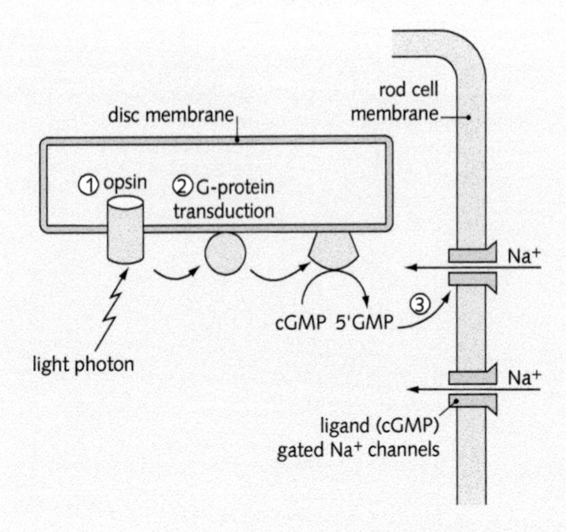

Fig. 8.9 Signal transduction of light impulses. (1) Conformational change. Afterwards, all-*trans* retinal no longer binds, which affects the G-protein transduction. (2) Increased activity of cGMP phosphodiesterase, which hydrolyses cGMP, reducing its intracellular level. (3) Low cGMP levels close the ligand-gated channels, and thereby hyperpolarize the rod.

the day depends primarily on cones (photopic vision). Cone cells contain one of three opsins that respond maximally to different wavelengths of light.

- The photopigment in rods is called rhodopsin and lies in the membrane of intracytoplasmic discs in the rod. It has seven membrane-spanning domains arranged around the retinal molecule, which attaches to the seventh transmembrane domain.

In cones, the variation in pigment is produced by different forms of opsin, each with their own specific interaction with retinal. The three opsins are sensitive to a particular wavelength of light. Only this wavelength of light will cause opsin 'activation':

- B cones at 420 nm (blue)
- G cones at 531 nm (green)
- R cones at 558 nm (red).

HINTS AND TIPS

Alterations in the photopigments within cone receptors lead to colour blindness.

HINTS AND TIPS

The cornea and lens yellow with age, and this filters out a lot of light in the blue wavelength band.

Connections in the retina

Figure 8.5 shows the neural circuits in the retina. In the outer plexiform layer each photoreceptor is in synaptic contact with two types of retinal neuron: bipolar and horizontal cells. Bipolar cells synapse with ganglion cells (the output cells of the retina) and horizontal cells feed information laterally so as to influence the activity of neighbouring bipolar cells.

Two types of bipolar cell exist, the activity of which in response to light is entirely governed by the type of glutamate receptor present on the bipolar cell:

- Excitatory (ON) bipolar cells: contain G-protein-coupled receptors which when glutamate binds lead to hyperpolarization of the cell. Thus cells are maximally active when light causes the reduction in glutamate release from photoreceptors which allows depolarization. ON refers to activity when they are exposed to light.
- Inhibitory (OFF) bipolar cells: contain classic glutamate-gated cation channels that produce classic excitatory postsynaptic potentials from an influx of Na^+. Thus these cells are maximally active in the dark and become hyperpolarized in the presence of light.

Again these cells release glutamate when they depolarize, which in turn depends whether light excites (ON cells) or inhibits (OFF cells) them.

The receptive field of a bipolar cell is the region of retina which when light falls on it affects the firing of the bipolar cell. Each bipolar cell receives direct synaptic input from a wide range of photoreceptors, the number of which reflect the type of information about the visual world being represented:

- If many receptors converge on a bipolar cell, its receptive field will be very large, condensing a lot of information into one signal – typical of rod cells.
- If a small number of photoreceptors converge on a bipolar cell, its field is smaller and less information is condensed into the information signal – typical of cone cells.

Bipolar cells are also connected via horizontal cells to a circumscribed ring of photoreceptors surrounding the central cluster of cells receiving direct synaptic input from photoreceptors; this surrounding ring is achieved by horizontal cells. Thus the receptive field has two parts, a receptive field centre, where the retinal photoreceptors provides direct photoreceptor input, and a receptive field surround, where the surrounding area of input arises from horizontal cells.

The response of the bipolar cell membrane potential to light in the receptive field centre is opposite to that of light in the surround (i.e. it is antagonistic), such that input from the surround will reduce the firing of the bipolar cell (Fig. 8.10). For instance, an ON bipolar cell centre will have an OFF surround.

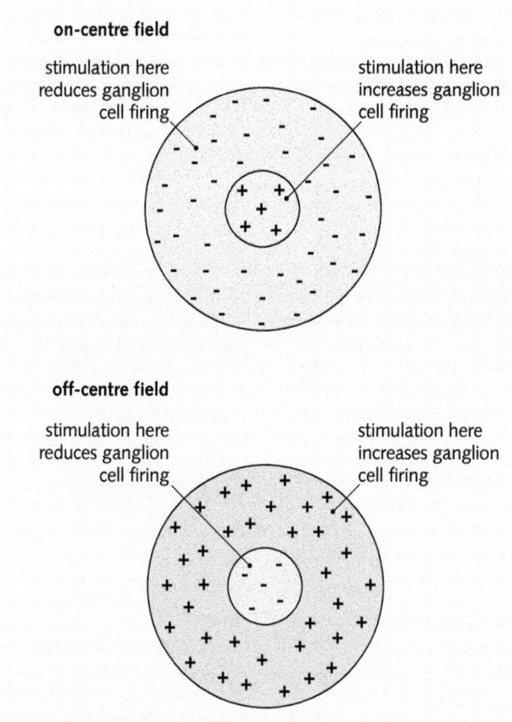

Fig. 8.10 Receptive fields of ganglion cells.

Horizontal integration

Boundaries between light and dark (i.e. the edges of objects) are enhanced by the horizontal connections provided by the horizontal cells in the plexiform layers. Horizontal cells cause a bipolar cell to be maximally activated when the surrounding photoreceptors are not activated. Conversely they inhibit the firing of the bipolar cells when there is photoreceptor activity in the 'surround' of its receptive field. This allows edges to be detected.

Now to bring all of these pieces together. There are two types of bipolar cell: ON (they become more active when light is shone on them) and OFF (they become less active when light is shone on them). The bipolar cells then have an antagonistic surround, which inhibits the firing of the bipolar cells when there is surround photoreceptor activity opposite to that of the centre (Fig. 8.10). Thus the activity of a bipolar cell will depend on the sum total photoreceptor stimulation in the centre and surround.

Amacrine cells relay signals from the rod bipolar cells (which do not directly contact the ganglion cells) to the cone bipolar cells (which do synapse with ganglion cells). This has the function of integrating rod and cone responses.

Ganglion cells

The centre–surround receptive field organization is passed from the bipolar cells to the ganglion cells via synapses in the inner plexiform layer. Amacrine cells also contribute to the amplification and modulation of ganglion cell receptive fields, but their exact function remains unclear.

Ganglion cells appear to be mainly responsive to differences in illumination that occur within a receptive field. The centre–surround organization of the receptive fields is thought be responsible for the neural response that exaggerates contrast at borders.

Three types of ganglion cell can be distinguished on the basis of their morphology, connectivity and electrophysiological properties (Fig. 8.11):

- M-type (magnocellular) cells, approximately 10% of the ganglion cell population
- P-type (parvocellular) cells, approximately 80% of the ganglion cell population
- Non-M-non-P cells.

Fig. 8.11 Retinal ganglion cell types

Ganglion cell	Structure	Receptive field	Response properties	Projection site	Function
M-type	Large cell, large dendritic arbour	Large	Conducts action potentials rapidly, with transient bursts. Sensitive to low-contrast stimuli	Thalamus, midbrain (superior colliculus)	Detection of stimulus movement and illumination
P-type	Small cell, small dendritic arbour	Small. Either detects movement or colour opponency (red and green)	Sustained discharge when centre is stimulated. can be wave length specific. Slowly adapting	Thalamus	Sensitive to stimulus form and fine detail. Colour detection
Non-M-non-P (koniocellular)	Small cell, small dendritic arbour	Small. Involved in detection of colour opponency (blue and yellow)	Wave length specific	Thalamus	Colour detection

P-type cells come in one of two flavours: they can either respond in an oppositional way (opponency) to different wavelengths of light (e.g. red stimulates and green inhibits) or they respond to achromatic (e.g. no colour) fine detail. Opposition is the colour version of the centre–surround. For instance it is possible to have a red ON cell with a green OFF surround and vice versa. P-cells can thus respond to the colour or the shape of an object.

CENTRAL VISUAL PATHWAYS AND THE VISUAL CORTEX

Central visual pathways

The major output from the ganglion cells (approximately 90%) forms the optic nerves, which emerge from the left and right eye from the optic discs, and travel to the lateral geniculate nuclei (LGN) of the thalamus. From here the cells project (as the optic radiation) onto the major target of the visual system: the primary visual cortex (V1).

A smaller projection (approximately 10%) also projects to the pretectal area of the midbrain (to control pupillary reflexes) and the superior colliculus (to provide information concerning eye movement).

The full visual field is the entire region of space that can be seen with both eyes looking directly ahead. If you fix your eyes on a particular point in space straight ahead of you, it is possible to pass an imaginary vertical line through that point, such that everything on the left of that line is in the left visual hemifield and everything in the right is in the right visual hemifield. The hemispheres process visual information from only the contralateral side of this visual axis (i.e. the opposite), however, each hemifield is constructed from both retinae (Fig. 8.12). For example, the right visual hemisphere is processed in the left visual cortex, but is constructed from the temporal (outside) portion of the left retina and the nasal (inside) portion of the right eye (Fig. 8.12). Clearly the nasal fibres will need to cross over so they can project onto the contralateral thalamus; this process occurs in the optic chiasm, which lies in front of the pituitary stalk (Fig. 8.12).

The central portion of the visual world can be viewed with both eyes separately. This corresponds to the binocular region and explains how we can see, for instance, a small nasal portion of the left hemifield when we close our left eye.

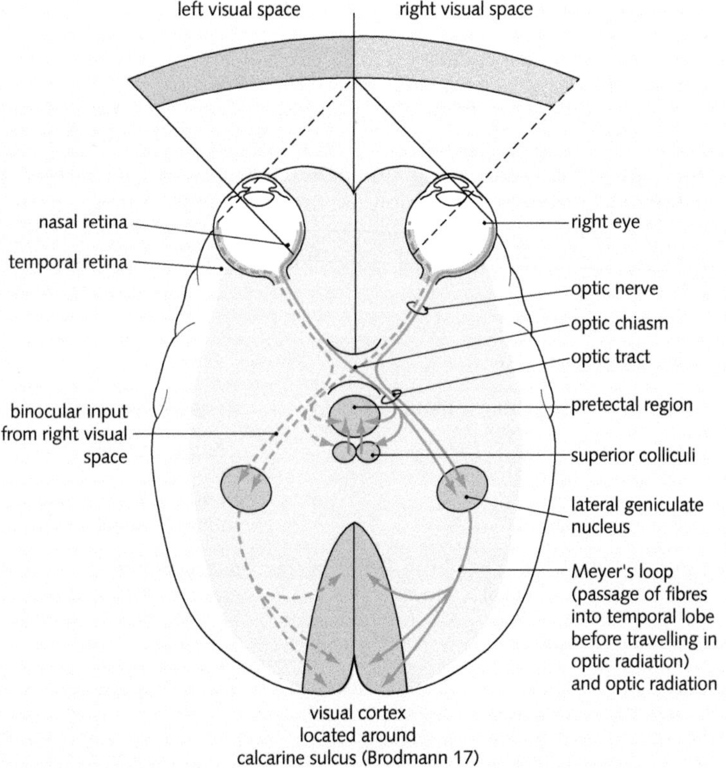

Fig. 8.12 Schematic representation of central visual pathways, showing the decussation of nasal fibres in the optic chiasm.

Thalamus and visual cortex

Lateral geniculate nucleus

The optic tract terminates in the lateral geniculate nucleus (LGN), where the information being carried by the different ganglion cell fibres becomes separated according to the eye and ganglion cell type of origin.

The retinal fibres terminate in six discrete layers which are stacked one on top of the other, with layer 1 the most ventral and layer 6 most dorsal. As mentioned above, there are three different types of ganglion cell in the retina (M-type, P-type and non-M-non-P) and that each retina contributes to the visual hemifield, thus in each optic nerve there are six distinct fibre tracts representing any one hemifield (the three types of ganglion cell from both eyes). Laminae 1, 4 and 6 of the LGN receive information from the contralateral eye and laminae 2, 3 and 5 receive information from the ipsilateral eye. Laminae 1 and 2 receive input from the M-type ganglion cells and laminae 3–6 are innervated by the P-type ganglion cells. The non-M-non-P cells innervate all six layers to form the koniocellular layers of each layer. In the LGN, therefore, the different information derived from the three categories of retinal ganglion cells from the two eyes remains separated, allowing the information they carry to be processed independently.

Cells in the LGN have the same response properties as the retinal ganglion cells that supply them – namely the centre–surround interactions and the electrophysiological responses. The responses to centre and surround visual stimuli here are much sharper than that of the retinal ganglion cells.

The LGN also has a retinotopic organization. Imagine the retina and LGN are both grids with x and y axes. Each point of space on the retinal map (e.g. 1, 2) will project to the same 'coordinates' on the LGN map (so 1, 2). In this way the representation of the visual world will remain consistent throughout central processing and reliably represent the experienced world.

There are non-retinal inputs to the LGN (from the visual cortex and the pontine reticular formation) that can alter the traffic of information to the visual cortex. This can be used to accentuate information of special interest, which is a mechanism of attention.

THE VISUAL CORTEX

The visual cortex lies along the calcarine sulcus on the medial aspect of the occipital lobe. As with other cortical areas there is a layered arrangement of neurons. Neurophysiological studies have further subdivided layer 4, as will be discussed below. The LGN projects a distorted retinotopic map onto what is known as the primary visual cortex (V1) or Brodmann's area 17. Those areas of the retina which contain large numbers of photoreceptors and, therefore, convey larger amounts of information concerning the visual world (e.g. the fovea) will have access to greater amounts of cortex for processing. In this scheme the peripheral retina will have much less cortex devoted to it (Fig. 8.13).

Three parallel pathways arising from the three retinal ganglion cell types, transport the visual information they represent to the final cortical destination for visual processing, the occipital lobe, via the LGN. These pathways are:

- Magnocellular pathway
- Parvocellular pathway
- Koniocellular pathway (the non-M-non-P pathway).

Each will be dealt with in turn below.

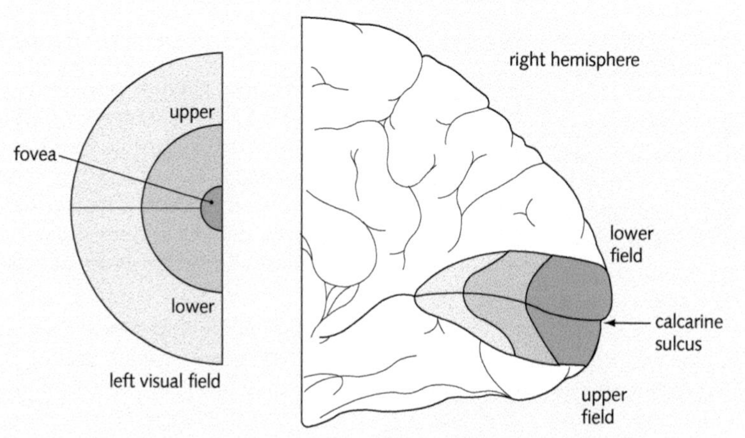

Fig. 8.13 Primary visual cortex – location and representation.

Magnocellular pathway

Magnocellular LGN neurons originate in laminae 1 and 2 and project to layer 4Cα of V1, but the left–right segregation remains. Input from the LGN from each lamina is not continuous, but projections from both laminae 1 and 2 are split up into a series of columns (called ocular dominance columns) as they arrive at layer 4Cα, much like zebra stripes. These stripes represent the M-cell visual inputs from either eye. The columns basically mean that as far as that particular region of cortex is concerned, it will only process visual information from the eye that feeds into that ocular dominance column, therefore either the left or right eye. The layer 4Cα neurons then project up to layer 4B.

At the first synaptic relay in layer 4Cα the receptive field structure of the magnocellular neurons changes, with many fields becoming elongated along a particular axis with the familiar ON/OFF centre-surround field. These cells probably receive input from three or more LGN cells with receptive fields aligned along one axis. These cells are simple cells: cells which respond best to a slit of light that is aligned with the long axis of the field and responds poorly to a slit of light perpendicular to the field. These layer 4Cα cells are said to be 'orientation selective cells'.

Layer 4B cells play the same role: orientation selection. However, layer 4Cα cells are monocular (they reside within ocular dominance columns) whereas layer 4B cells have binocular receptor fields which construct a retinotopic binocular image of the world. Layer 4B cells are also important for direction selectivity, that is these receptive fields respond strongly to stimulus travelling across the visual field in a particular direction (i.e. left to right). Thus, the M-type ganglion cells are used for the analysis of motion.

Parvocellular pathway

Parvocellular pathway neurons originate from P-type neurons of the retina and travel to V1 via laminae 3, 4, 5 and 6 of the LGN. The parvocellular LGN sends axons to layer 4Cβ of V1, which then project to the blob and interblob regions of layer 3.

Blobs are areas of cortex that contain high levels of cytochrome oxidase, the cytochrome staining of which has been found to run the depth of the cortex (through the full thickness of layers 2 and 3, and 5 and 6). The blobs are organized in rows across the cortex and each blob centres on an ocular dominance column from layer 4. Interblob regions are simply the spaces in between the blobs.

The interblob cells in layer 3 are known as complex cells because their receptive fields are more complex as they do not have distinctive ON and OFF regions, instead they give ON and OFF responses to stimuli throughout the receptive field. Complex cells are mostly binocular and highly selective to the orientation of the stimulus. As complex cells are highly responsive to orientation and have small receptive fields, it is likely that these cells (and the parvocellular neurons that feed them) are involved in the analysis of object detail and shape.

These interblob regions are akin to 'orientation' ocular dominance columns as they will only process information provided it occurs within a particular orientation (i.e. vertical or horizontal). The adjacent column of cortex will only analyse information provided it is rotated further around than that of the neighbouring cortex. In this scheme the first column will only process, say, a vertical line, the next column will only process stimuli with a 15° tilt and the next column will only process stimuli with a 30° tilt and so on. This trend ensures that for every stimulus orientation occurring within any given point of the visual field, it will be analysed by a bit of cortex devoted to that orientation (Fig. 8.14). The cortex maintains the distorted retinotopic map projecting from the LGN.

Koniocellular pathway

Most blob cells are sensitive to the wavelength of light and are monocular, just like the koniocellular and some parvocellular layer 4Cβ neurons that give rise to them. It appears that these blob regions are likely to be involved in the analysis of colour.

Figure 8.14 shows the organization of inputs and outputs into the striate cortex (V1). A 2 × 2 mm section of cortex contains two complete sets of ocular dominance columns (i.e. two from the left eye and two from the right), 16 blobs and in the interblob region two whole samples of all the 180° of possible line orientations. This amount of cortex is sufficient for the analysis of any given point of the visual world.

Progression of visual processing

As with other functions of the nervous system the primary visual cortex is part of a complex system of information interpretation, there being a number of supplementary visual cortices. The processing circuits are formed by pathways through distinct areas of the visual cortex each of which contain a retinotopic map. This allows representation of different types of activity in the visual field:

- V2 has an unknown function, but possibly acts as a processing and relay station for higher areas.
- V3 may have a role in depth perception and visual acuity.
- V4 has a role in colour perception.

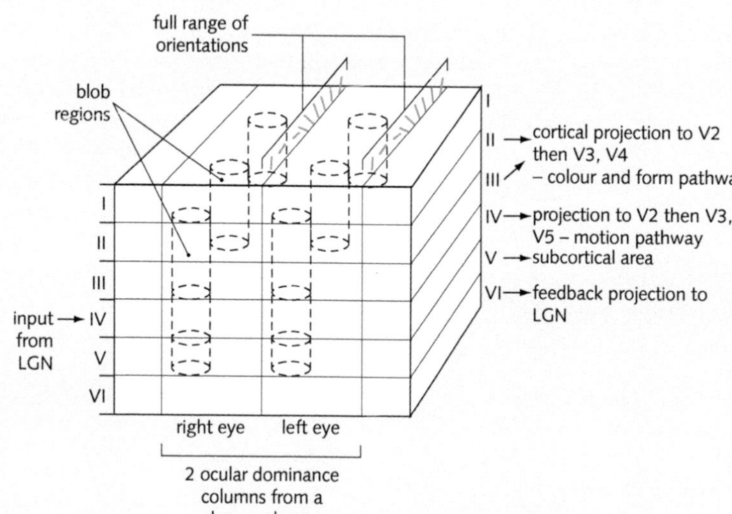

Fig. 8.14 Organization of inputs and outputs in the striate cortex. Diagram shows ocular dominance columns, blob regions and orientation selectivity. LGN, lateral geniculate nucleus.

- V5 is concerned with motion detection.
- Inferotemporal areas have complex cells which respond to particular stimuli such as faces.

Three parallel pathways process colour, motion and form. Each takes its 'job' from the type of ganglion cell and V1 cell layer from which its afferent projection arise. This is summarized in Fig. 8.15.

Fig. 8.15 Causes of visual loss

Acute	Chronic
Retinal detachment	Refractive error
Acute closed-angle glaucoma	Cataracts
Retinal artery occlusion (if temporary known as amaurosis fugax)	Corneal disease and oedema
Optic neuritis	Primary open-angle glaucoma
Stroke affecting central visual pathways	Age-related macular degeneration
Migraine	Diabetic retinopathy
	Hereditary retinal disease
	Compression of central visual pathways, e.g. tumour
	Drugs: alcohol, methanol, chloroquine

ATTENTION AND PERCEPTION

Attention

The process of attention is the active pursuit of a focus from sensory information in order to process it further. A certain amount of processing of all information has to occur before attentional mechanisms select the appropriate information.

Attending to a part of our environment involves visual and motor mechanisms to orient the body in space, allowing us to scan the visual field more fully with the fovea or interact with the environment in motor tasks.

The factors that determine where attention is directed are novelty (brightness, colour and change in orientation) and relevance to current tasks.

The pre-attentive process is a rapid scanning of a scene to detect objects/gross form. The attentive process focuses on specific features of a part of the scene.

Perception

The process of perception involves representing the contents of the environment and then making sense of the representation (e.g. by organizing visual information into objects and background, and then identifying the objects).

Representation of the environment in the visual cortex is achieved by the retinotopic maps. Higher centres know that, if a certain population of V1 neurons are firing, then specific boundaries are present in a specific part of the visual field.

The segregation of visual information into objects and background relies on certain features of the visual scene. Objects are picked out using the following characteristics:

- Common shape, colour or texture
- Continuity
- Proximity
- Common size
- Closure
- Depth, which can be worked out from:
  - Monocular information about size, texture, perspective, overlap, movement parallax
  - Binocular information about the difference between the view from the eyes and about how the eyes move to focus on the same part of space.

The identification of objects, once picked out from the environment, relies on comparison with memories of objects. This occurs in the visual association cortex at the occipitotemporal junction.

Eye movements

Eye movements are important in attentional mechanisms as they direct the fovea onto points of interest in the visual scene quickly and accurately. There are five types of eye movement, two of which stabilize the eye when the head moves:

- Vestibulo-ocular – this uses vestibular input to hold the retinal image stable during brief or rapid head rotation. For horizontal movements, lateral rectus motor neurons (VI nucleus) are influenced by vestibular nuclei cells and medial rectus motor neurons (III nucleus) are driven by interneurons in the contralateral abducens nucleus.
- Optokinetic – this uses visual input to hold the retinal image stable during sustained or slow head rotation. The underlying pathway comprises a retinal projection via the tectum to the vestibular nucleus and a cortical component from V1.

The remaining three eye movements keep the fovea on a visual target:

- Saccade – this brings new objects of interest onto the fovea. Saccades are very fast and occur every 300 ms. The pattern of saccadic eye movements is guided by current cognitive tasks, as shown by recordings of eye movements when pictures are scanned for details. Horizontal saccadic movements are generated in the pontine reticular formation, and vertical ones in the midbrain, under influence from a circuit involving the frontal eye fields (in the frontal lobes), the pulvinar nucleus of the thalamus and the superior colliculus.
- Smooth pursuit – this holds the image of a moving target on the fovea. This type of movement is controlled by visual and frontal cortical areas, relaying information to the vestibulocerebellum.
- Vergence – this adjusts the eyes for differing image distances. This movement is controlled by midbrain neurons near the oculomotor nucleus. Convergence/divergence of the eyes is induced by blur, and is important in accommodation.

Smooth pursuit movements and saccadic eye movements can alternate (e.g. when looking out of a train window) and this combination of movements is termed optokinetic nystagmus.

HINTS AND TIPS

When examining a patient with nystagmus then the fast phase of the movement defines its direction.

Strategies in visual processing

The visual system employs two strategies to make sense of the visual environment:

- Bottom-up processing occurs when a visual scene is analysed purely in terms of the incoming visual information, without searching visual memory for similar scenes that might help with making sense of the scene.
- Top-down processing occurs when visual memory influences the way in which the current visual scene is processed, so that some sort of sense can be made of the way in which objects are distinguished from their background.

Disorders of attention and perception

In the condition of neglect, patients fail to turn their attention to areas in the visual scene on one-half of space, typically the left-hand side of space following a right parietal lobe lesion. They will usually ignore the left-hand side of their visual axis (e.g. eating only the right half of the food on a plate) or describing only the right half of a visual scene (when looking at it and when recollecting it from memory).

In the condition of agnosia, patients cannot recognize and name objects from visual examination, despite being able to fully describe the physical features of the object as well as being able to recognize it from tactile information. Here, there is a failure of the higher processes of perception that integrate all the visual information about an object and compare it with visual memory. Bilateral visual cortex disease usually produces agnosia.

These conditions differ in important respects:

- In agnosia, there is a failure of recognition of an object usually in the left-hand side of the visual field.
- In neglect, there is a failure to attend to one-half of space, whatever the objects.

LOSS OF VISION

Glaucoma

There are two types of glaucoma, both of which are characterized by funduscopic changes, visual field loss and raised intraocular pressure. Acute closed-angle glaucoma is a sight-threatening emergency, whereas primary open-angle glaucoma runs a more chronic and insidious course.

Acute closed-angle glaucoma

This presents as a painful red eye, and may be associated with vomiting. Blurred vision and the appearance of light objects having a 'halo' are common in the evenings (when the pupil is dilated). The cause of the rise in intraocular pressure is shown in Figure 8.16.

Treatment aims to lower the pressure within the eyeball – first medically (e.g. with a pupil constrictor such as pilocarpine), then flow should be restored surgically or with a laser. The other eye should be treated prophylactically.

Primary open-angle glaucoma

This is more common than closed-angle glaucoma, and the third commonest cause of blindness in the UK. The intraocular pressure rises slowly due to a blockage in the trabecular meshwork, which drains the aqueous humour. Symptoms may not be present until severe damage has occurred, so screening programmes exist for high-risk patients (older people and those of Afro-Caribbean origin). Signs may include:

- Visual field loss
- 'Cupping' of the optic disc on funduscopy
- Haemorrhages on the optic disc.

Medical treatment includes the use of:

- β-Blockers (topical) – reduce the secretion of aqueous humour
- Parasympathomimetic agents (e.g. pilocarpine drops) – constrict the pupil.

Laser treatment and surgery may ultimately be appropriate.

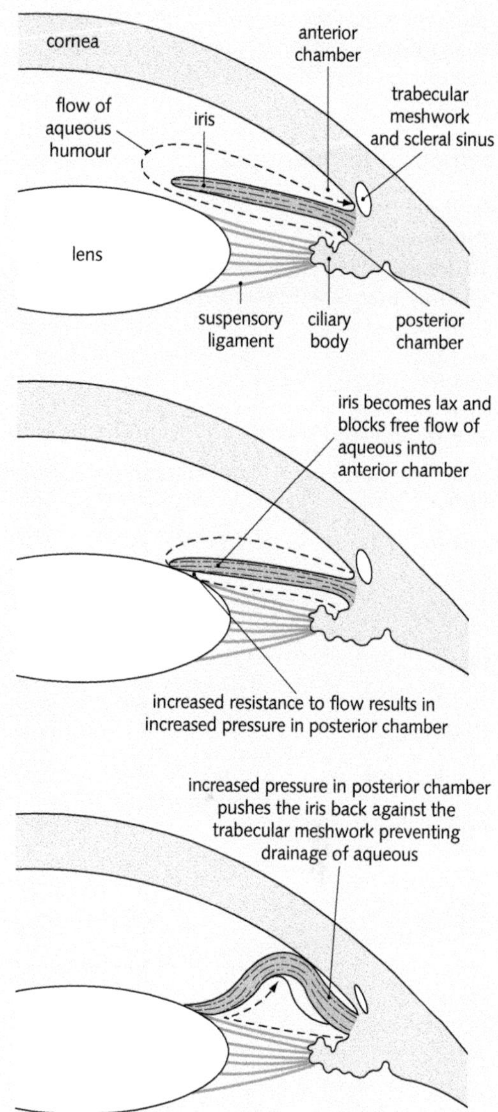

Fig. 8.16 Acute closed-angle glaucoma – mechanism.

Damage to the central pathways for vision

The patterns of visual loss following central lesions depends on the location of the lesion. These are summarized in Chapter 17 (Fig. 17.18). Three common types of visual loss are outlined below.

Monocular visual loss

Caused by:

- Amaurosis fugax (optic nerve ischaemia)
- Migraine

- Temporal arteritis leading to optic nerve infarction
- Optic neuritis (may be part of multiple sclerosis)
- Rare things – methanol poisoning, hereditary optic atrophy neurosyphilis.

Bitemporal hemianopia

Pressure on the optic chiasm due to:

- Pituitary adenoma
- Other tumours (e.g. meningiomas)
- Carotid artery aneurysms.

Homonymous hemianopia

This is caused by posterior cerebral artery occlusion and infarction of the occipital cortex. There may be macular (central) sparing.

Lesions affecting the optic radiations and internal capsule may cause variable degrees of visual loss, for example the fibres conveying the superior and inferior regions of space (causing homonymous visual impairment affecting just one quadrant).

Other causes of visual loss are summarized in Figure 8.17.

Fig. 8.17 The three parallel visual pathways

Basic function	Ganglion cell	Visual cortical region in pathway	Response of cells	Perceptual role	V1 cortical destination
Motion	M-type	V1, V2, V3, V5, then to the parietal lobe	Rapid responses for moving stimuli; no sensitivity to colour	Direction of motion and arrangement of objects	Layer 4Cα into the ocular dominance columns. They then project to layer 4B
Form	P-type	V1, V2, V4, then to parietal and temporal lobes	Slowly adapting, some colour sensitivity. Sensitive to orientation of edges	Detection of shape and stationary objects	Layer 4Bβ and then onto the blob and interblob areas of layer 3
Colour	Non-M-non-P	V1, V2, V4, then to temporal lobe	Colour sensitive	Direction of colour	Layer 3 (blob region)

Hearing, speech and language

Objectives

In this chapter you will learn about:

- The anatomy of the outer, middle and inner ear.
- The process of auditory signal transduction.
- The functions of inner and outer hair cells.
- The central pathways of hearing.
- The term 'tonotopic organization'.
- The function of special speech areas.
- The differences between sensorineural and conductive deafness.
- The neural basis of speech.

THE EAR AND CONDUCTION OF SOUND

Sound is the oscillation of molecules in a medium. As the medium (e.g. air) is alternately compressed and rarified energy is transmitted as a longitudinal wave.

Sound is principally defined in terms of its amplitude (loudness) and frequency (pitch):

- Amplitude is measured on a logarithmic scale – the decibel (dB) – as the human ear can detect a wide variation in sound intensities. For human hearing, dB $= 20 \times \log_{10} (P/P_o)$ where $P =$ sound pressure; $P_o =$ the average auditory threshold for frequencies from 1000 Hz to 3000 Hz (20 mPa or 0.002 dynes/cm^2). Thus, a 20 dB change is equal to a 10-fold increase (+20 dB) or decrease (–20 dB) in loudness. Sound pressures greater than 100 dB may damage the cochlea.
- Frequency is measured on a linear scale (cycles/sec or hertz, Hz). Normal hearing occurs over the range from 20 Hz to 20000 Hz, whereas greatest auditory acuity occurs in the frequency range of 1000 Hz to 4000 Hz.

The auditory system consists of the hearing apparatus (outer ear, middle ear and inner ear) and a pathway from the inner ear to the brainstem and auditory cortex.

The anatomy of the auditory apparatus

Figure 9.1 depicts the auditory apparatus.

Outer ear

The pinna and external ear canal form a tube closed at one end by the tympanic membrane. This tube has a resonant frequency of 3 kHz. The threshold for hearing in the frequency range 2.5–4 kHz is therefore decreased by –15 dB (i.e. these frequencies are easier to hear).

HINTS AND TIPS

Tensor tympani and stapedius are activated milliseconds before speech to protect the ear from the high sound intensities created within the head.

Middle ear

Alternating air pressure (the sound wave) makes the tympanic membrane vibrate. The ossicles vibrate along with it. The ossicles are:

- The malleus (hammer) which is attached to the tympanic membrane itself
- The incus (anvil) which provides a bridge across the middle ear
- The stapes (stirrup) whose base plate sits in the oval window at the entrance to the cochlea.

Figure 9.2 illustrates the relationship between the three auditory ossicles.

The surface area of the base plate is 17 times smaller than that of the tympanic membrane. Together with the mechanical advantage of the lever system of the incus and malleus (at frequencies near 1000 Hz), this amplifies the pressure changes by 1.3 × 17 or 22-fold

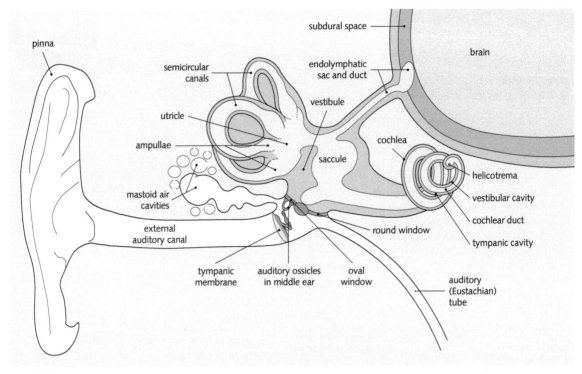

Fig. 9.1 Components and relations of the outer, middle and inner ear.

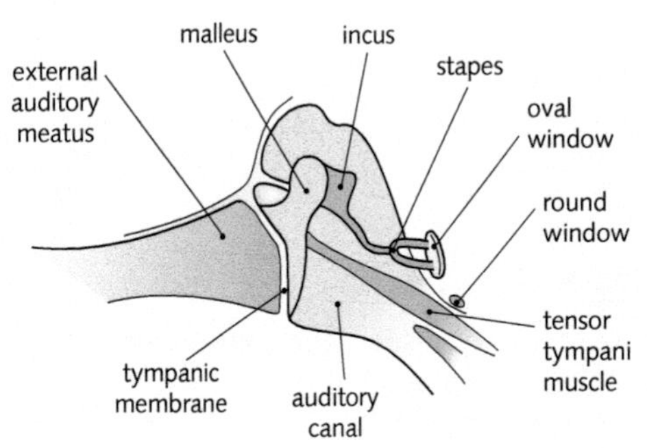

Fig. 9.2 Anatomical relations of the auditory ossicles.

(+28 dB). This ensures that sound waves are transmitted efficiently from air to the fluid-filled cochlea.

Vibrations of the ossicular chain are dampened down when they become extreme. Two muscles perform this function:

- Tensor tympani muscle on the malleus
- Stapedius muscle on the stapes.

The reflex contraction of these muscles has a delay of 40–60 ms and cannot protect the cochlea from a sudden loud explosion. This reflex suppresses low frequencies more than high frequencies and may explain how we understand speech in a noisy environment.

For maximum efficiency, the pressure on either side of the eardrum needs to be equal. The middle ear mucosa constantly absorbs air, and therefore the pressure in the middle ear gradually drops below atmospheric pressure. The Eustachian tube connects the middle ear to the pharynx and allows the pressure to equilibrate when it is opened (by swallowing or yawning). Blockage of this tube leads to a relative hearing defect.

Inner ear

The cochlea is a spiral tunnel (with 2.5–3 turns, 32 mm long with a diameter of 2 mm) divided into three compartments running the whole of its length. The upper compartment (scala vestibuli) and lower compartment (scala tympani) communicate at the apex of the spiral (at the helicotrema). They contain a fluid called perilymph which resembles cerebrospinal fluid. Vibration of the base plate of the stapes causes movement in the perilymph in the scala vestibuli.

The scala media (cochlear duct) lies between the scala vestibuli and the scala tympani, and contains a fluid called endolymph. Endolymph has a high potassium concentration and therefore a positive potential (80 mV) with respect to the perilymph. The organ of Corti rests on the basilar membrane inside the cochlear

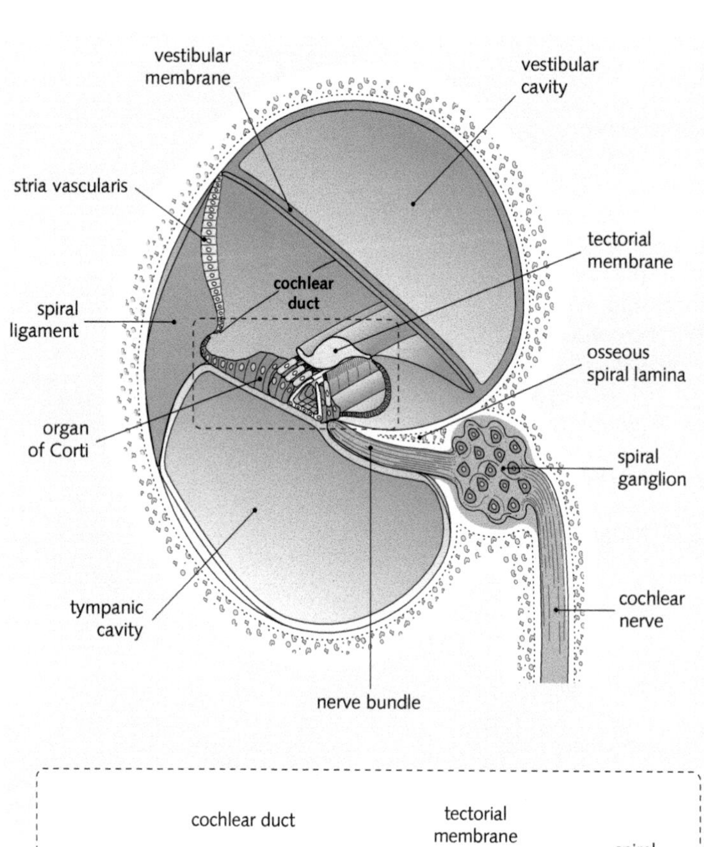

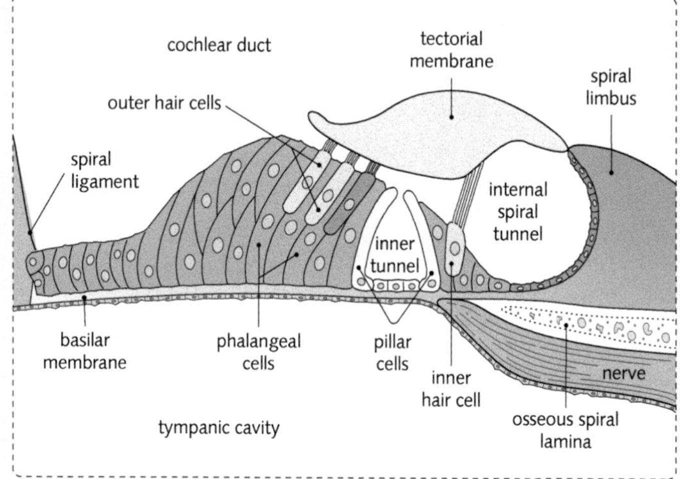

Fig. 9.3 The organ of Corti in the cochlea.

duct. The cochlear duct is separated from the scala vestibuli by Reissner's membrane and from the scala tympani by the basilar membrane (Fig. 9.3).

Movement of the perilymph following displacements of the oval window makes the basilar membrane vibrate. This is then transmitted to the hair cells in the organ of Corti, which convert vibrations of their cilia into oscillating changes in their membrane potential. Cranial nerve VIII afferent neurons, whose cell bodies lie in the bony spiral lamina, contact the hair cells and send auditory information to the cochlear nuclei in the lateral medulla.

The organ of Corti

The properties of the basilar membrane and the hair cells enable different frequencies of sound to be detected.

The basilar membrane increases in width as it winds round the cochlea so that its transverse fibres are longer at the apex (500 μm) than at the base (100 μm). Longer fibres have a lower resonant frequency and shorter ones have a higher resonant frequency. This is accentuated because the stiffness of the basilar membrane also decreases 100-fold from base to apex.

The electrical and mechanical properties of the hair cells also vary along the basilar membrane. At the base, the hair cells and their stereocilia are short and stiff whereas at the top the hair cells and their stereocilia are more than twice as long and less stiff. The hair cells are thus tuned mechanically. They are also tuned electrically and their ability to generate electrical oscillations matches their mechanical tuning.

The afferent fibres from the apical part of the cochlea, therefore, carry low-frequency sound signals, whereas those from the basal part of the cochlea carry high-frequency signals.

Transduction of vibration

The hair cells convert the oscillating movements of stereocilia into neuronal signals.

Vibrations of the basilar membrane result in oscillating movement of the hair cells (Fig. 9.4). The stereocilia projecting from the upper surface of the hair cells are fixed at their extracellular end to the immobile tectorial membrane. They sway with the same frequency as the part of the basilar membrane that the hair cells rest upon. This results in oscillating changes in the physical arrangement of the hair cell membrane and, consequently, changes in the structure of membrane ion channels. Fluctuations in ion permeability are produced, leading to oscillations of membrane potential with the same frequency as the basilar membrane (note that the maximum firing rate of a nerve fibre has an upper limit of around 500 Hz so that the transduction process is not linear). For frequencies above 4000 Hz, interpretation of the signals from the cochlea is probably due to the tonotopic organization of the auditory pathway. Below 4000 Hz, temporal coding is pivotal and uses the property that afferents fire with maximum probability during a particular phase of a sound wave (phase-locking).

Control over sensitivity

Hair cells are arranged in rows on either side of the pillar cells – three rows of outer cells and one row of inner cells. The inner and outer rows have different functions based on the different proportions of output-signalling fibres and input-controlling fibres that contact them.

As a general rule, afferent neurons contact the base of the inner cells and efferents (from the superior olivary complex) contact the base of the outer cells. Inner hair cells are responsible for the detection of sound. The outer hair cells are contractile, and may alter the mechanical properties of the tectorial membrane. In this way they may provide a mechanism for 'tuning' the ear to sounds of particular interest.

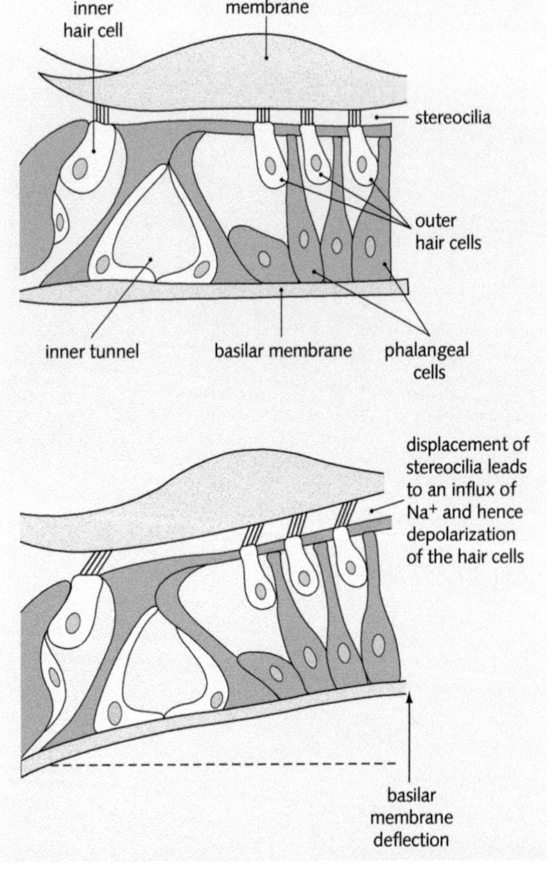

Fig. 9.4 Vibration of the organ of Corti causes bending of hair cell stereocilia, resulting in an oscillating depolarization/hyperpolarization.

Tonotopic mapping

The spatial separation of frequencies in the cochlea (i.e. each auditory fibre conveys information relating to a restricted part of the auditory spectrum) leads to frequency selectivity of the cells to which the VIIIth nerve fibres project. Tonotopic mapping occurs as early in the pathway as the projection to the cochlear nucleus. Afferent fibres which arise from the base of the cochlea (high-pitched sounds) penetrate deeply into the nucleus. In contrast, fibres which originate at the apex of the cochlea (low-pitched sounds) terminate in more superficial regions. This is analogous to other mapping systems in other sensory systems (e.g. somatotopy).

Sound can be conducted through bone. Thus, after middle ear damage, some hearing may be preserved by relying on bone conduction.

Central auditory pathways and the auditory cortex

Central auditory pathways

The pathways are organized so that:

- Tonotopic organization is retained throughout the pathways to different areas of the primary auditory cortex.
- Inputs from both ears interact with each other in the process of sound localization.

Figure 9.5 shows that VIIIth nerve afferent fibres terminate in the dorsal and ventral cochlear nuclei, at the level of the inferior cerebellar peduncle. From here, there are two main pathways:

- Fibres from the dorsal cochlear nucleus pass in the dorsal acoustic stria, then cross to the opposite side to join the lateral lemniscus and terminate in the contralateral inferior colliculus.
- Most fibres from the ventral cochlear nucleus pass ventrally and cross to the opposite side in the trapezoid body. Some fibres end in the superior olivary complex on both sides. Others continue upwards in the lateral lemniscus to the contralateral inferior colliculus. The medial part of the superior olive receives information from both ears. This is believed to be important for sound localization. Fibres from the superior olive project to the inferior colliculi, on both sides, via the lateral lemnisci.
- Fibres from the inferior colliculus project, bilaterally, to the medial geniculate nuclei of the thalamus and, from there, to the ipsilateral primary auditory cortex, on the superomedial aspect of the temporal lobe.

HINTS AND TIPS

Damage to one side of the central auditory pathway at any level (other than the cochlear nerve) will not result in deafness in one ear. This is because of the bilateral projections to the auditory cortex, both directly and by communication between pathways.

Auditory cortex

The auditory cortex is functionally organized into tonotopic maps of the frequency range that we can hear, with low frequencies represented rostrally and laterally and high frequencies caudally and medially. This gives rise to isofrequency bands of cells running mediolaterally across the primary auditory cortex.

Cells responding to input from both ears to varying degrees are arranged into columns. Cells in a column have a similar frequency response and the same binaural response properties. There are two types of column, which alternate across the cortex:

- Suppression columns – cells in this column respond more strongly to input from one ear, and these may be involved in sound localization.
- Summation columns – cells in this column respond more strongly to stimulation of both ears than either ear separately.

The cortex uses differences in sound intensity and time of arrival at each ear to localize sounds, and the function of each hemisphere is to localize sound from the contralateral side of space.

- From 200 Hz to 2000 Hz, the process involves the delay between a sound reaching one ear then the other (interaural delay).
- From 2000 Hz to 20000 Hz, it involves the difference in sound intensity perceived in each ear (interaural intensity differences).

Speech processing

In most people, one hemisphere carries out language processing and is called the dominant hemisphere; this is usually the left hemisphere for both right-handed and left-handed people.

Wernicke's area is in the temporal lobe on the dominant side. It is an auditory association area which integrates sound information so that meaningful speech can be recognized (Fig. 9.6). It codes sounds into phonemes, the most basic sound units of spoken language.

Speech processing involves other areas such as the frontal lobe.

Localization of sound

A sound source is localized in the vertical plane (elevation) and in the horizontal plane (azimuth). The pinna of the outer ear is crucial in determining elevation. Sound waves enter the ear either directly or are reflected from the pinna and are slightly delayed in arriving at the tympanic membrane (Fig. 9.7). Due to the peculiarities of the shape of the pinna, sounds arising from different directions in the vertical plane are reflected differently. Differences in delay times are used to determine the sound's position in the vertical plane.

The superior olivary nucleus is involved in the localization of sound in the horizontal plane. When the head is positioned so that one ear is closer to the sound source, the head forms a shadow which decreases the sound intensity reaching the contralateral ear. For higher frequencies, the discrepancy in sound level between the ear nearest and furthest from the sound is

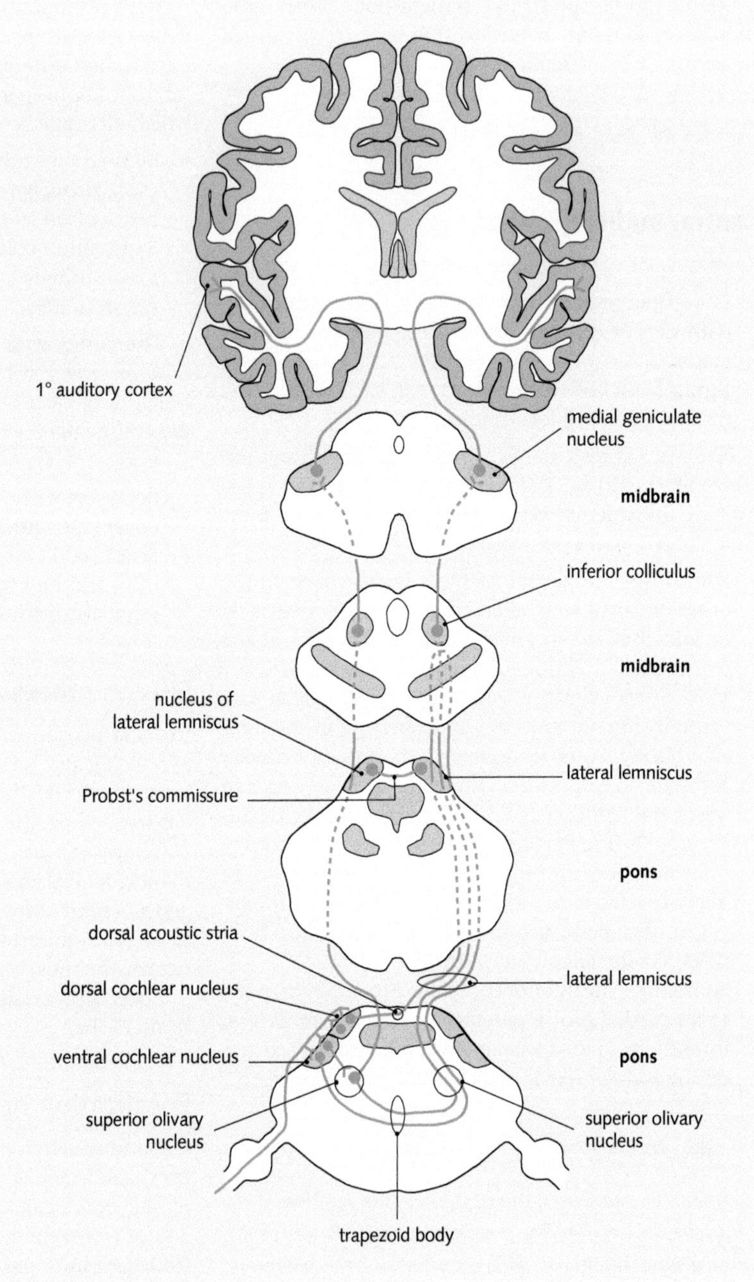

Fig. 9.5 Central auditory pathways.

calculated by neurons in the lateral superior olivary nucleus. This nucleus sends projections to the tectum which controls eye and head reflexes in response to sound. For lower frequencies, neurons in the medial superior olivary nucleus calculate the phase difference, which is a result of sound entering the ear furthest from the source being slightly delayed. A topographic map of these time differences exists in the medial superior olivary nucleus, enabling determination of azimuth.

LOSS OF HEARING

Testing

Hearing is tested by pure-tone audiograms (Fig. 9.8). Hearing loss may be either:

- Conductive – caused by failure of sound to reach the inner ear

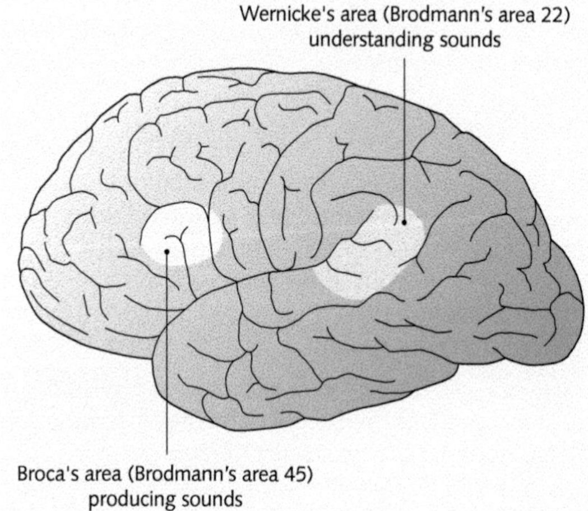

Fig. 9.6 Location of Broca's and Wernicke's areas in the dominant hemisphere.

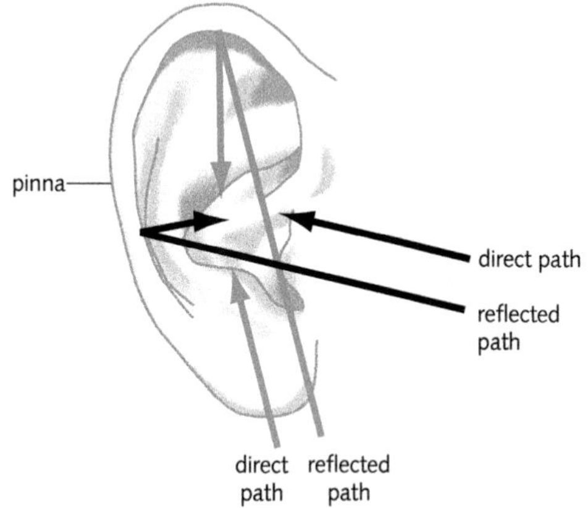

Fig. 9.7 Role of the pinna in determining a sound direction in elevation.

or

- Sensorineural – caused by a failure at the level of the cochlea or more centrally.

HINTS AND TIPS

Rinne's test distinguishes between the two forms of deafness. A tuning fork is used to test each ear separately. In conductive hearing loss, sound is perceived more clearly if the base of the tuning fork is placed against the mastoid process. This overcomes the conduction deficit, and allows vibrations to reach the ossicular chain.

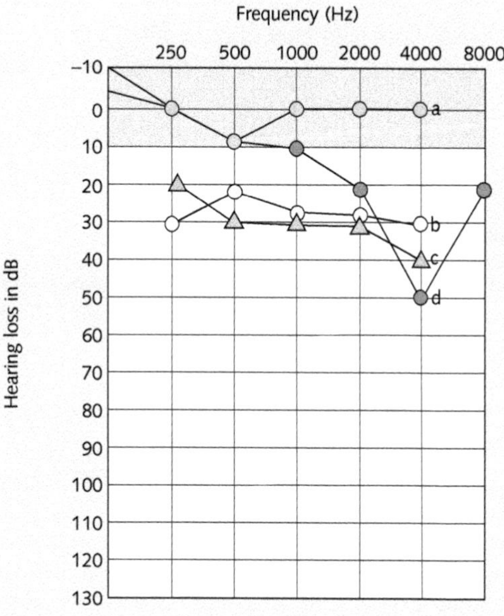

Fig. 9.8 Pure-tone audiograms – circles, air conduction; triangles, bone conduction.
(a) Normal
(b) Conductive hearing loss
(c) Sensorineural hearing loss
(d) Noise induced high-frequency loss.

Sensorineural deafness

- Lesions within the cochlea itself (Fig. 9.9)
- Lesions within the petrous temporal bone (trauma, complications of middle ear infection, tumours)
- Lesions at the cerebellopontine angle (particularly acoustic neuromas, but also meningiomas and inflammatory damage such as meningitis)
- Cortical or pontine lesions causing deafness are rare.

Fig. 9.9 Sensorineural deafness – causes within the inner ear
Ménière's disease
Drugs (e.g. gentamicin)
Congenital infection (rubella, syphilis)
Trauma (excessive exposure to noise, birth asphyxia)
Advancing age (presbyacusis)

HINTS AND TIPS

Excessive exposure to some ototoxic drugs, e.g. streptomycin and aminoglycosides (especially gentamicin) can cause sensorineural deafness. These antibiotics exclusively damage the outer hair cells in the cochlea.

Ménière's disease

This is a disease of uncertain aetiology – probably due to a build-up of endolymph. Characteristic symptoms are:

- Sensorineural deafness
- Ringing in the ears (tinnitus)
- Vertigo with vomiting, balance disturbance and nystagmus.

It tends to be a recurrent disease and the vertigo, in particular, may be disabling.

Management includes rest, antipsychotic drugs for the acute attack (prochlorperazine) and histamine analogues for prophylaxis (e.g. betahistine). Ultimately, surgical drainage of endolymph, destruction of the labyrinth or section of the vestibular nerve may be required.

Conductive hearing loss

Causes include:

- Perforation of the tympanic membrane
- Fluid or infection in the middle ear
- Disorders of the ossicles.

Cochlear implants

This relatively new technique is designed to provide benefit to those people with profound deafness, who do not benefit from a traditional amplification hearing aid. It comprises:

- An electrode which is surgically inserted into the cochlea
- An external processing device (which may be subcutaneous)
- An external microphone.

Patients hear sounds which are very different from normal hearing. Approximately 50% will be able to discriminate speech without having to lip-read. Their own speech also generally improves. It may be particularly successful in children.

SPEECH AND LANGUAGE

The driving force behind human language is to communicate ideas to the people around us. Speech production normally only exists when someone else is around to engage in the complementary process of speech recognition. Therefore, it is helpful to consider the two processes together.

The neural basis of speech

The comprehension of speech utilizes multiple regions of the brain. The left hemisphere appears dominant for language in almost all right- and left-handed people. The anatomical localization of speech centres around the perisylvian area (which surrounds the sylvian fissure).

There are three main regions to language:

- Broca's area in the inferior frontal lobe, required for fluent language production (the motor programmes that underlie the production of words)
- Wernicke's area in the posterior superior temporal lobe, required for language comprehension
- The arcuate fasciculus – the white matter tract that connects Broca's and Wernicke's areas.

It is important not to forget other areas of the brain required for speech. These areas include:

- The ear and auditory nerve (cranial nerve VIII): these are required for hearing speech
- Cerebellum: involved in the coordination of muscles used to articulate speech
- Motor output pathways – these include the nerves that control the muscles of articulation, all of which arise from the brainstem. These nerves are the facial (VII), hypoglossal (IX), vagus (X) and the hypoglossal (XII)
- The larynx (innervated by the vagus nerve) – this is involved in producing intonation required for speech.

Speech production

Speech production involves the transformation of thoughts into sentences and words and, ultimately, a series of articulatory commands sent to the vocal apparatus.

Broca's area is in the frontal lobe on the dominant side and processes the motor programmes that are sent to the vocal muscles, producing speech. It matches up a desired phoneme with the motor commands to produce that phoneme.

Connections between Wernicke's area and Broca's area ensure that the sounds that we wish to make are actually made.

Disorders of speech

Damage to any one of the three main areas of language results in characteristic verbal deficits:

- Broca's – damage reduces motor output for speech which becomes effortful and dysfluent, but with well-preserved comprehension.
- Wernicke's – damage reduces the comprehension of speech, which is fluent but a stream of grammatically incoherent words (often called a 'word salad').

- Arcuate fasciculus – damage produces conduction aphasia in which the speech is normal but repetition is markedly defective.

Lesions to other structures required for speech also produce characteristic clinical signs:

- Auditory (VIII) nerve – lesions produce deafness so the patient will not be able to understand speech into the damaged ear.
- Facial (VII) nerve – lesions produce weakness of the muscles of the face, some of which are important in speech production. This results in dysarthria.
- Glossopharyngeal (IX), vagus (X) and hypoglossal (XII) nerves – lesions in these nerves result in the weakness of the muscles of articulation and therefore produce dysarthria.
- Larynx – nervous innervation to the larynx arises from the vagus nerve. Dysfunction of the larynx produces dysphonia or an altered quality in the tone of the voice.

Other disorders of speech (dysphonia, dysphasia, dysarthria) as well as methods of assessing speech are covered in Chapter 17.

Olfaction and taste (gustation) 10

Objectives

In this chapter you will learn about:

- The process of olfactory transduction.
- The process of taste transduction and how signal transduction varies for the four taste modalities.
- The central pathways of olfaction.
- The central pathways of gustation.

RECEPTORS FOR SMELL AND TASTE

Olfactory receptors

Olfactory receptors are located in the dorsal epithelial lining of the nasal cavity (Fig. 10.1).

Mechanisms of the sense of smell

Odours (usually small, lipid-soluble, volatile molecules) enter the mucous film of the olfactory epithelium and diffuse to the receptor cell cilia. Interaction with specific binding proteins on the ciliary surface results in changes in a second-messenger pathway. Most odorant receptors are coupled to cyclic adenosine monophosphate (cAMP). On binding of an odorant molecule, the resultant rise in cAMP opens a cation channel causing depolarization that is proportionate to the concentration of the odorant.

Each olfactory sensory neuron expresses only a single type of odorant receptor which binds a range of related molecules with varying affinities. There are many olfactory receptor proteins, which allow recognition of thousands of different odorants and at very low concentrations (parts per 10^{12}).

Taste receptors

Clusters of gustatory receptors (50–150) are found in the 2000–5000 taste buds in the epithelial layer of the tongue, palate and pharynx. Gustatory receptor cells are continually replaced by cells from the basal layer every 10 days. The base of each receptor cell is innervated by a branch of a primary afferent fibre, forming a type of synapse. Their superior surface is covered in microvilli (the site of taste transduction) and mucus. Hydrophobic compounds can, therefore, reach the receptors by dissolving in the mucus, whereas hydrophilic substances dissolve in the saliva.

In the tongue, taste buds are located on different types of papilla (Fig. 10.2). Signal transduction varies for the four primary taste modalities:

- Saltiness is detected by Na^+ ions passing through an amiloride-sensitive channel to depolarize the receptor cell membrane, resulting in release of a transmitter that activates the primary afferent fibre.

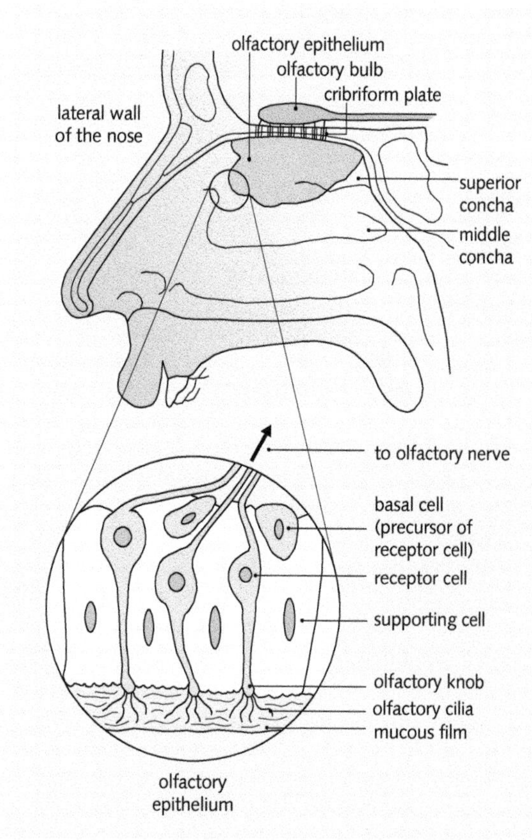

Fig. 10.1 Location and structure of the olfactory epithelium.

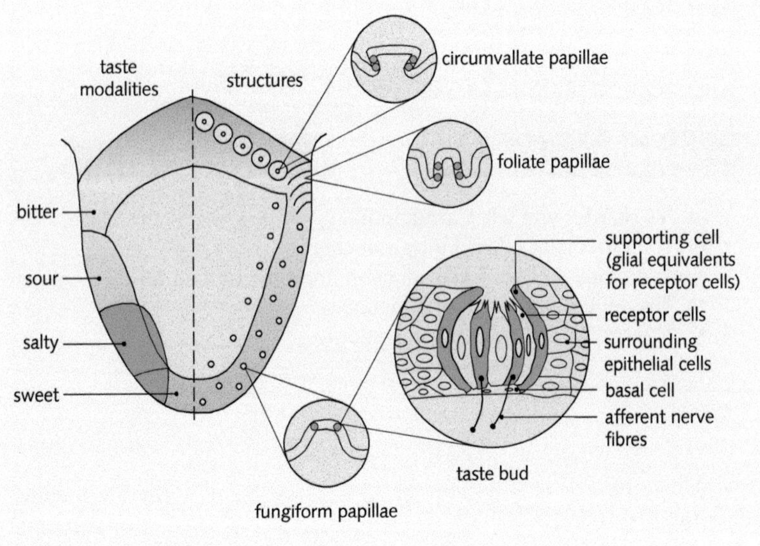

Fig. 10.2 Structure of a taste bud and location of different papillae and taste modalities on the tongue.

- Sourness results from H^+ ion production by acids. H^+ ions depolarize the cell in two ways: directly by passing through amiloride-sensitive Na^+ channels causing an inward current, and indirectly by binding to and blocking K^+ channels.
- Sweetness is signalled when molecules bind to a specific receptor site coupled to a G-protein (gustducin). This triggers an increase in cytoplasmic cAMP, which then activates protein kinase A. This phosphorylates K^+ channels, which become blocked, leading to depolarization.
- Bitterness receptors are essentially poison detectors. Some bitter compounds (e.g. quinine and divalent salts) bind directly to and block K^+ channels, producing depolarization by reducing an outward potassium current. Other compounds bind to specific bitter membrane receptors that activate G-protein second-messenger cascades. One type of bitter receptor produces an increase in intracellular inositol triphosphate (IP_3), causing intracellular Ca^{2+} release. This leads to transmitter release and afferent nerve activation.
- A fifth taste modality, umami (savouriness), produced by monosodium glutamate has recently been defined. Transduction of the umami taste involves metabotropic glutamate receptors of the mGluR4 subtype.

Taste afferent neurons are less specific than the receptors because one afferent can innervate several papillae and, in the solitary nucleus, a single cell can receive synapses from many taste afferent neurons. Therefore, taste has to be interpreted from broadly tuned input channels.

The brain may interpret taste using other inputs such as smell, temperature and texture.

CENTRAL PATHWAYS OF SMELL AND TASTE

Central pathways of smell

The fibres of the olfactory nerve (cranial nerve I) pass through the roof of the nose, which is formed by a perforated bone called the cribriform plate. They synapse in the olfactory bulb at the base of the frontal lobe in regions called 'glomeruli'. Glomeruli are odour-specific functional units, each receiving approximately 25000 olfactory receptor neurons which respond to the same odours. Glomeruli are made up of the diffusely branching dendritic networks of mitral cells, tufted cells (output cells projecting to higher olfactory areas) and periglomerular cells (local inhibitory neurons).

The circuitry in the olfactory bulb allows higher olfactory areas to have an influence on output cell activity; also, output can be inhibited by the incoming olfactory information (Fig. 10.3). The complexity of this circuit allows olfactory processing to begin in the bulb. Lateral inhibition increases the contrast between glomeruli that respond to similar odorants. Connections from the brainstem modify the responsiveness of mitral and tufted cells with respect to the behavioural state (e.g. hungry versus sated).

From the olfactory bulb, mitral and tufted cells project in the olfactory tract to the olfactory cortex and beyond (Fig. 10.4):

- Anterior olfactory nucleus, where olfactory input from both sides is connected through the anterior commissure

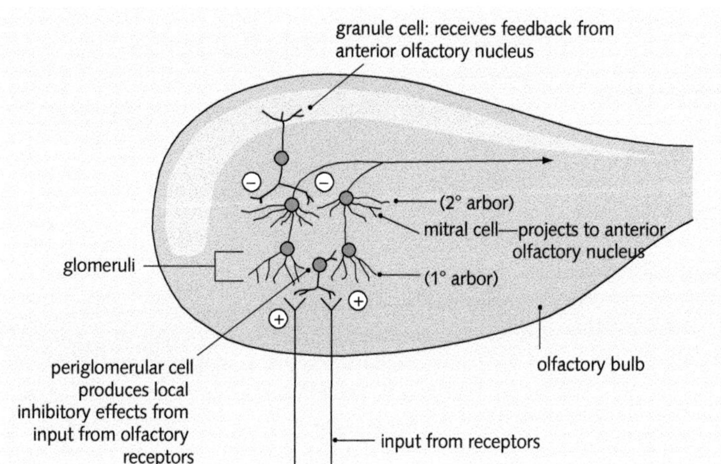

Fig. 10.3 Influences on the efferent fibres from the olfactory bulb.

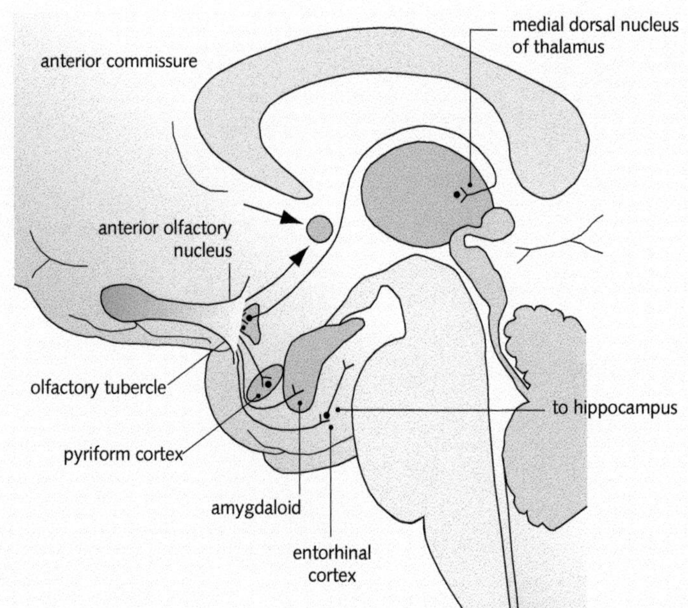

Fig. 10.4 Central pathway of smell.

- Olfactory tubercle, which has connections with the thalamus (medial dorsal nucleus)
- Pyriform cortex, which processes the discrimination between odours
- Amygdala, which is concerned with motivational and affective aspects of olfaction
- Entorhinal cortex (parahippocampal gyrus), which projects to the hippocampus and most probably encodes olfactory aspects of episodic memories.

HINTS AND TIPS

Damage to the cribriform plate (e.g. due to trauma) may section the olfactory nerve and result in anosmia. In addition, when inserting a nasogastric tube, it should be aimed straight towards the back of the head, and not upwards. Otherwise, the tube may pierce the cribriform plate and damage tissue posterior to it. It may be preferable to avoid nasogastric feeding.

Central pathways of taste

The taste pathway does not cross over the midline and so the hemispheres have ipsilateral gustatory perception.

Taste receptors synapse on afferent neurons of cranial nerve VII, IX or X, depending on their location. Taste signals from the anterior two-thirds of the tongue are transmitted in the chorda tympani (cranial nerve VII). Taste from the posterior one-third of the tongue is relayed in cranial nerve IX. Cranial nerve X sends information only from the top of the pharynx. The afferent neurons pass into the medulla where they synapse in a part of the nucleus of the solitary tract called the gustatory nucleus.

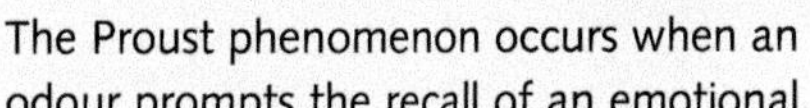

The Proust phenomenon occurs when an odour prompts the recall of an emotional, autobiographical memory. Most likely, it is the direct pathway between the olfactory tract and amygdala, together with connections to the entorhinal cortex and hippocampus, which initiates this experience.

Some cells from the gustatory nucleus project to the hypothalamus and are involved in autonomic responses to feeding. Others project first to the thalamus (ventroposterior medial nucleus) and then to ipsilateral cortex taste area I (Brodmann's area 43) and taste area II in the insula (Fig. 10.5). Taste area I mediates conscious taste perception whereas taste area II is believed to be involved in emotional aspects of taste.

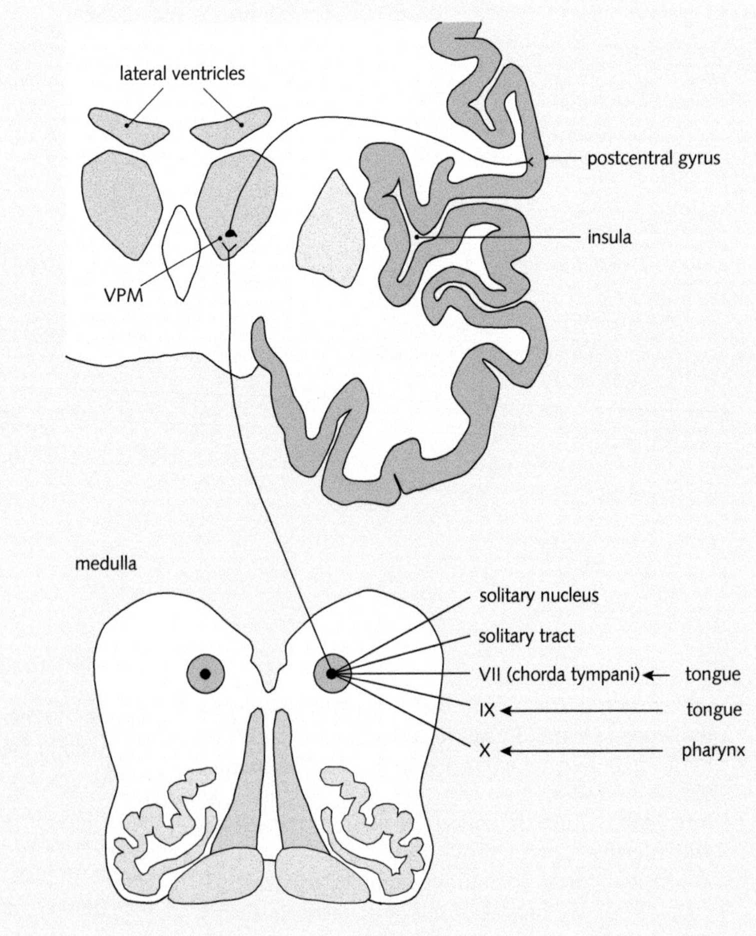

Fig. 10.5 Central pathway of taste. VPM, ventral posterior medial nucleus.

The brainstem 11

Objectives

In this chapter you will learn about:

- The anatomy of the brainstem, including the brainstem nuclei.
- Which cranial nerves leave the brain in the pons, medulla and midbrain.
- The location, organization and function of the reticular formation.
- The principles behind the diagnosis of brainstem death in the UK.
- The stages of sleep and how the electroencephalogram (EEG) appearance varies between sleep and wakefulness.
- Sleep disorders.

THE BRAINSTEM NUCLEI

This section describes the anatomy of the brainstem by relating cross-sectional appearance to overall structure. A knowledge of the functions of the cranial nerves is essential in medical practice and in understanding the reasoning behind the diagnosis of brain death. The trochlear nerve (IV) is the only cranial nerve to leave via the dorsal aspect of the brainstem. It has a tortuous intracranial course, and is particularly susceptible to damage in head injuries.

Figure 11.1 shows where each of the cranial nerves leaves the brainstem and the levels of the cross-sectional views of the brainstem are illustrated in Figures 11.2–11.8.

Figure 11.2 shows the appearance of the medulla oblongata just above its connection with the spinal cord. At this level, two 'pyramids' can be seen as enlargements of the dorsal part of the medulla. This is where the motor fibres decussate before continuing down the spinal cord in the corticospinal tracts. The gracile and cuneate sensory relay nuclei are also found at this level, along with the spinal trigeminal nucleus (cranial nerve V).

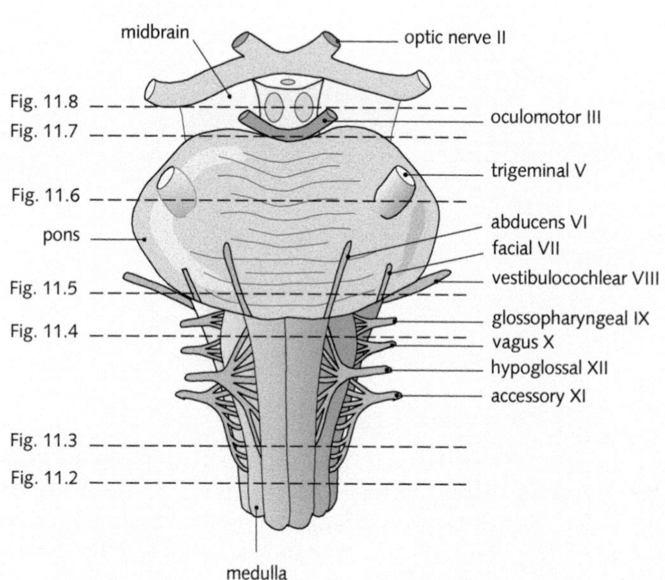

Fig. 11.1 Cranial nerves as they leave the brainstem.

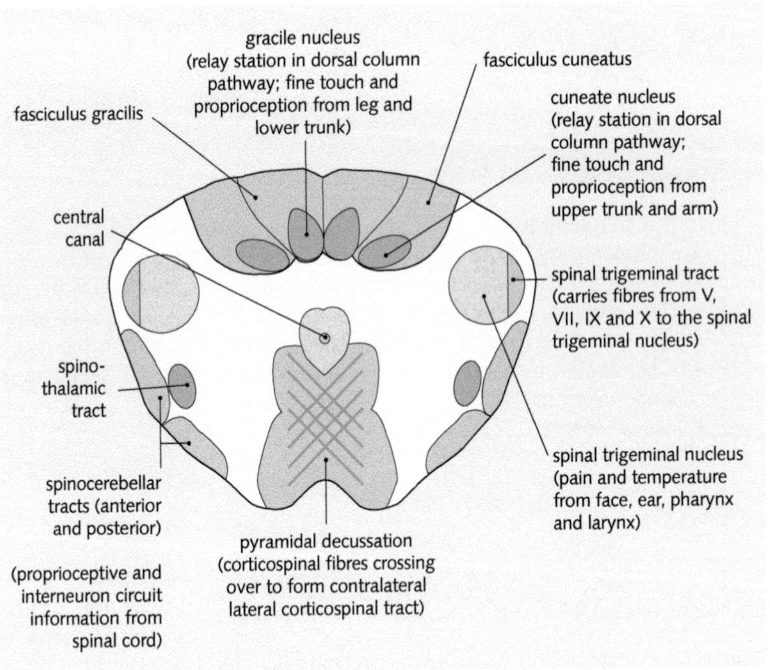

Fig. 11.2 Section through lower medulla (level of motor decussation).

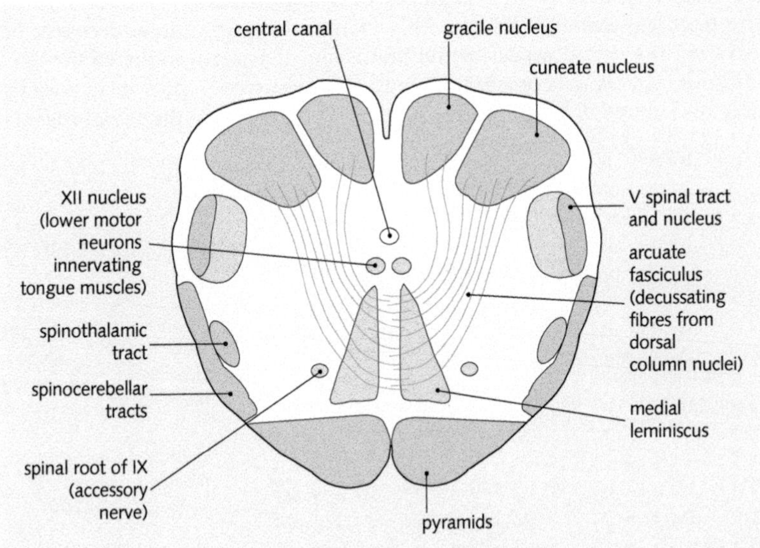

Fig. 11.3 Section through mid-medulla (level of sensory decussation).

Figure 11.3 shows a section through the middle of the medulla, illustrating the decussation of the medial lemnisci. This is the crossing of sensory (internal arcuate) fibres between the gracile and cuneate nuclei. The spinal trigeminal tracts and nuclei, hypoglossal (XII) nuclei and dorsal motor nuclei of the vagus can also be seen at this level (Fig. 11.4).

The upper medulla (Fig. 11.4) forms the floor of the fourth ventricle. There is much more grey matter at this level, as demonstrated by the number of nuclei here. The reticular formation is found anterior to the cranial nerve nuclei, on either side of the medial longitudinal fasciculus.

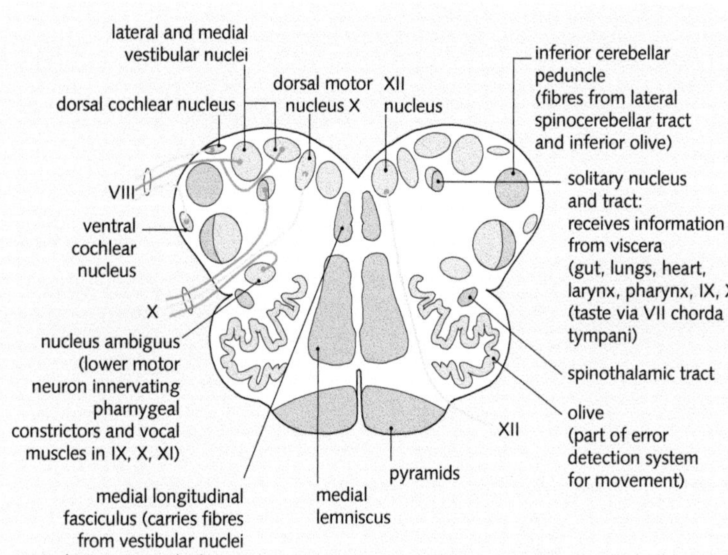

Fig. 11.4 Section through upper medulla (level of inferior olive).

> **HINTS AND TIPS**
>
> Raised intracranial pressure can push the medulla and cerebellar tonsils downwards towards the foramen magnum. Symptoms may include headache, neck stiffness and paralysis of cranial nerves IX–XII. Lumbar puncture is very dangerous in these patients as it may lead to further herniation of the brain through the foramen magnum and ischaemia of the compressed areas. This process is often referred to as 'coning'.

Figure 11.5 shows a section through the lower pons. The medial lemnisci can still be seen but have rotated 90° to lie transversely. The medial longitudinal fasciculi lie just beneath the floor of the fourth ventricle and form the pathways connecting the vestibular and cochlear nuclei with those controlling eye movements.

The upper part of the pons (Fig. 11.6) is similar to the lower part but, in addition, contains the motor and principal sensory nuclei of the trigeminal nerve (V).

The anterolateral aspect of the midbrain is made up of the two cerebral peduncles (Fig. 11.7). Through each of these runs a pigmented area – the substantia nigra. The cerebral aqueduct connects the third and fourth ventricles. Just posterior (dorsal) to it lies the tectum, which consists of the inferior and superior colliculi (Fig. 11.8).

> **HINTS AND TIPS**
>
> The cerebral aqueduct in the midbrain is narrow and vulnerable to blockage by tumours. This can cause a non-communicating hydrocephalus.

THE RETICULAR FORMATION

Location and organization

Once all the nuclei and tracts have been identified in the brainstem, a central core of cells remains. This loosely arranged network is called the brainstem reticular formation. Cellular connectivity in the reticular formation is characterized by a considerable degree of convergence and divergence such that a single cell may respond to many different sensory modalities. Although involved in several quite different functions there is considerable overlap of the areas involved. Closest to the midline lie the raphe nuclei, with the large cell region adjacent to it and the small cell region more laterally.

In this central core, cell groupings can be identified on the basis of their specific neurotransmitters. These are: noradrenaline (norepinephrine), 5-hydroxytryptamine (5-HT), acetylcholine and dopamine. These neurochemical groups project extensively, with the exception of the dopaminergic system which projects to the striatal system, limbic areas, prefrontal cortex and anterior cingulate cortex.

Fig. 11.5 Section through lower pons (level of the facial colliculus). Superior cerebellar peduncle and vestibular nucleus not shown (they lie on the lateral aspects of the fourth ventricle).

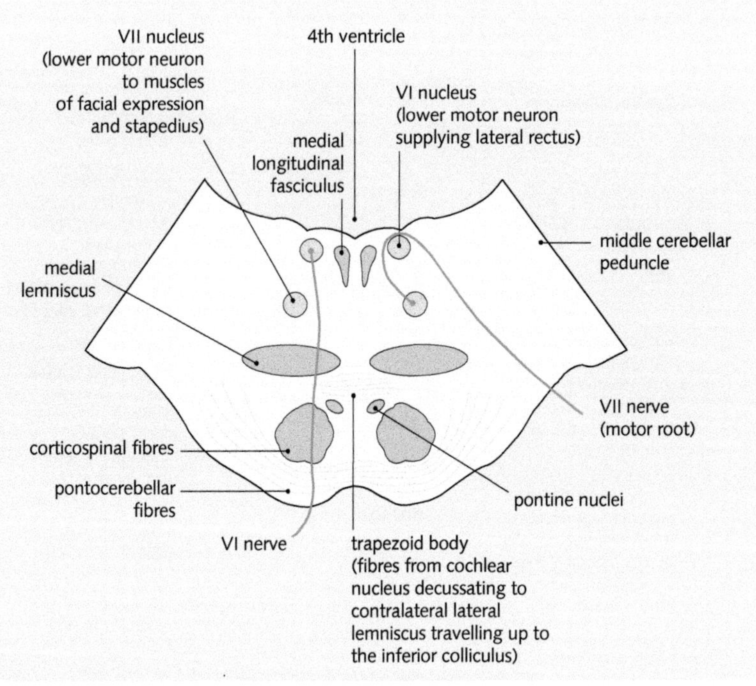

Fig. 11.6 Section through upper pons (level of the trigeminal nuclei).

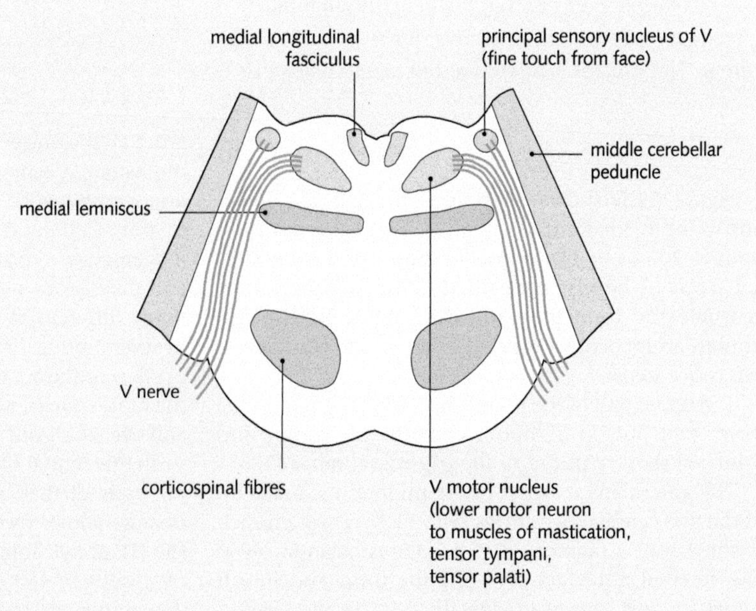

inferior colliculus (auditory pathway relay station)
periaqueductal grey (antinociceptive neurons)
IV
lateral lemniscus
IV nucleus (lower motor neuron to superior oblique)
aqueduct
spinothalamic tract
medial longitudinal fasciculus
substantia nigra (dopaminergic input to striatum)
medial lemniscus
decussation of superior cerebellar peduncle fibres (dentothalamic tract)
cerebral peduncle (corticopontive, corticospinal, and corticobulbar fibres)

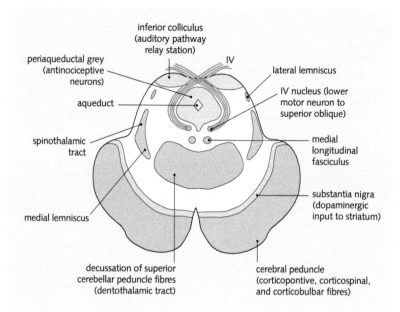

Fig. 11.7 Section through lower midbrain (level of inferior colliculus).

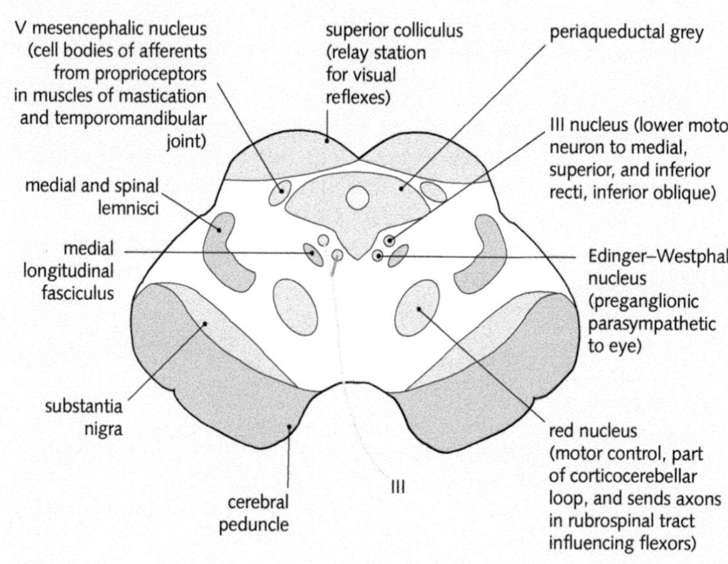

Fig. 11.8 Section through upper midbrain (level of superior colliculus).

The remainder of the reticular core can be partially defined according to function:

- A sensory portion in the lower medulla and lower pons (receiving spinoreticular fibres)
- A motor portion in the upper medulla and upper pons (receiving fibres from the corticospinal tract giving rise to the reticulospinal tracts).

The pontine and medullary neurons project into the midbrain reticular formation, which in turn, projects mainly to the hypothalamus and also the thalamic reticular and intralaminar nuclei. There is also a large projection from the hypothalamus and prefrontal association cortex to the reticular formation.

The cells of the reticular formation can be histologically differentiated from other neurons in that:

- They have large laterally oriented dendritic trees which receive information from many sources.
- They project diffusely either to higher parts of the nervous system or to the spinal cord (most reticular cells have an upward and downward projection).

Function of the reticular formation

The functions of the reticular formation are:

- Sleeping and waking – some parts of the reticular formation are involved in producing sleep states and others in awakening mechanisms. This is related to behavioural arousal and awareness, and is thought to be mainly due to activity in the noradrenergic system. This is referred to as the reticular activating system.
- Modulation of sensory information across the thalamic relay nuclei. This includes the modulation of pain – the reticular system may have a role in the 'gating' mechanism.
- Motor control via modulation of spinal interneurons and transmitting information to the cerebellum (lateral parts of the reticular formation).
- Modulation of respiration – centres controlling inspiration, expiration and the normal rhythm of breathing have been identified physiologically in the medulla and pons.
- Modulation of responsiveness of hippocampal neurons.
- Integration of autonomic functions, particularly cardiovascular. Centres controlling heart rate and blood pressure have been identified in the medullary reticular formation. During sleep, heart rate and respiration slow down and blood pressure falls; before awakening, they are adjusted so that the transition from horizontal to vertical does not cause fainting.
- Control of endocrine functions via the hypothalamic nuclei.
- Possible role in cognition.
- Motor acts involving motivation and reward (dopaminergic system, particularly the mesolimbic projections from the midbrain to the ventral striatum).

BRAIN DEATH

Usually, death is diagnosed by the absence of a pulse, the absence of heart sounds and fixed pupils. However, if the patient is on life support, these may not be appropriate markers. In these cases, brain death may be declared according to the UK brain death criteria, even if the heart is still beating. The criteria are:

- Deep coma with absent respiratory effort
- Absence of drug intoxication and hypothermia
- Absence of hypoglycaemia or ion imbalance
- Any drug which could mask the situation must have been allowed an adequate opportunity to be metabolized and excreted, e.g. thiopentone.

It is diagnosed by testing brainstem function systematically or, more logically, the function of the cranial nerves:

- Fixed pupils (II/III)
- Absent corneal blink reflex (V)
- No vestibular-ocular reflexes (tested by injecting ice cold water into the external meatus, and looking for eye movement towards that ear) (VIII)
- An absence of motor responses within all cranial nerve distributions
- Absence of a gag reflex (IX)
- No spontaneous respiration after turning off the respiratory pump, even when extreme levels of hypercapnia are reached (medulla respiratory centres).

SLEEP AND THE ELECTROENCEPHALOGRAPH

Sleep is defined as a readily reversible state of decreased responsiveness to, and interaction with, the environment. We spend approximately one-third of our lives sleeping. Of that time, one-quarter is spent actively dreaming. The observation that lesions in the brainstem of humans can cause sleep and coma suggests that the brainstem contains neurons whose activity is essential to remaining awake.

The EEG is a record of the electrical activity produced by the brain. It is obtained by attaching electrodes to the skull and connecting them to a suitable amplifier. In an awake, resting subject with the eyes open, the EEG shows a high frequency (13–30 Hz), low voltage pattern called 'beta activity'.

Two states of sleep can be distinguished according to EEG and other physiological measures. Non-rapid eye movement (NREM) sleep has high-voltage, low-frequency EEG and is characterized by decreased cerebral blood flow and brain glucose utilization, with maintenance of muscle tone. As an individual falls asleep they pass through four stages of NREM sleep (see Figure 11.9). Subsequently, REM sleep begins after about 90 minutes with the EEG exhibiting a waveform similar to that seen in the awake state. During REM sleep muscle tone is absent (apart from brief twitches of limb muscles and rapid eye movements), autonomic functions become irregular and dreaming occurs. During sleep, we cycle through the different stages tending to awaken just after an REM phase.

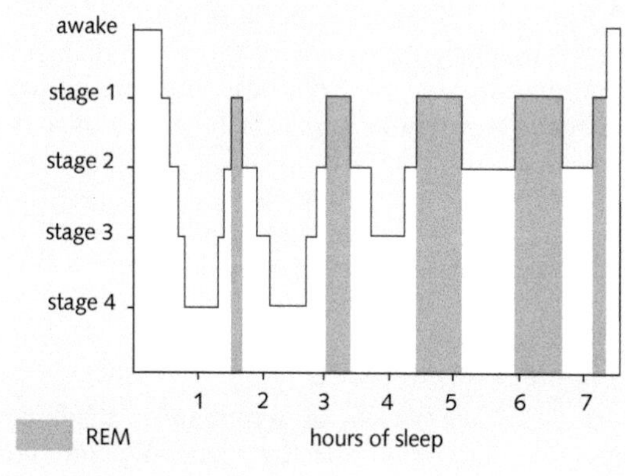

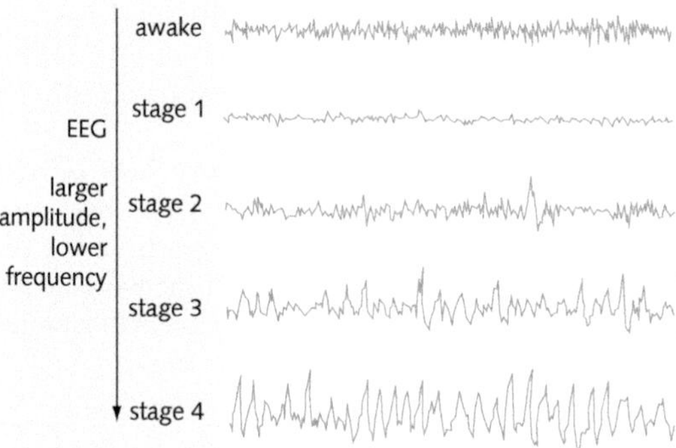

Fig. 11.9 Stages of sleep and the sleep cycle with electroencephalograms (EEGs).

Three hypotheses have attempted to explain the purpose of sleep:

- An ecological hypothesis suggests that sleep allows animals to remain quiet and hidden during periods of highest risk of predation.
- A metabolic hypothesis argues that sleep enables correction of chemical imbalances that accrue during the awake state.
- A learning hypothesis suggests that sleep is needed either to unlearn false memories (and so prevent neural networks from becoming saturated) or to consolidate true memories.

SLEEP DISORDERS

Wake/sleep complaints are second only to complaints of pain as a reason to seek medical attention. Sleep disorders are generally split into the hypersomnias, insomnias and parasomnias.

Hypersomnias

Obstructive sleep apnoea

This is the most common medical disorder causing hypersomnia. It is characterized by the collapse of the upper airway during sleep (believed to be due to obesity). This collapse results in a fall in blood oxygenation causing repetitive arousals (up to 100 per hour of sleep), disrupting the quality of the sleep. This disruption is not noted by the patient during sleep, but manifests as daytime tiredness.

Obstructive sleep apnoea (OSA) is a risk factor for hypertension (during night-time wakening sympathetic activation occurs, constricting blood vessels increasing vascular resistance) and is associated with heart disease and type 2 diabetes mellitus (presumably due to obesity).

Narcolepsy

This is a rare neurological condition that is characterized by the tendency for patients to fall asleep during the day, especially if they are not active or are engaging in non-stimulating activities. This is despite achieving normal levels of sleep the night before. Other symptoms include cataplexy (paralysis following emotional arousal, e.g. laughing or being scared), hypnagogic (occurring at sleep onset) or hypnopompic (occurring at awakening) hallucinations, sleep paralysis (one wakes to find they cannot move their body, but can breathe and move the eyes), automatic behaviours and disrupted night-time sleep.

Narcolepsy is believed to represent a breakdown in the boundaries between wakefulness and sleep. Narcoleptics have been found to lack hypocretin-1 (also known as orexin) in their hypothalamus, perhaps through an immune-mediated mechanism (90% of patients carry either the *HLA-DR15* or *HLA-DQ6* gene). How hypocretin-1 deficiency links to hypersomnia is unclear.

Treatment options usually include stimulant medicines (e.g. amfetamines). Animal studies have found that systemic administration of hypocretin-1 reduces narcolepsy and could, therefore, suggest a future development in treatment.

Insomnias

This is the most prevalent sleep condition in the population and is defined as an inability to sleep sufficiently long enough or have a satisfying sleep. Untreated insomnia is a major risk factor for the development of psychiatric problems (including depression and substance misuse) and a risk factor for road traffic accidents. It is important to remember that insomnia may be a presenting symptom of psychiatric illness (e.g. depression).

Insomniacs show increased adrenocorticotropic hormone (ACTH) and cortisol levels and increased arousal patterns on sleep electroencephalograms (EEGs), suggesting that insomnia may just represent a disorder of hyperarousal.

Treatment options include:

- Behavioural techniques – relaxation techniques and setting bedtime routines so the brain 'knows' that it should be getting ready for sleep.
- Medication – including low-dose benzodiazepines; this must be carefully monitored because of risks of dependency. Melatonin is a night-hormone which may be used in a subpopulation of melatonin-deficient elderly people with insomnia. Melatonin-agonists are being investigated as potential treatment options.

Circadian rhythm disorders

These are covered in Chapter 12.

Parasomnias

Parasomnias are defined as unpleasant or undesirable behavioural or experiential phenomena that occur predominantly during sleep. Most parasomnias represent the simultaneous combination of wakefulness and:

- Non-REM sleep: presenting with disorders of arousal such as sleep-walking, sleep terrors and confusional arousals. They usually arise from slow-wave sleep, therefore presenting in the first third of the sleep cycle. Aetiological factors are those that disrupt the normal sleep neural patterns in already susceptible patients (e.g. febrile illness, alcohol, emotional stress or medication).
- REM sleep: presenting with sleep behaviour phenomena usually in men aged 50 or older. This results in the failure of muscle paralysis during sleep, allowing patients to 'act out' their dreams (e.g. punching out) with sometimes violent or injurious results.

Acute behaviours can be secondary to medication especially serotonin selective reuptake inhibitors (SSRIs). Chronic behaviours can be idiopathic or associated with neurodegenerative disorders, especially the synucleinopathies (e.g. Parkinson's disease, Lewy body dementia).

Treatment for both types of associations is with clonazepam, which is highly effective.

These conditions are likely to occur when the brain crosses from one state to another during the wake–sleep cycle. The primary dysfunction here is believed to be a breakdown in the synchronous neural network activity and neurotransmitter system activity needed for either wakefulness or sleep.

Neuroendocrinology

Objectives

In this chapter you will learn about:

- The anatomy and afferent and efferent projections of the hypothalamus.
- The neuroendocrinological basis of the stress response.
- How feeding is regulated by the hypothalamus.
- Circadian rhythms: functions, mechanisms and disorders.
- The limbic system.
- The function of the cingulate gyrus.

THE HYPOTHALAMUS

The hypothalamus sits adjacent to the third ventricle and is uniquely poised as a centre that integrates information from the nervous system and peripheral homeostatic signals (e.g. blood pressure, fluid and electrolyte balance). This function relies on three features of the hypothalamic anatomy (Fig. 12.1):

- A lack of the blood–brain barrier at the circumventricular organs (nuclei adjacent to the ventricles) permitting blood-borne substances to modulate hypothalamic activity via projections to the hypothalamus. The organum vasculosum of the lamina terminalis (OVLT) is sensitive to changes in osmolarity and the area postrema is sensitive to toxins in the blood and can induce vomiting via hypothalamic projections.
- Several connections with many brainstem sensory nuclei including the nucleus of the solitary tract (sensory information from the vagus concerning blood pressure and gut distension), reticular formation (several sensory domains from the spinal cord), the retina (via retinohypothalamic connections; see later) and limbic and olfactory systems (such as the amygdala, hippocampus and olfactory cortex to control autonomic nervous system output associated with emotion).
- The hypothalamus also has some intrinsic receptors including thermoreceptors and osmoreceptors that monitor temperature and ion balance, respectively.

Output from the hypothalamus comes in the form of:

- Neural signals via the autonomic system (see Ch. 7).
- Endocrine signals to the pituitary gland. Groups of neurons surrounding the third ventricle send axons to the posterior pituitary to cause the release of oxytocin and antidiuretic hormone (ADH). Smaller neurons send axons to the base of the pituitary gland where they secrete several different releasing factors (e.g. corticotropin-releasing factor and thyroid-releasing factor) into the capillary system of the anterior pituitary gland.
- Outputs within the brain to 'inform' the rest of the brain what the hypothalamus has done. This is via releasing-factor neurons and is best illustrated with corticotropin-releasing factor (CRF; see below).

THE SECRETORY HYPOTHALAMUS

The brain has several secretory functions most of which originate in the hypothalamus. Two examples of how the brain can influence the rest of the body via secretory changes from the hypothalamus are:

- The stress response and the activation of the hypothalamic–pituitary–adrenal (HPA) axis
- The neuroendocrinology of feeding.

The stress response

Stress is usually defined as a coordinated reaction to threatening stimuli and is characterized by avoidance behaviour, increased vigilance and arousal, activation of the sympathetic nervous system and release of cortisol from the adrenal gland.

The hypothalamus plays a pivotal role in orchestrating the appropriate humoral, visceromotor and somatic motor responses to any given stressor.

Central to the physiological response to stress is the brainstem (see Ch. 11). The brainstem receives and integrates somatosensory, humoral, metabolic, visceral

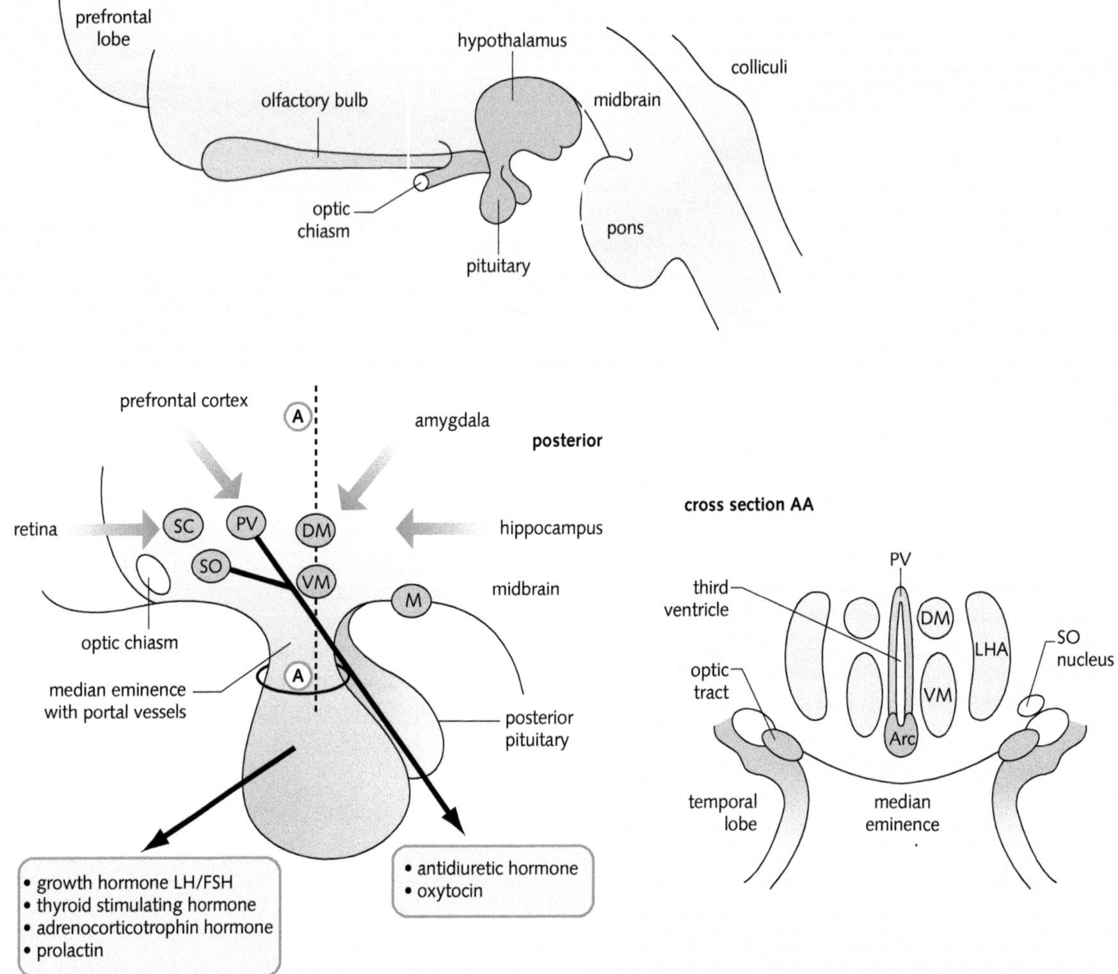

Fig. 12.1 Anatomy and connections of the hypothalamus. SC, suprachiasmatic nucleus; PV, paraventricular nucleus; SO, supraoptic nucleus; DM, dorsomedial nucleus; VM, ventromedial nucleus; M, mamillary bodies; Arc, arcuate nucleus; LHA, lateral hypothalamic area.

and pain information from the rest of the body (Fig. 12.2). After integration the information is sent to the hypothalamus to trigger the appropriate response (in this case the 'stress response').

This, however, is only half the story. We have all experienced the increase in heart rate associated with anticipated fear (e.g. when watching horror movies). This situation arises because we are able to influence the activity of the fear response via 'higher centres', predominantly through the amygdala (described later). These higher centres receive information from several modalities (more simply different senses), process the emotional content and present any resulting emotion to 'consciousness'. Should we think that something is harmful or scary then the thought can activate the stress response via descending connections with brainstem nuclei. Central to this process is the limbic system.

When the hypothalamus has received information that the body is under stress it initiates the HPA axis stress response (Fig. 12.2). Central to this response is the paraventricular nucleus (PVN). The parvocellular region of the PVN secretes CRF into the portal circulation of the anterior pituitary. CRF binds to its receptor on corticotropes – cells which reside in the anterior pituitary gland and release ACTH into the systemic circulation. ACTH travels through the systemic circulation until it reaches the adrenals, where it stimulates release of cortisol from the adrenal cortex.

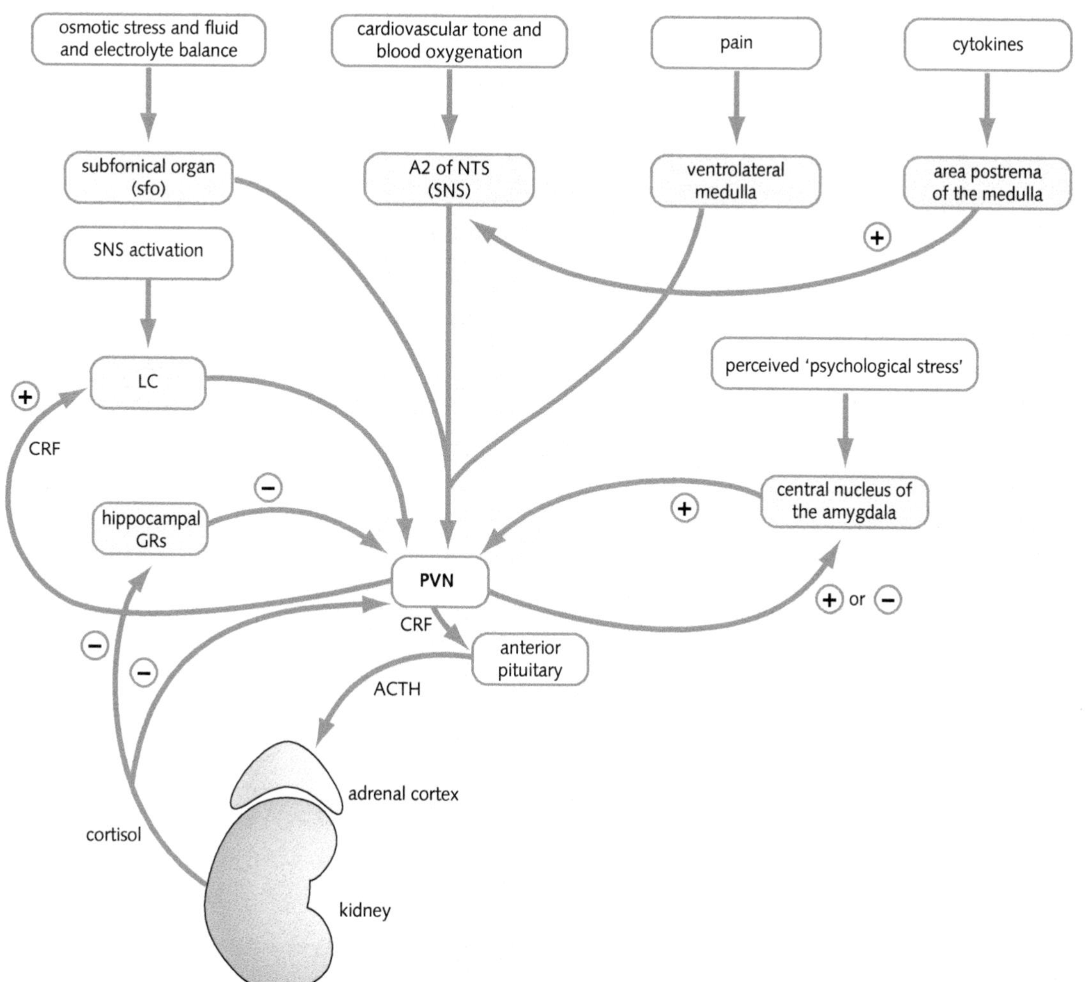

Fig. 12.2 Pathways leading to hypothalamic–pituitary–adrenal axis activation. ACTH, adrenocorticotropin hormone; CRF, corticotropin-releasing factor; GR, glucocorticoid receptors; LC, locus coeruleus; NTS, nucleus of tractus solitarius; PVN, periventricular nucleus; SFO, subfornical organ; SNS, sympathetic nervous system.

HINTS AND TIPS

Cushing's disease is due to hyperadrenocorticism. Often this is iatrogenic, as a result of administration of systemic corticosteroids (e.g. prednisolone), or due to a pituitary gland tumour producing excessive ACTH. Symptoms include central obesity, round ('moon') face, striae, high blood pressure, hair loss, thinning of the skin, diabetes and osteoporosis.

CRF also acts as neurohormone and can influence a number of other centres via projections throughout the brain. CRF projections connect cognitive (the neocortex) and emotional (the amygdala) processing centres with autonomic centres (the locus coeruleus and raphé nuclei) to produce an integrated response to stress. Of note is the connection between CRF neurons from the PVN and the locus coeruleus. Activation of this pathway stimulates the sympathetic nervous system within seconds. Again we have all experienced a racing heart when we have been scared. Thus, perhaps it is appropriate to think that whenever CRF has been or is being released, it is effectively coupling both the unconscious 'flight or fight' autonomic nervous system and our higher function centres (i.e. our conscious selves) together so we can identify and best cope with the stressor (e.g. avoidance).

Negative feedback for the HPA axis arises through glucocorticoid receptors located in the PVN itself or in the hippocampus (which send projections to the PVN). Activation of these receptors curtails CRF activity in the PVN.

The neuroendocrinology of feeding

The hypothalamus is also the brain's feeding centre. However, unlike the stress response, feeding is not confined to one particular nucleus, but it is a more widespread event involving large portions of the hypothalamus.

Several neuropeptides take part in the regulation of feeding and hunger. However, there are a few 'major players'. These can be split into two groups:

- The orexigenic molecules: neuropeptide Y (NPY) and Agouti-related protein (AgRP)
- The anorexigenic molecules: α-melanocyte stimulating hormone (α-MSH) and cocaine- and amfetamine-related transcript (CART).

HINTS AND TIPS

Why did David manage to defeat Goliath? Goliath was said to be 3 m (9 feet 10 inches). This gigantism could be due to a growth-hormone secreting macroadenoma of the pituitary gland, causing optic chiasm compression and therefore bitemporal hemianopia. Goliath never saw the stone coming!

The two groups are constantly opposing each other in the control of appetite and hunger.

When we eat and are becoming 'full' several events occur:

- Gastric distension occurs causing the activation of mechanosensitive receptors on the axons forming ascending vagal (cranial nerve X) fibres. The ascending fibres terminate in the nucleus of the tractus solitarius (NTS).
- Gastric distension and fat digestion also causes the release of cholecystokinin (CCK), which augments the ascending vagal inputs to the NTS.
- Adipocytes release the hormone leptin, which travels through the systemic circulation to the median eminence of the hypothalamus. Once there, leptin crosses the blood–brain barrier to activate leptin receptors in the arcuate nucleus of the hypothalamus.

These 'satiety' signals commence the neuroendocrine response to feeding which ends in the termination of feeding behaviour. Principally, the activation of leptin receptors in the arcuate nucleus stimulates the release of α-MSH and CART from their respective neurons. These neurons then project to several regions of the nervous system to reduce feeding behaviour (Fig. 12.3) by altering the motivation to feed, altering sympathetic nervous activity and stimulating hormone release, including TSH and ACTH.

What about when we are hungry? As leptin levels fall, release of orexigenic molecules (NPY and AgRP) from a separate population of arcuate nucleus neurons increases. These molecules inhibit ACTH and TSH release thereby reducing the metabolic response. In the lateral hypothalamic area, AgRP blocks the MC4 receptor increasing the desire to eat. Normally these two groups are in a state of dynamic flux, in which one gains 'power' over the other and in doing so exerts its behavioural consequence on our food-seeking activities.

HINTS AND TIPS

Diabetes insipidus (DI) is a condition characterized by excessive thirst and excretion of large volumes of dilute urine. The most common cause is a lack of antidiuretic hormone (ADH) production by the hypothalamus due to either a hypothalamic tumour or head trauma (central or neurogenic DI). The second commonest cause is an insensitivity of the kidneys to ADH (e.g. due to renal failure) – so-called nephrogenic DI.

THE CIRCADIAN RHYTHM

The term circadian rhythm refers to the coordination of behaviour and physiology to the daily cycles of daylight and darkness. Some animals are more active during the day and some are more active at night, it just depends on whether they are 'geared up' for the night or day.

Physiological and biochemical processes rise and fall with the circadian rhythm; in humans these processes include body temperature, blood flow, urine production, hormone levels and metabolic rate (see Fig. 12.4).

Biological clocks

The circadian rhythm is controlled by an internal clock, which has its anatomical foundation in the suprachiasmatic nuclei (SCN) of the hypothalamus. Electrical stimulation of the SCN causes the shift of circadian rhythms, and lesions of the SCN abolish circadian

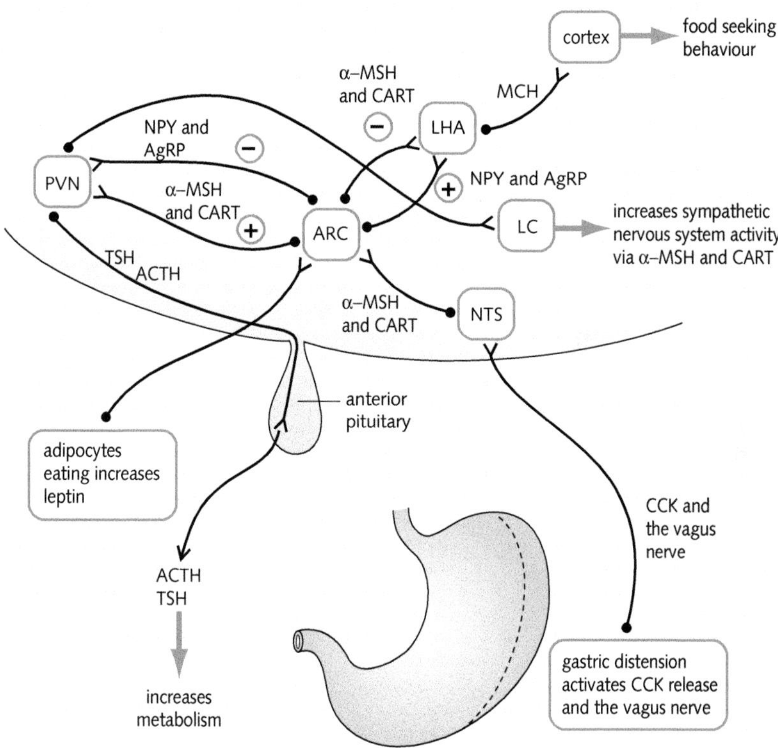

Fig. 12.3 Neuroendocrinological regulation of feeding. α-MSH, α-melanocyte-stimulating hormone; ACTH, adrenocorticotropin hormone; AgRP, Agouti-related protein; ARC, arcuate nucleus; CART, cocaine- and amfetamine-related transcript; CCK, cholecystokinin; LHA, lateral hypothalamic area; LC, locus coeruleus; MCH, melanin-concentrating hormone; NTS, nucleus of the solitary tract; NPY, neuropeptide Y; PVN, periventricular nucleus; TSH, thyroid-stimulating hormone.

rhythms all together. However, transplantation of SCN from one animal to another resurrects circadian rhythms, suggesting that the intrinsic properties of SCN neurons are able to govern circadian rhythms.

SCN rhythmicity with light depends on another, previously unmentioned, type of photoreceptor in the retina. These photoreceptors express a different type of photopigment called melanopsin. Melanopsin is not present in rods and cones and is very slowly excited by light. Axons from these photoreceptors form the retinohypothalamic tract which travels directly to the SCN from the retina. Information from these photoreceptors is able to reset the circadian clock residing within the SCN.

Output from the SCN is much less clear, but mainly innervates the surrounding hypothalamus as well as some diencephalic and midbrain areas. The principal neurotransmitter of projections from the hypothalamus is GABA (although there are some glutamatergic fibres as well); presumably the SCN coordinates the effects of the circadian rhythm by inhibiting the neurons they innervate.

Biological clock mechanisms

It appears that each SCN neuron acts as a clock. The rhythmicity of SCN cells relies not on connections or action potentials but rather on genes and gene products. The central gene in this process is known as *clock* (an acronym for *circadian locomotor output cycles kaput*). This gene, when translated from mRNA into its protein form, feeds back and interacts with the transcription mechanisms underlying its expression. This interaction decreases gene expression, effectively switching off the gene. Gradually as levels of protein decrease (because less protein transcription is occurring) the genes are switched back on, causing an increase in *clock* gene

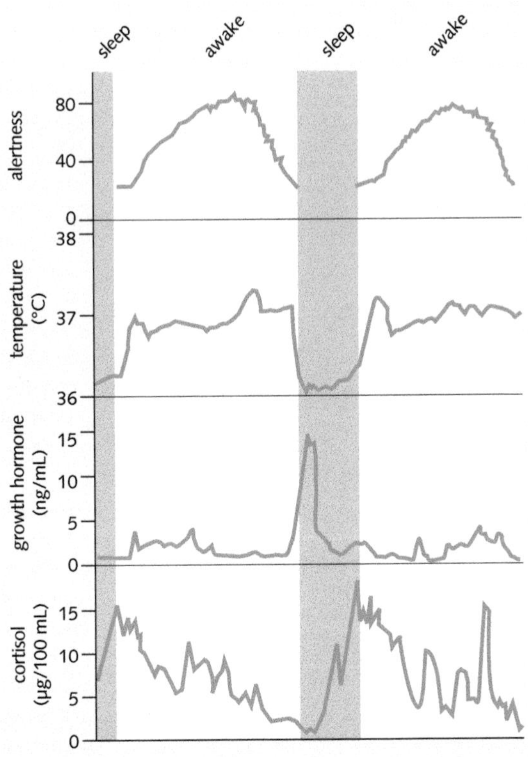

Fig. 12.4 Circadian rhythm of various physiological functions. Note how cortisol and growth hormone levels are highest during the night when compared with body temperature and alertness.

product expression. This ebb-and-flow cycle of protein expression takes about 24 hours, building the foundation on which circadian rhythms are founded. *Per1*, another timekeeping gene, helps regulate circadian rhythms in a similar way.

Light from the retina serves to reset the clocks in the SCN neurons each day, but SCN cells can reset each other via cell–cell interactions, gap junctions and glial cells interactions.

Melatonin

Melatonin is a sleep-promoting hormone secreted by the pineal gland, which is located at the base of the brainstem. Melatonin is synthesized and secreted during the dark period of the light–dark cycle. It is believed that melatonin release is associated with the initiation of sleep, but its exact role is unclear.

The SCN has direct connections with the pineal gland via *N*-methyl-D-aspartate (NMDA)-gated glutamate pathways. Activation of these fibres by light causes a reduction in melatonin release; thus melatonin release is maximal during the night.

A good example of circadian rhythms in action is jet-lag. Previously in another time zone we have trained our circadian rhythms to respond to the 24-hour cycle of our 'home' light–dark cycle. As one travels across time zones and the light–dark cycle changes, circadian rhythms still cycle in the 'native' (or original) cycle. Thus, a person's light–dark cycle and the light–dark cycle of the new time zone are no longer synchronized, resulting in difficulty going to sleep. This occurs because melatonin levels will not be maximal whenever darkness ensues in the new time zone, but they will be maximal whenever our home time zone turns dark, which may occur in the middle of the new time zone's day. This is why you may sleep during the day.

Treatment for jet-lag is with bright light as it helps to reset the circadian rhythm to the light–dark cycle of the new time zone. Many believe that melatonin supplements help with jet-lag, which in theory they should. However, efficacy of melatonin supplements has not been demonstrated.

Circadian rhythm disorders

The primary symptom of circadian rhythm disorder is the inability to sleep during the desired sleep time. Once patients manage to get to sleep there is no further abnormality. It is believed the problem lies with an inability for an individual's biological clock to adjust to the demands of the geophysical environment.

Circadian rhythm disorders can be split into two groups:

- Primary – this is the malfunction of the biological clock itself. These are difficult to diagnose and may present as other sleep, medical or psychiatric disorders (e.g. hypersomnia, insomnia, substance misuse).
- Secondary – these result from environmental effects on the underlying clock system such as jet-lag or shift-work. These are usually discovered during the history.

Mainstays of treatment include:

- Chronotherapy – the patient trains their body to go to bed progressively earlier and to sleep for only a pre-determined number of hours
- Phototherapy – exposure to bright light can influence the underlying physiology of the circadian rhythm and attempts to treat the 'dysrhythmia'.

THE LIMBIC SYSTEM

The limbic system is a complex system of fibre tracts and grey matter. It was introduced above, lying in the medial aspect of each temporal lobe, encircling (limbus = border) the upper part of the brainstem. This serves as the 'nervous system' for emotion and behaviour. It also has extensive connections to both lower and higher parts of the central nervous system, allowing it to integrate a wide variety of stimuli.

Structure of the limbic system

Figure 12.5 shows the arrangement of the limbic structures. This complicated system can be considered as two simpler circuits:

- A system primarily involved in learning and memory
- A system involved with processing of emotion, especially its behavioural and endocrine aspects.

The hippocampal circuit

The medial temporal lobe contains the structures primarily involved with learning and memory. Output from the hippocampus arises from axons which form the fornix, most of which project to the mamillary bodies of the hypothalamus. Mamillary body neurons then project to the anterior nucleus of the thalamus which in turn projects to the cingulate cortex. The dorsomedial nucleus of the thalamus also receives input from other temporal lobe structures including the amygdala and inferotemporal cortex and projects to virtually all of the frontal cortex (Fig. 12.6).

This circuit also has connections with polysensory association cortical regions in the frontal, temporal and parietal lobes via the entorhinal cortex (the major input structure into the hippocampus). The hippocampus,

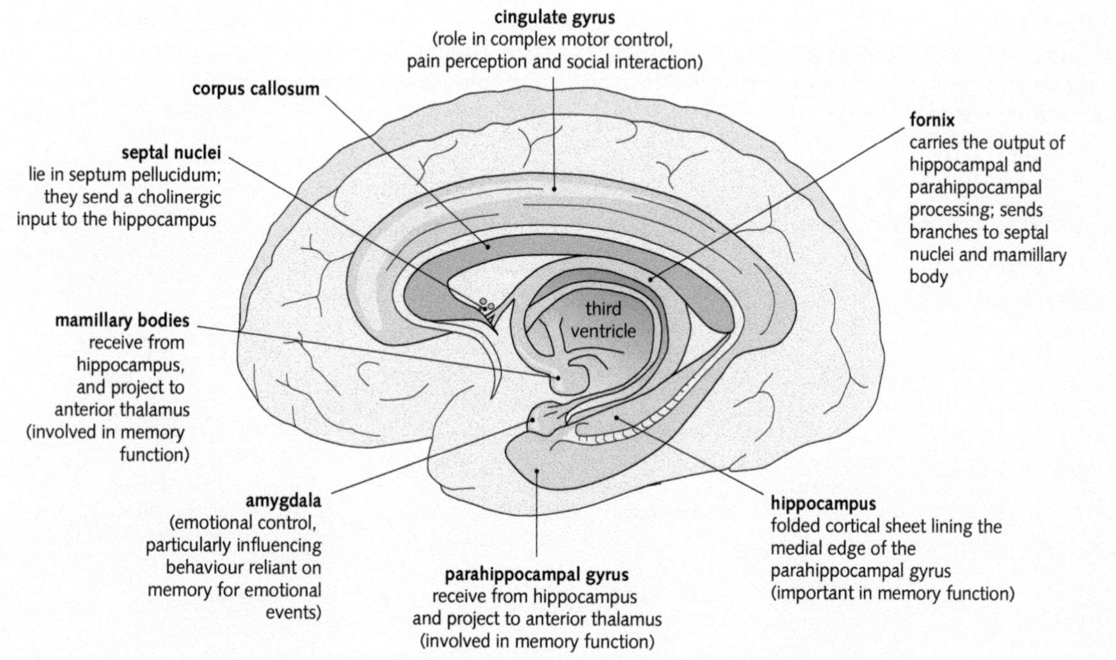

Fig. 12.5 Outline of the limbic system.

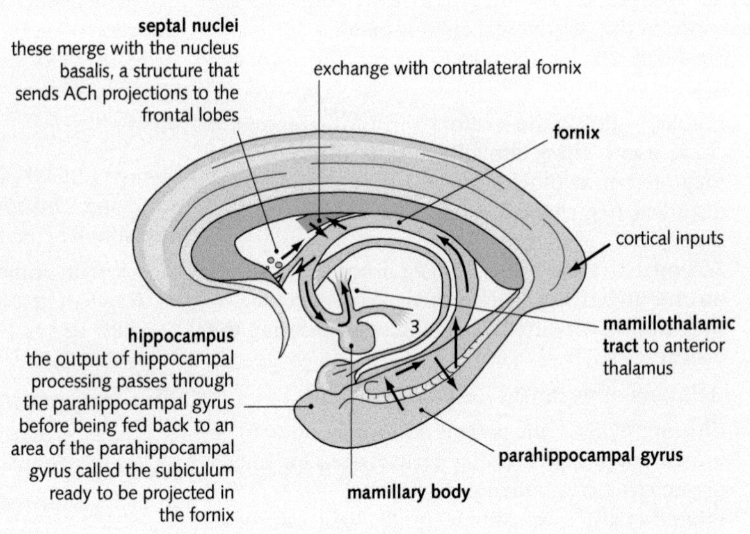

Fig. 12.6 Processing in the hippocampal circuit. To trace the pathway start at the hippocampus and follow the arrows. ACh, acetylcholine.

therefore, receives highly processed information from the cortex. The hippocampus also receives efferents from the amygdala via the entorhinal cortex and by projections into the hippocampus proper.

Brainstem nuclei also have inputs to the hippocampus, such as the locus coeruleus (noradrenergic transmission) and the raphé nuclei (serotonergic transmission), both of which modulate hippocampal function.

The amygdala

This almond-shaped collection of subcortical nuclei lies in the anterior pole of each temporal lobe. There are three main groups of nuclei:

- The deep nuclei (including the lateral and basal nuclei; otherwise known as the basolateral nucleus)
- The superficial nuclei and area (which includes some cortical components; also known as the corticomedial nuclei)
- The central nucleus.

The amygdala has interconnections with several cortical and subcortical areas. Subcortical projections contact with autonomic and visceral centres in the diencephalon and brainstem, while the cortical projections travel via the external capsule. These connections are shown in Figure 12.7.

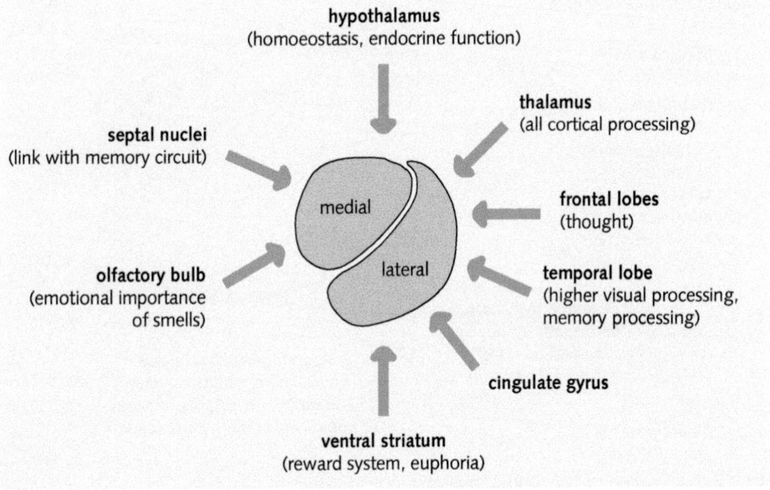

Fig. 12.7 Connections of amygdala.

Each of these nuclei has extensive connectivity with other areas of the brain:

- The central nuclei have two major outputs – one to the hypothalamus (known as the stria terminalis) and one to the dorsomedial nucleus of the thalamus (the ventral amygdalofugal pathway).
- The deep nuclei send projections to the nucleus accumbens, striatum, hippocampus and surrounding cortex.
- The superficial nuclei receive higher-order uni- and polymodal sensory information from widespread cortical areas, the PFC and the cingulate cortex. These nuclei appear to form the principal input to the amygdala.

The amygdala projects to several cortical areas including, for example, those underlying early stages of visual processing in the occipital lobe. This suggests that some amount of processing occurs in the amygdala, which then modulates the early stages of cortical sensory input. Furthermore, it seems that the amygdala is critical to the processing of emotional features in sensory input and, therefore, determines the emotional significance of sensory information. When the amygdala is stimulated patients report strong feelings of fear along with a sympathetic autonomic response. Lesions here can cause impaired recognition of emotional facial expressions of other people.

It appears that each of the nuclei play a specific role in the fear response:

- The central nucleus appears to orchestrate the behavioural/motor responses via projections to the periaqueductal grey matter (the ventral amygdalafugal pathway) and also by activating the autonomic system via projections to the lateral hypothalamus (the stria terminalis).
- The deep nuclei project to the cerebral cortex where emotion is experienced. It is interesting to note that these neurons receive direct innervation by cholinergic neurons, suggesting these neurons help us focus attention on the stimulus when this circuit is activated (for attention see Ch. 13).

The cingulate cortex

The cingulate gyrus loops around the limbic system and the lateral ventricles. The cingulate gyrus can be split into two general regions:

- The anterior cingulate cortex, which supports executive behaviour (e.g. social interaction)
- The posterior cingulate cortex, which supports evaluative and memory function.

Furthermore, the anterior cingulate can be split into three further subdivisions running rostral-caudally. These are:

- An emotional subdivision (most rostral)
- A cognitive subdivision
- A motor function subdivision (most caudal), which is adjacent to the more superior motor areas.

Functional imaging tasks show that more rostral areas are activated in tasks involving emotion, whereas more caudal regions are activated with cognitive-motor tasks. It is suggested that the cingulate cortex underlies social interaction, such that patients with cingulate lesions become socially isolated and may be so withdrawn that they are akinetic and mute.

Memory and the higher functions 13

Objectives

In this chapter you will learn about:
- Mechanisms of learning and memory.
- Amnesia.
- The anatomical and functional basis of the higher functions.
- Disorders of the higher functions.
- Cognitive development.
- Cognitive degeneration with ageing.

MEMORY

Declarative and non-declarative memory

Before 1958, it was unclear which part of the brain was responsible for memory. Everything changed after a patient called HM underwent surgery to remove his temporal lobes in order to treat his intractable epilepsy. Soon after the surgery, which involved the removal of both hippocampi, it was discovered that HM was profoundly amnesic, with limited memories of his life prior to the surgery (retrograde amnesia) and an inability to form new memories (anterograde amnesia).

Some time later though, it was discovered that, in fact, HM could learn. In a series of famous experiments, HM was found to be able to learn and perform several motor tasks (for example, drawing a star in a mirror) with great precision, although he could never remember the conscious experience of having learnt the task. This finding gave rise to the first distinction of memory: the difference between explicit (or declarative) and implicit/procedural (or non-declarative) memory:

- Declarative memories are those one can 'declare' to others and includes autobiographical and factual memories.
- Implicit memories are those which cannot be consciously recalled and include such things as motor skills, conditioning (remember Pavlov's dog) and priming (where our memories are 'jogged' into remembering from a cue).

These differences are described in more detail in Figure 13.1.

After HM, several other patients began to emerge, all with temporal lobe damage and with declarative memory defects. These findings suggested that it was the medial temporal lobe structures in particular (e.g. the hippocampus and limbic system) where explicit memories were formed and stored.

However, further tests revealed that these patients could use their working memory, which is our ability to use the information we are currently processing 'right now'. This memory is closely related to attention (we try to keep our attention focused on the information by mental rehearsal; like trying to remember a phone number). Working memory relies on pathways within the frontal lobes, not medial temporal lobe structures. This anatomical distinction allows explicit memory to be subdivided into short-term (STM) and long-term memory (LTM). STM is synonymous with working memory, lasting for only a few seconds. Working memory is discussed more fully later.

LTM itself is further subdivided into episodic memory (autobiographical; the 'episodes' in our life) and semantic memory (e.g. facts about the world we know). Both of these are formed in the hippocampus, but semantic memory migrates to the overlying medial temporal cortex. It is likely that semantic facts begin as episodic memories, but degrade with time into facts instead of 'events'.

The above developments can be brought together as a 'taxonomy of memory' (Fig. 13.2), all subtypes of which rely on different anatomical areas.

Sensory memory

This is part of declarative memory and is a store of all the sensory information that has just been processed. It is held in stores that are modality specific (e.g. visual stores, tactile stores) with a very high capacity, but are limited in the time which information can be held (fading after 0.5 s).

Fig. 13.1 Types of memory and their functions and location

Type of memory	Subdivision	Anatomical localization	Function or example
Declarative/ Explicit	Episodic	Hippocampus	Long-term memory. Usually includes the events/episodes of our lives
	Semantic	Parahippocampal gyrus	Remembering the facts of the world (e.g. Britain is an island)
	Short-term memory/ working memory	Prefrontal cortex	Retention of information to guide ongoing behaviour
Nondeclarative/ Implicit	Conditioning	Distributed	Associating a stimulus that evokes a reasonable response from a second stimulus
	Procedural	Striatum	Forms behavioural habits and allows us to remember tasks
	Motor skills/memory	Learnt in the cerebellum then stored in the cerebellum and another unknown site (perhaps the cortex)	The memory of learned motor skills

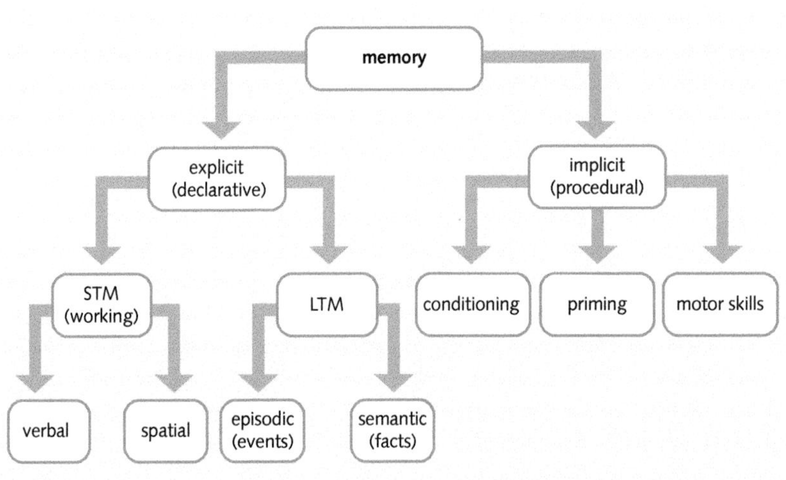

Fig. 13.2 The taxonomy of memory. Many believe that there should be an arrow from episodic memory to semantic memory, demonstrating the development of semantic memory. Each branch represents a different anatomical location.

There is no conscious access to sensory memory. Its function is in selective memory, filtering the inputs that will be consciously processed by working memory. Sensory memory also forms part of the input into working memory.

Working memory

This is the retention of information needed to guide ongoing behaviour. Working memory appears to rely on functions of the prefrontal cortex (PFC), especially attention, problem solving and the planning of behaviour. An example of working memory is with verbal fluency tasks where subjects must remember words they have said while saying others, so as to not repeat already said words. The subjects must dynamically remember what they have said along with the ongoing task. Lesions of the PFC render people unable to use recent information and to use stored memory to guide ongoing behaviour.

During working memory tasks, some PFC neurons demonstrate increased firing patterns (the representation of information in a 'language' the brain understands) during delays between trials, suggesting these neurons keep recent memories 'active' and 'to hand' by keeping the firing pattern representing that information 'online'.

Key features of working memory are:

- Its span (maximum capacity) is typically less than a dozen units of information, usually 7 ± 2 units (e.g. numbers or words).
- It functions as a push-down stack, so that new units of information displace the oldest units from the working memory store. Units are usually only stored for a few minutes at most, unless mental rehearsal is performed.
- It has a visual and a verbal store where visuospatial and verbal information is held, and the central executive which manipulates the information.

Long-term memory mechanisms

Learning seems to rely on the unique physiological properties of cells in the hippocampus.

When we learn, the brain converts the 'fact' into a unique pattern of electrical activity (similar to a unique binary code). This electrical activity excites particular synapses throughout the hippocampus, so that should this 'code' or 'fact' pass once more through the hippocampus those synapses will fire reliably and strongly, but only when the input matches that of the 'fact'. This electrical phenomenon is known as long-term potentiation (LTP).

LTP occurs when the patterned input causes the release of glutamate which activates AMPA (α-amino-3-hydroxy-5-methyl-4-isoxazolepropionic acid) receptors (see Ch. 3), allowing the influx of Na^+ into the cell and depolarization of the membrane. NMDA (*N*-methyl-D-aspartate) receptors are key to LTP. Activation of NMDA receptors requires binding of glutamate and the co-agonist glycine as well as the removal of the Mg^{2+} block (which occurs with membrane depolarization). Once the NMDA receptors are open high levels of Ca^{2+} flow into the cell, initiating LTP. Sufficient glutamate is available for this to happen when several presynaptic neurons fire at once (which occurs during learning) (Fig. 13.3).

This increase in electrical activity is not permanent, so how does the memory become consolidated into long-term memory? The high levels of Ca^{2+} activate two protein kinases which phosphorylate other intracellular proteins that facilitate structural changes in the post-synaptic neurons underlying the memory. These changes include the insertion of new AMPA receptors into the postsynaptic membrane and optimization of function of pre-existent AMPA receptors. These structural changes are the basis of long-term memory, such that whenever we need to recall the 'fact' and the

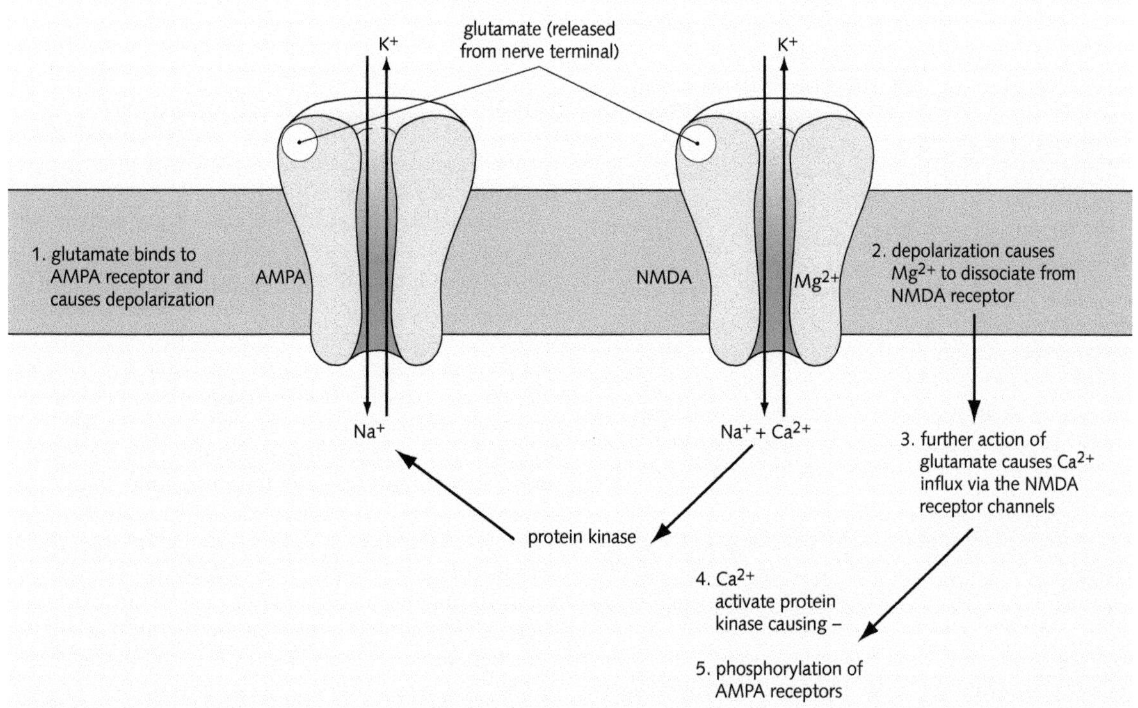

Fig. 13.3 Proposed mechanism of long-term potentiation.

patterned input for that 'fact' enters the hippocampus, it will robustly activate these 'primed' synapses allowing the memory to be recalled.

DISORDERS OF MEMORY

Amnesia

Amnesia is defined as an abnormal mental state whereby memory and learning are affected out of proportion to other cognitive functions in an otherwise alert and responsive patient. Several amnestic syndromes exist:

- Transient global amnesia – severe forgetfulness and confusion with total episodic memory loss and disorientation. Patients usually remembers their identity. This state is presumed to be due to transient ischaemia of the temporal lobes or diencephalon.
- Post-traumatic amnesia – this occurs after a severe blow to the head, resulting in a dense retrograde amnesia that resolves with time such that only the incident itself is not remembered. Duration of coma following brain injury is the best predictor of the severity of memory loss and cognitive deficit.
- Korsakoff's syndrome – this may follow Wernicke's encephalopathy (a triad of loss of memory, ataxia and nystagmus). This syndrome is due to thiamine deficiency secondary to chronic alcoholism. Thiamine deficiency leads to the degradation of the mamillary bodies in the hypothalamus (one of the structures involved in the limbic system) resulting in a dense retrograde amnesia. Patients classically confabulate (report events that never happened, mistaking their guesses or imagination for actual memories). Patients must be given thiamine in the acute situation.
- Other amnestic syndromes exist and also include the dementias.

'Clinical' memory is best tested with the Mini-Mental State Examination MMSE, which examines short-term/working memory and long-term memory. Clinically, episodic memory can be examined by asking the patient if they are able to successfully navigate around their last school. This is a feature of the navigational function of the hippocampus in forming episodic memories.

THE HIGHER FUNCTIONS AND THEIR DISORDERS

Memory is only one of the higher functions. The following sections outline the anatomical and functional bases for the clinical higher functions as well as what happens when they are disrupted.

Wakefulness/consciousness

This is maintained by the brainstem and thalamic reticular activating system. Consciousness appears to rely especially on acetylcholine and noradrenaline (norepinephrine).

Coma and persistent vegetative state

A coma is a profound state of unconsciousness and usually represents dysfunction of the reticular activating network. The patient cannot be awakened, does not respond to pain or execute voluntary movements.

A persistent vegetative state is one in which there is a non-functional cortex with a functional reticular activating system. Patients lose higher brain function, but 'lower' functions (i.e. those controlled by the brainstem, such as breathing and circulation control) remain intact. Their eyes may open spontaneously. However, these patients are not able to be roused and are unable to respond to commands.

Orientation

This requires several cognitive functions and, therefore, has a diffuse anatomical location. A diagnosis of disorientation suggests impairment in several cognitive domains.

Delirium

Orientation is usually tested by asking the patient what time of day it is, who they are and where they are (time, person, place). Disorders of orientation require widespread cortical dysfunction, because it relies on so many cognitive processes to work together. The principal example of disorientation is delirium.

Patients with delirium become acutely confused and disorientated, hence its other name: acute confusional state. This condition is common in the inpatient (medical and surgical) population and especially among elderly people. Delirium is believed to arise due to a lack of cholinergic transmission following changes in cerebral homeostasis. This renders the patient unable to concentrate, which precipitates confusion. Other signs include miniature visual hallucinations ('lilliputian'), disorientation to time and place, disrupted sleep–wake cycles and a fluctuating symptom level. Treatment is conservative with orientating instruments (e.g. a large clock, glasses if needed) and nursing with the same member of staff (if possible). These efforts attempt to re-orientate the patient to time, person and place while the cerebral homeostatic challenge wanes. Haloperidol can be used as a sedative if conservative measures fail to calm and reorientate the patient.

Attention

Attention can be classified into several different categories (e.g. selective, divided or preparatory) or in terms of its object (e.g. spatial and non-spatial). Clinically, sustained attention is probably the most relevant category.

Attention has a diffuse anatomical location, which generally centres on the PFC. Attention is mediated by several neurotransmitter systems, all of which add their 'flavour' to build up the whole experience of attention. Central to attention is acetylcholine (ACh), noradrenaline (NA) and dopamine (DA). ACh mediates attention by increasing the signal-to-noise ratio for any given neuron, meaning that information being conveyed by neurons in the PFC has less chance of being disrupted by the transmission across surrounding synapses. NA seems to work by 'notifying' the brain of interesting stimulus in our experienced world. Both NA and DA reinforce the transfer of information through the PFC by optimizing the transmission of action potentials to the cell body carrying the information, which again prevents the disruption of information. Attention is said to be mediated by either:

- Top-down mechanisms – that is to say we can 'choose' to focus our attention, e.g in an exam. This is mediated by the PFC
- Bottom-up mechanisms – where we are alerted to potentially interesting or dangerous stimuli in our nearby environment. Ascending brainstem connections mediate this.

Sustained attention is best tested with MMSE tasks, such as reciting the months of the year backwards, spelling 'world' backwards or subtracting 7 from 100 sequentially ('serial 7's').

Inattentive disorders typically present as neglect (Ch. 8).

Executive function

Executive functions refer to the range of abilities which allow us to plan, initiate, organize and monitor our thoughts and behaviours. These tasks are served mainly by the frontal lobes and are essential for social performance. A number of functional subdivisions exist within the frontal lobes, each serving a specific domain that contributes to executive function. Motor and premotor areas direct movement (see Ch. 6). The dorsolateral PFC, lying anterior to the premotor cortex is especially involved in attention, working memory and organization of thought and behaviour. The orbitofrontal cortex concerns itself with the regulation of social behaviour. The medial frontal cortex (including the anterior cingulate with its connections to the limbic system) mediates motivation and arousal.

While disorders of the frontal lobes can be hard to diagnose, they often become apparent when one interviews a patient with frontal damage. Specific tests include:

- Verbal fluency (list as many animals or words beginning with 'P' in a minute as possible)
- Motor sequencing (the Luria three-hand movement test: fist, edge, palm)
- Tests of abstraction.

One should also note the manner of the patient during the interview, especially if there has been a change in previously normal behaviour. For example:

- Disorders of attention, working memory and thought could be due to premotor dysfunction.
- Poor social behaviour could be due to orbitofrontal dysfunction.
- Apathy may be due to medial frontal or cingulate gyrus dysfunction.

Language

The main areas of language and the result of damage to these areas is described in Chapter 9.

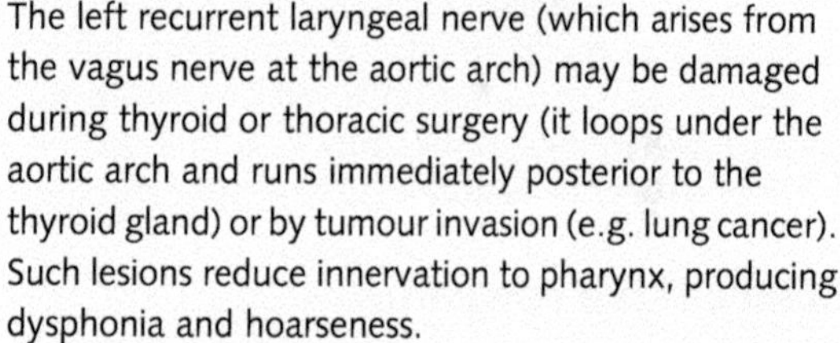

HINTS AND TIPS

The left recurrent laryngeal nerve (which arises from the vagus nerve at the aortic arch) may be damaged during thyroid or thoracic surgery (it loops under the aortic arch and runs immediately posterior to the thyroid gland) or by tumour invasion (e.g. lung cancer). Such lesions reduce innervation to pharynx, producing dysphonia and hoarseness.

Arithmetic

These skills are located in the dominant hemisphere particularly in the angular gyrus of the inferior parietal lobe.

Dyscalculia can be diagnosed by asking the patient to perform simple arithmetic tasks. This may be a hard sign to elicit.

Praxis

Praxis is the ability to perform skilled actions and relies not only on intact motor pathways from the cortex to the muscle, but also on the prefrontal and parietal cortices. This is discussed more fully in Chapter 6.

Dyspraxia is the inability to perform skilled actions despite intact basic motor and sensory abilities. The problem is with the planning and initiation of movement, which depends on the frontal and parietal lobes (see Ch. 6).

Dressing apraxia is difficulty in dressing caused by an inability to successfully navigate the spatial arrangement of clothes in relation to the body. This is a problem with perception rather than a motor dysfunction and, therefore, has a different anatomical basis.

Perception

Essentially perception involves the successful deduction of what is being represented in all sensory domains. It is covered more fully in Chapter 8.

Deficits are usually seen in visual perception. This includes the neglect syndromes also described in Chapter 8.

COGNITIVE DEVELOPMENT

Cognitive development

Cognitive development in children is assessed by learning tests and by observation of their behaviour. There are set 'milestones', which children should have achieved by certain ages.

Many factors influence the rate of cognitive development and the level that an individual ultimately achieves. The chemical environment is crucial both in utero and in early childhood, as is nutritional status during this period. Depending on how cognitive function is assessed, the amount and quality of education will influence final performance.

Ability of the newborn

The newborn's cognitive abilities include:

- Auditory discrimination as well as localization of the sound source. This is tested by observing head movements.
- Operant learning where, if certain responses are rewarded, babies will be more likely to make those responses.
- The production of smooth pursuit eye movements.
- Preferential interest in certain stimuli (e.g. human faces).

The newborn's motor capabilities are basic motor programmes (e.g. reaching movements if body-weight is supported).

The social behaviour of the newborn is to interact with the primary care-giver by imitation of facial movements.

Motor changes

New motor abilities emerge in a set pattern, with the rate of appearance varying according to stimulation and encouragement of the child. Certain conditions (e.g. Down's syndrome) will adversely affect the attainment of these milestones.

Visual input is crucial to the natural development of reaching movements. Babies who are congenitally blind need special devices, such as echo locators, to develop appropriate reaching movements.

The fundamental changes in motor development as the child gets older are greater control over fine movements and greater fluidity of a series of movements.

Perceptual changes

Changes in perceptual ability involve learning how to interpret sensory information. One milestone is the development of depth perception shown by Gibson's visual cliff experiment. An infant is allowed to freely explore a table, part of which is transparent revealing a drop to floor level. In very young infants, there is no sign of fear to the apparent risk of falling. During the period of crawling, however, infants will not cross the visual cliff onto the transparent area.

The rate of acquisition of knowledge about the environment limits the development of perceptual abilities and will also affect attentional mechanisms.

Overall scheme of cognitive development: Piaget's theory

Sensorimotor stage: 0–2 years

During this stage exploration of the environment occurs and children learn to distinguish themselves from it (the beginnings of self-awareness). This stage is also characterized by the development of object permanence, where infants understand that objects still exist when they can no longer perceive them (e.g. after removing them from the visual field). For Piaget, this was the basis of thought because it demonstrates that infants can hold representations of objects in their minds.

Preoperational stage: 2–7 years

Children at this stage are able to engage in symbolic play – using language and pictures to represent experiences. There is a decline in egocentricity and they can empathize with others.

Concrete operational thought: 7–11 years

This stage is characterized by the development of conservation, where children can appreciate that some aspects of objects remain the same, despite changes in appearance. This is displayed with the pencils test. Two identical pencils are placed so that they have their bases and tips aligned. One is then moved relative to the other so that it looks longer than the other (if one ignores the fact that the bases have moved relative to each other). Children who conserve will not infer that, when the pencils have moved, one must be longer than the other. Children at this stage are capable of logical thought – seeing relations between things and applying rules to new situations – but they cannot undertake tasks involving abstract reasoning.

Formal operational thought: 11–15 years

At this stage, the ability of abstract reasoning develops.

Language acquisition

The process of language acquisition is not well understood, but current thinking (based on the theories of Chomsky and Pinker) is that there is a pre-programmed way of understanding language construction.

This inbuilt understanding of the workings of language allows rapid learning at a young age, no matter how that language is presented (i.e. learning and ease of use is the same for verbal and sign systems; deaf children learn sign language more quickly and use it in a far richer fashion than their hearing parents).

Children with delayed speech should undergo urgent investigation for hearing deficits, as language may be more difficult to acquire as the child gets older.

COGNITIVE DEGENERATION

The ageing brain

The gross changes in the brain include reductions in total volume, weight, size of gyri and an increase in ventricular size. This is due to atrophy (i.e. shrinkage of the brain) associated with nerve cell loss. There are also changes in the distribution of cell types. There is a steady decrease in the number of large neurons, accompanied by an increase in both small neurons and glial cells from the age of 20 years onwards.

Neuronal death may be due to pre-programming, sensitivity to certain factors or accumulated mutations.

Successful ageing

A decline in mental function is not an inevitable consequence of ageing. Compensatory sprouting of dendrites by remaining neurons can help to maintain the total number of synaptic connections. This process is called reactive synaptogenesis.

Reactive synaptogenesis explains why there is an increase in the length of dendrites in hippocampal granule cells between middle and old age. The mean dendritic length begins to fall back after 80 years, suggesting that there is a limit to how long this process can continue protecting against the effects of cell loss.

Psychological aspects of ageing

The normal changes in cognitive function begin at between 50 and 60 years of age and comprise:

- Reduction in the ability to perform problem-solving tasks, particularly if the problems are very novel or involve switching between different types of response.
- Slowing of responses in certain cognitive tests, due to reductions in decision speed rather than motor function.
- Memory function decreases, affecting visual information more than verbal information, and recall more than recognition.
- Alterations of motor functions (particularly proprioceptive dysfunction, changes in gait and muscle weakness).

Often, there are changes in social functioning, so-called disengagement behaviour, where there is withdrawal from social contact. This may be caused by a lack of opportunity for social contact due to physical limitations on travel or financial limitations.

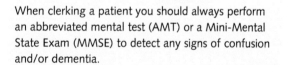

HINTS AND TIPS

When clerking a patient you should always perform an abbreviated mental test (AMT) or a Mini-Mental State Exam (MMSE) to detect any signs of confusion and/or dementia.

Mood changes after the age of 60 years typically include depression and anxiety as reactions against a perceived loss of a role in society, loss of social support and bereavement. This should not be assumed to be 'normal'.

Basic pathological processes within the central nervous system

Objectives

In this chapter you will learn about:

- The clinical features of raised and low intracranial pressure.
- The difference between vasogenic and cytotoxic oedema.
- The principles and primary types of cerebral herniation.
- The pathological processes underlying demyelinating and degenerative diseases in the nervous system.
- The pathophysiology and classification of epilepsy and the mechanism of action of common antiepileptic drugs.
- How malignancy can affect the nervous system.
- How infection manifests in the nervous system.
- How metabolic disorders affect the nervous system.

INTRACRANIAL PRESSURE CHANGES AND CEREBRAL BLOOD FLOW

The bones of the cranium fuse in the first 2 years of life, making the skull a rigid structure with a fixed volume. Intracranial pressure is determined by the volume of the three contents of the skull – brain, cerebrospinal fluid and blood. None of these are compressible or expandable. Therefore, for intracranial pressure to remain stable a change in the volume of any one of them must be accompanied by an equal and opposite change in the other two. This compensatory mechanism has a limited capacity in terms of speed and magnitude (Fig. 14.1), and its failure results in an increase or decrease in the intracranial pressure (Fig. 14.2). Cerebral blood flow depends on vascular resistance and blood pressure. Within the fixed volume of the skull, intracranial pressure must be considered. Normally, cerebral blood flow changes in response to the energy requirements of brain tissue. There are two types of regulatory mechanism that serve to maintain cerebral blood flow at an appropriate level:

- Chemoregulation – build-up of metabolic by-products, decrease in extracellular pH, decreased $P\text{O}_2$ and increased $P\text{CO}_2$ all result in cerebral vasodilatation. Conversely, increased extracellular pH, decreased $P\text{CO}_2$ and decreased metabolic by-products result in vasoconstriction.
- Autoregulation – a change in cerebral perfusion pressure results in an appropriate compensatory change in vessel calibre (i.e. decreased cerebral perfusion pressure causes cerebral vasodilatation whereas increased cerebral perfusion pressure results in vasoconstriction).
- Autoregulation means that cerebral perfusion pressure can fluctuate within certain limits without causing a significant change in cerebral blood flow. This system fails when cerebral perfusion pressure exceeds 160 mm Hg or falls below 60 mm Hg.
- Autoregulation is impaired in the damaged brain (e.g. after subarachnoid haemorrhage or trauma). Consequently, a decrease in cerebral perfusion pressure is more likely to result in reduced cerebral blood flow and secondary ischaemia. Equally, high cerebral perfusion may increase cerebral blood flow, damage the blood–brain barrier and cause cerebral oedema.

Physiological compensatory mechanisms for an expanding intracranial mass lesion:

- Immediate – cerebrospinal fluid outflow to the lumbar theca and decreased cerebral blood flow
- Delayed – decreased extracellular fluid.

Cerebral oedema

The skull contains approximately 900–1200 mL of intracellular and 100–150 mL of extracellular fluid. An increase in the volume of either of these two components results in cerebral oedema.

The pathogenesis of cerebral oedema can be divided into vasogenic, cytotoxic and interstitial. These types usually coexist to variable degrees, depending on the primary pathology.

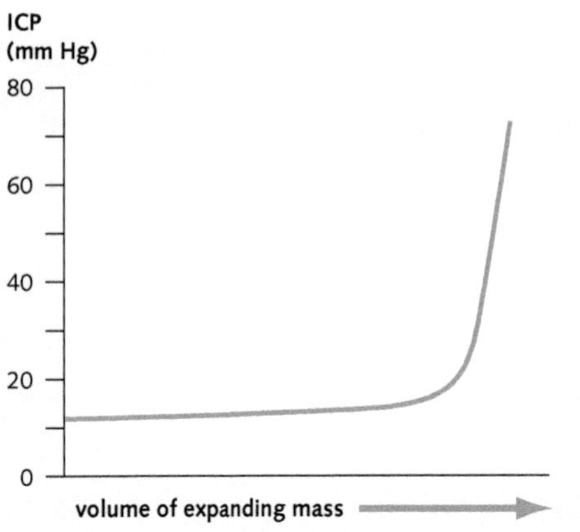

Fig. 14.1 Graph of intracranial pressure against volume of an expanding mass. Compensatory mechanisms initially maintain a normal intracranial pressure. Later, these mechanisms fail and small increases in volume result in larger and larger increases in intracranial pressure.

Vasogenic oedema is usually responsive to treatment with corticosteroids, osmotic diuretics and hyperventilation, whereas cytotoxic oedema is often resistant to these therapies. Ultimately, successful treatment relies on identifying and treating the underlying cause.

Vasogenic oedema

This is intercellular oedema that results from increased permeability of the capillary endothelial cells. It is caused either by defects in tight endothelial cell junctions or increased active transport, allowing protein-rich plasma to enter the extracellular space.

Vasogenic oedema develops around tumours, abscesses and plaques of multiple sclerosis and predominantly affects white matter. It may also be seen in trauma, infection and ischaemic areas.

Cytotoxic oedema

This is an intracellular oedema resulting from damage to the ATP-dependent sodium pump, leading to the accumulation of sodium, calcium and water within neurons and glia. Cytotoxic oedema affects both grey and white matter and is commonly seen early in ischaemic brain damage and dilutional hyponatraemia.

Interstitial oedema

This is an extracellular oedema seen particularly in hydrocephalus. It results from the extravasation of the cerebrospinal fluid through the ependymal cells into the extracellular space of the periventricular white matter.

Hydrocephalus

This is covered in Chapter 1.

Clinical effects of raised intracranial pressure

- Headache – worse in mornings and aggravated by stooping/bending
- Vomiting – occurs with sudden rise in intracranial pressure
- Papilloedema – occurs in a proportion of patients.

Raised intracranial pressure produces symptoms and signs, but does not cause neuronal damage until cerebral blood flow is compromised. However, damage does result from brain shift and subsequent herniation.

HINTS AND TIPS

Cushing's triad is the triad of widening pulse pressure (with a rising systolic BP and a diastolic that remains the same or rises slightly), change in respiratory pattern (irregular respirations), and bradycardia. It is sign of increased intracranial pressure.

Fig. 14.2 Clinical features of raised and low intracranial pressure

	Causes	Symptoms and signs
Raised intracranial pressure	Space-occupying masses (e.g. tumour, haematoma, abscess), increase in brain water content (oedema), increase in cerebral blood flow volume (e.g. vasodilatation, venous outflow obstruction), increased CSF volume (excessive production, impaired absorption)	Early morning headache and vomiting (often without nausea), dizziness, blurred vision, diplopia (usually caused by VI nerve palsy as a false localizing sign), papilloedema, focal sensory and motor neurological signs, depressed consciousness, coma, falling pulse rate and rising blood pressure
Low intracranial pressure	Decrease in cerebral blood flow volume (e.g. dehydration, blood loss), decrease in CSF volume (e.g. CSF otorrhoea and rhinorrhoea, lumbar puncture, surgical CSF shunting)	Headache and nausea mainly on sitting or standing

CSF, cerebrospinal fluid

Cerebral herniation

The brain is divided into semi-separate compartments by the following dural infoldings:

- The falx cerebri (which extends in the midline between the two cerebral hemispheres)
- The tentorium cerebelli (the posterior bifurcation of the falx extending laterally over the superior face of the cerebellum with an elongated opening through which the brainstem passes).

When intracranial volume increases, either due to increased intracranial pressure or to a space-occupying lesion, the surrounding brain tissue is pushed away and forced to herniate into an adjacent compartment. Cerebral herniation is divided into four types, as shown in Figures 14.3 and 14.4.

Treatment of raised intracranial pressure

The aim is to treat the cause. If this proves unsuccessful there are several methods of artificially reducing intracranial pressure. Treatment is started when mean intracranial pressure (measured by ventricular catheter or a surface pressure recording device) exceeds 25 mm Hg:

- Mannitol infusion – reduces intracranial pressure by producing an osmotic gradient between plasma and brain tissue. Best reserved for emergency situations.
- Cerebrospinal fluid withdrawal – difficult to achieve in practice.
- Sedatives (e.g. propofol) – if standard methods fail, sedation may help in carefully controlled situations.
- Controlled hyperventilation – lowering $P\text{CO}_2$ to below 3.5 kPa causes vasoconstriction and a consequent reduction in intracranial pressure. Caution is required as the resultant reduction in cerebral blood flow may aggravate ischaemic brain damage.
- Decompressive craniectomy – this technique is associated with high morbidity.
- Hypothermia – cooling to 34°C lowers intracranial pressure.
- Steroids – help to decrease intracellular pressure by stabilizing cell membranes. Useful for treating patients with oedema surrounding intracranial tumours.

HINTS AND TIPS

Lumbar puncture should not be performed if there is clinical suspicion of raised intracranial pressure. If intracranial pressure is raised, lumbar puncture causes rapid decompression which may cause herniation of the cerebellar tonsils ('coning') with consequent brainstem haemorrhage and death. If in any doubt, a computed tomography scan or magnetic resonance image of the head should be obtained first.

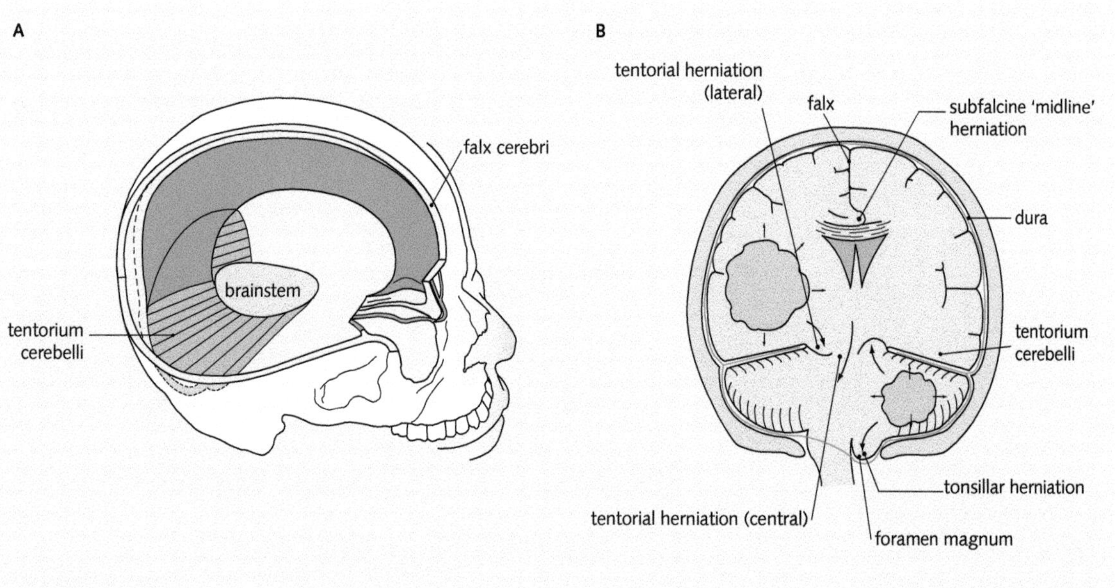

Fig. 14.3 A, Infoldings of the dura mater which compartmentalize the brain tissue. B, Cerebral herniation. (Modified from Lindsay KW, Bone I (1991) *Neurology and Neurosurgery Illustrated.* Churchill Livingstone).

Fig. 14.4 Types of cerebral herniation

Clinical type	Aetiology	Clinical signs
Type 1: subfalcine herniation	Unilateral hemispheric SOL causing that hemisphere to be compressed beneath the falx	Frequently seen radiologically, does not usually cause any clinical signs
Type 2: lateral tentorial herniation	Unilateral hemispheric SOL causing the uncus of the temporal lobe to herniate through the tentorial hiatus; may progress to type 3	Ipsilateral third nerve palsy, ipsilateral hemiplegia (contralateral cerebral peduncle compression)
Type 3: central tentorial herniation	Midline SOL, very large unilateral hemispheric SOL, or bilateral hemispheric diffuse swelling causing a vertical displacement of the diencephalon through the tentorial hiatus; may progress to type 4	Impaired upward gaze (pretectum and superior colliculi compression), hemianopia (occipital lobe infarction), hemi/quadriparesis (cerebral peduncle compression), rising blood pressure and bradycardia (aqueduct compression and hydrocephalus), depressed consciousness and respiration (brainstem compression), coma
type 4: tonsillar herniation	Unilateral subtentorial SOL causing herniation of the cerebellar tonsils through the foramen magnum	Neck pain, tonic extension of the limbs, cardiac arrhythmia and rising blood pressure, depressed consciousness and respiration, coma

SOL, space-occupying lesion

DEMYELINATION

In demyelinating disorders of the central nervous system, myelin and/or oligodendroglia are affected, whereas axons are spared.

In myelinated axons, sodium channels are only present at the nodal regions with the rest of the axon electrically insulated. If myelin is removed, the current density at the nodal regions is reduced because current escapes across the bare membrane (see Fig. 14.5).

A decreased current density depolarizes the nodal region more slowly than normal, leading to reduced conduction velocity. Normal activation of the target site depends upon the timing as well as the number of action potentials in a population of fibres. Therefore, any disruption in timing leads to disruption of function.

If more than one node is demyelinated, the severe decrease in longitudinal current may cause the current to fade along the length of the axon as more and more is lost across the membrane. This will stop the axon

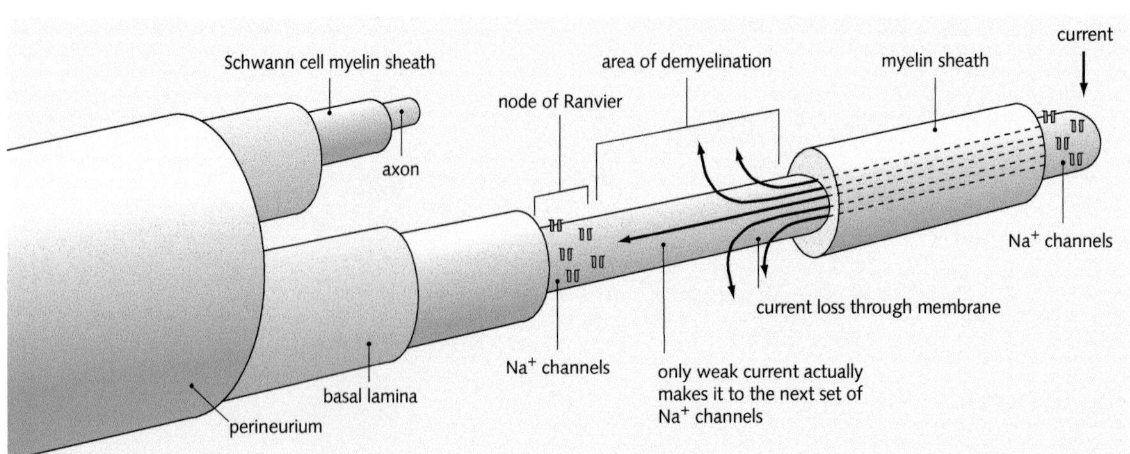

Fig. 14.5 The effect of demyelination on current flow in an axon.

from depolarizing to its threshold level, leading to conduction block.

Myelin disorders can be classified into two types:

- Myelin is inherently abnormal or was never formed appropriately (e.g. leukodystrophy). These diseases tend to present during infancy or early childhood.
- Normal myelin breaks down due to a pathological insult (e.g. multiple sclerosis).

Multiple sclerosis

Multiple sclerosis is a chronic disorder in which episodes of inflammatory demyelination affect any part of the central nervous system (CNS). It has an extremely variable course with a tendency towards progressive disability. Multiple sclerosis cannot be diagnosed until the patient has suffered multiple attacks at different neuroanatomical sites.

Incidence and prevalence

The incidence and the prevalence of multiple sclerosis vary markedly between different geographical areas and different population groups. The UK annual incidence is about 1 per 20 000 and the prevalence is about 1 per 1000. Multiple sclerosis occurs most commonly in temperate climates with prevalence varying according to latitude (in Shetland [60°N] the rate is 309/100 000 where as in Cornwall [51°N] it is 63/100 000). Peak age is 20–40 years and women are affected more than men.

Aetiology

The aetiology of multiple sclerosis is unknown, but is likely to involve environmental factors (e.g. a viral infection) in genetically susceptible patients. There is a weak human leukocyte antigen association, leading to theories of an autoimmune basis. The pathological hallmarks are scattered demyelinating lesions ('plaques') in perivascular areas of the white matter of the brain and the spinal cord.

Symptoms and signs

Depending on the anatomical location of the plaques, four main groups of symptoms are recognized:

- Optic nerve – attacks of optic neuritis presenting with blurring of vision associated with periorbital and retro-orbital pain exacerbated by eye movements, reduced visual acuity, central scotoma, afferent pupillary defect and a pink and swollen optic disc (which becomes pale and atrophic at a later stage).
- Brainstem – diplopia; dysconjugate eye movements, particularly internuclear ophthalmoplegia; limb and gait ataxia, titubation, tremor, dysarthria and vertigo.
- Spinal cord – sensory symptoms including Lhermitte's phenomenon (electric shock-like sensation extending down the spine into the limbs on neck flexion); spastic weakness; bladder, bowel and sexual dysfunction.
- Other clinical features – dementia, euphoria and emotional lability; facial pain; painful tonic spasms; Uhthoff's phenomenon (transient worsening of symptoms following a hot bath or exercise).

Figure 14.6 relates demyelination of axons in the CNS to the clinical features of multiple sclerosis.

Investigations

Multiple sclerosis is a clinical diagnosis and no test is pathognomonic. Cerebrospinal fluid (CSF) shows oligoclonal bands in almost all cases. Evoked potentials (visual, auditory and somatosensory) may be prolonged. Magnetic resonance imaging is abnormal in almost all patients.

Treatment

Acute relapses are treated with oral or intravenous steroids. Analgesia and baclofen may reduce spasticity. Bladder symptoms may require specialist referral. Interferon beta is effective in reducing relapse rate, but has no proved effect on long-term disease progression. It is not effective in all patients and is expensive.

Prognosis

The progression of multiple sclerosis cannot be predicted, although different patterns of disease exist:

- Relapsing and remitting – 70% move through this stage during which attacks are punctuated by virtually complete recovery.
- Secondary progressive and relapsing/remitting secondary progressive – there is incomplete recovery between attacks with cumulative loss of function and increasing disability.
- Primary progressive – common in late-onset multiple sclerosis, symptoms and signs are usually spinal. There is insidious progression with no periods of remission.

Overall, about 50% of patients need help with walking after 15 years.

Other demyelinating conditions

Acute disseminated encephalomyelitis may follow many common viral infections, and causes focal brainstem and spinal cord demyelination that resembles multiple sclerosis. The prognosis is variable – from complete recovery to 25% mortality in severe cases.

Central pontine myelinolysis is associated with alcoholism and hyponatraemia. It presents acutely with pontine and medullary symptoms. Extra-pontine lesions are not uncommon. It is treated by slow correction of underlying metabolic abnormalities. Prognosis is poor.

Fig. 14.6 Pathophysiology of multiple sclerosis symptoms

Symptoms	Cellular explanation
Blindness, numbness, weakness, paralysis	Block in conduction of action potential caused by dissipation of current after demyelination
Paraesthesia (tingling)	Extracellular potassium builds up at sites of demyelination as channels exposed leak potassium. This raises membrane potential to threshold and action potential generated spontaneously (Nernst equation)
Remission of symptoms	Caused by: (a) Remyelination by oligodendrocytes (b) Use of alternative neural pathways (c) New sodium channels produced
Relapse	(a) Extension of existing lesion with exposure of membrane with few sodium channels (b) New lesion site
Lhermitte's sign (feeling of electric shock in limbs upon stretching	Lesions often form in areas of the central nervous system that are constantly being moved, such as the part of the spinal cord in the region of the cervical vertebrae. When lesioned axons are stretched they generate impulses. (A similar problem occurs in the optic nerve and flashes are seen at night when there is much less light to mask the effect of these spontaneous impulses.)

DEGENERATION

Proteinopathies

Abnormal protein aggregation is a common characteristic of many neurodegenerative diseases of the brain.

Tauopathies

Filamentous deposits made of an abnormally phosphorylated form of the microtubule-associated protein tau constitute a major defining characteristic of several neurodegenerative diseases known as tauopathies, with Alzheimer's disease being the most common example. Other tauopathies include corticobasal degeneration (CBD), progressive suranuclear palsy (PSP) and some of the recently described frontotemporal dementias (FTD).

Alzheimer's disease is the most common cause of dementia, accounting for 80% of all cases of dementia in the community. The incidence increases with age; familial cases are occasionally seen. The female:male ratio is 3:1. There is a cognitive decline affecting all aspects of cognition and personality (e.g. memory, attention, orientation, etc.). The pathology is characteristic, with intraneuronal tau aggregates (neurofibrillary tangles) and extra-cellular accumulation of ß-amyloid. Neuritic plaques are ß-amyloid deposits surrounded by degenerate neuronal processes filled with abnormal tau protein (neuritic processes).

HINTS AND TIPS

Alzheimer's disease is typified by the inability to form new memories, and is due to the deposition of neurofibrillary tangles and ß-amyloid plaques in the parahippocampal areas.

There is a characteristic decrease in brain weight and cortical atrophy (most evident in the superior and middle temporal gyri). There is marked loss of neurons, usually most prominent in the hippocampus, parahippocampal gyrus and the frontal, anterior temporal, and parietal cortices (mainly affecting glutaminergic pyramidal neurons).

Cell loss also occurs in the basal forebrain complex notably the basal nucleus (of Meynert), which gives rise to a diffuse acetylcholine projection to most of the neocortex and the medial septal nuclei, which give a diffuse cholinergic innervation to the hippocampus.

HINTS AND TIPS

Vascular dementia (so-called 'multi-infarct dementia') is characterized by a stepwise (stroke-by-stroke) deterioration in cognitive function. It accounts for $<10\%$ of cases of dementia. Diagnosis is suggested by the history and confirmed by CT scan. Treatment involves adequate blood pressure control and antiplatelet drugs such as aspirin.

Clinical features include:

- Memory impairment (particularly of recent events), apathy, poor reasoning and judgement
- Behavioural disturbance (aggression is often prominent)
- Aphasia, apraxia and spatial disorientation
- Eventually patients become mute, bedfast and incontinent.

Investigations are largely undertaken to exclude other (treatable) causes of dementia:

- Imaging (CT, MRI) which shows brain atrophy, flattening of the gyri, widening of the sulci and dilatation of the ventricles will also help to exclude vascular causes of dementia that can be prevented from progressing
- B_{12}/folate levels and thyroid function tests.

Treatment involves:

- Maintenance of general health – concurrent illnesses (including affective disorders) may exacerbate symptoms
- Avoidance of sedative drugs
- Consider using acetylcholinesterase inhibitor (e.g. donepezil) which may slow cognitive decline in some patients.

Most patients die from the complications of immobility within 5–10 years of diagnosis.

Synucleinopathies

Synucleinopathies are a diverse group of neurodegenerative disorders characterized by the development of intracellular fibrillary aggregates of α-synuclein. Examples include idiopathic Parkinson's disease (Ch. 6), dementia with Lewy bodies and multiple system atrophy (MSA). The pathogenetic mechanisms underlying these neurodegenerative disorders are unknown. Clinically, they are characterized by a chronic and progressive decline in motor, cognitive, behavioural and autonomic functions, depending on the anatomical distribution of the lesions.

Prionopathies: transmissible spongiform encephalopathies

Transmissible spongiform encephalopathies (TSEs) are characterized histopathologically by spongiform changes, neuronal cell loss and gliosis in the grey matter of the brain. In association with these changes there is deposition of amyloid composed of an altered form of a naturally occurring protein (prion protein). TSEs can be transmitted by inoculation (vCJD, kuru) but may also occur spontaneously (CJD) or as an inherited disorder (fCJD, GSS). The most common TSE in humans is Creutzfeldt–Jakob disease (CJD).

Sporadic CJD most often occurs in middle-aged to elderly people. Clinical features include a rapidly progressive dementia, characteristic EEG changes and myoclonus. Death occurs after 4–6 months on average. There is currently no effective treatment.

Variant CJD (vCJD) has been found in a small number of (mostly UK-based) patients. The causative agent appears to be the same as that which causes bovine spongiform encephalopathy (BSE) in cows. vCJD patients are typically younger than those with sporadic CJD and present with neuropsychiatric changes and sensory symptoms in the limbs. Later, there is ataxia, dementia and death (mean time to death is over 1 year). Brain pathology illustrates florid plaques containing prion proteins.

Other proteinopathies

Other proteinopathies associated with adult-onset neurodegenration include TDP-43 proteinopathy amyotrophic lateral sclerosis (ALS) and trinucleotide repeat disorders (Huntington's disease).

EPILEPSY

An epileptic seizure (fit) is a paroxysmal alteration in nervous system activity that is time limited and causes a clinically detectable event. Types of epileptic seizure are described in Figure 14.7.

Epilepsy is a condition in which more than one seizure has occurred, in the absence of abnormal metabolic states (most people will develop seizures if you make them sufficiently hyponatraemic!). Incidence is greatest in early and late life, with a prevalence of approximately 0.5%. Febrile convulsions in childhood are not classed as epilepsy although, if prolonged, they may predispose to epilepsy in later life.

Epilepsy is a clinical diagnosis and the patient is often normal on examination; a careful history is vital. It is particularly useful to obtain a history from a witness. A patient who has had a seizure with loss of consciousness may remember feeling odd (an aura) before the event (e.g. strange smells, metallic taste), and may remember feeling confused, disorientated and sleepy afterwards (the postictal phase), but will have no memory of the fit itself. Tongue-biting and urinary incontinence are infrequently seen.

Risk of another seizure within 1 year of the first is 40%, rising to 50% within 3 years.

Status epilepticus is defined as seizures occurring in series with no recovery of consciousness, or a seizure lasting more than 30 minutes. It constitutes a medical emergency, as there is a high risk of brain damage and death.

Partial (focal) epilepsy

Focal epilepsy may arise from an intracerebral structural defect and causes motor or sensory symptoms localized to one body part. This may then spread to adjacent areas as the electrical activity moves to contiguous regions of the cortex (e.g. jacksonian march). These are simple partial seizures. An underlying structural defect may be found.

Complex partial seizures usually arise in the temporal lobe. They are 'complex' because they are associated with disturbance of consciousness.

Seizures arising in the medial temporal lobe may cause disturbances of smell and taste, visual hallucinations and a sense of déjà vu. They may evolve to a tonic–clonic seizure (secondary generalization). Weakness following the event may continue for minutes to hours (Todd's paresis).

Primary generalized epilepsy

Any of the seizure types described in Figure 14.7 may occur in one patient. In a generalized tonic–clonic seizure, the tonic (increased tone) phase is a sudden tonic contraction of muscles usually with upward eye deviation. The clonic (with clonus-type activity) phase follows. Initial EEG changes are often bilateral. This condition usually has its onset in childhood. Absence (or petit mal) attacks usually consist of a brief interruption of activity, sometimes with complex motor activity (such as fumbling with clothes), but without collapse. EEG during this event shows a three-per-second spike-and-wave activity.

Epilepsy syndromes

- Benign childhood epilepsy with centrotemporal spikes
- Lennox–Gastaut syndrome - this is characterized by frequent seizures and is difficult to manage
- Infantile spasms - characteristic brief episodes with shock-like flexion of arms, head and neck and drawing up of the knees (called a salaam attack). It is associated with progressive mental handicap
- Juvenile myoclonic epilepsy – a familial late-childhood-onset disease with myoclonic jerks, tonic–clonic seizures ± absence seizures, with typical interictal EEG.

Pseudoseizures

Pseudoseizures (simulated seizures) occur in up to 20% of patients referred for 'intractable epilepsy'. They may occur in association with real epilepsy or as a result of psychological disturbance.

HINTS AND TIPS

A normal interictal EEG does not exclude a diagnosis of epilepsy as 50% may be normal. CT and/or MRI is used to search for a provoking structural lesion. Blood tests to identify reversible causes, along with a toxic screen and electrocardiogram (to identify long Q-T syndromes) are important in all patients.

Antiepileptic drugs

The main epileptic drugs are outlined in Figure 14.8.

First fits are often not treated but, unless seizures are years apart, most neurologists would treat after the second event. There is a wide range of antiepileptic medications and choice depends mostly on seizure type. A major reason for differentiating partial from generalized seizures is that different drugs are effective for each. Some patients may benefit considerably from surgical removal of an epileptogenic focus in a temporal lobe. In 70% of patients epilepsy eventually remits. Trials of treatment withdrawal should be considered at an appropriate time.

Fig. 14.7 Types of epileptic seizure

Primary generalized epilepsy	Absence seizures; primary generalized tonic–clonic seizures; others: myoclonic, atypical absences; tonic, clonic and atonic seizures
Partial (focal) epilepsy ± secondary generalization	Simple partial seizure (without loss of consciousness), complex partial seizures (with disturbed consciousness)
Secondary generalized epilepsy	Due to underlying generalized cerebral abnormality
Epilepsy due to underlying focal or metabolic cause	Primary intracranial lesions (tumour, stroke, infections, trauma), metabolic (hypoglycaemia, hypomagnesaemia, liver failure), drugs (and most in overdose), drug withdrawal (alcohol, benzodiazepines), toxins (alcohol, carbon monoxide)

Fig. 14.8 Antiepileptic drugs

Drug	Indications	Mechanism of action	Side effects	Notes/cautions
Phenytoin	All forms of epilepsy except absence seizures; status epilepticus	Blocks voltage-gated Na^+ channels. It has a higher affinity for channels in the inactivated state. This state is prolonged, preventing the channel from opening and stopping the neuron from firing rapidly. Channel block is use-dependent. At higher frequencies more channels are cycling through the inactivated state. Consequently the block is more likely to occur in neurons within a seizure focus. It does not prevent the onset of an epileptic discharge, but stops it from involving other areas	Nausea, dizziness, nystagmus, ataxia, slurred speech, gum hypertrophy, allergic reactions (rash, hepatitis, lymphadenopathy), megaloblastic anaemia, hirsutism, teratogenesis (cleft palate)	Hepatic P_{450} enzyme inducer (increases the metabolism of oral contraceptives, anticoagulants, dexamethasone and pethidine). Variable oral absorption. It has a narrow therapeutic index and the relationship between dose and plasma concentration is non-linear; small dose increases in some patients may produce large rises in plasma concentrations with acute toxic effects. Monitoring plasma concentration assists dosage adjustment
Carbamazepine	Partial and secondary generalized tonic–clonic seizures, primary generalized tonic–clonic seizures	As for phenytoin	Nausea, rash, dizziness, visual disturbances, ataxia, leucopenia, cholestatic jaundice, hepatitis, cardiac conduction disturbances, gynaecomastia	Well absorbed orally. Half life 25–60 hours when first given. P_{450} enzyme inducer (similar interactions to phenytoin). Induces its own metabolism, hence half-life decreases if taken regularly
Sodium valproate	Drug of choice in primary generalized epilepsy, generalized absences and myoclonic seizures	As for phenytoin. It also increases GABA content and GABA action	Nausea, weight gain, transient hair loss, thrombocytopenia. Rarely, hepatic dysfunction	Well absorbed orally (half-life 10–15 hours). Interacts with other central nervous system depressants (e.g. alcohol), potentiating their effects
Ethosuximide	Absence seizures	Unclear	Nausea, vomiting, diarrhoea, anorexia, weight loss, drowsiness, dizziness, ataxia, irritability	May make tonic–clonic seizures worse
Lamotrigine	Monotherapy and adjunctive treatment of partial seizures and primary and secondary generalized tonic–clonic seizures	Inhibits voltage-sensitive Na^+ channels, thereby stabilizing neuronal membranes and modulating presynaptic transmitter release of excitatory amino acids	Skin rash, hypersensitivity syndrome, hepatic dysfunction, blood disorders, tremor, agitation, nystagmus, arthralgia	Valproate increases plasma-lamotrigine concentration whereas enzyme inducing antiepileptics reduce it

Continued

Fig. 14.8 Antiepileptic drugs – cont'd

Drug	Indications	Mechanism of action	Side effects	Notes/cautions
Levetiracetam	Monotherapy and adjunctive treatment of partial seizures. Adjunctive therapy of myoclonic and tonic–clonic seizures	Unknown	Dyspepsia, weight changes, cough, ataxia, tremor, depression, visual disturbances, thrombocytopenia	
Phenobarbital	All forms of epilepsy except absence seizures; status epilepticus	Barbiturate. Binds to $GABA_A$ receptors, potentiating the effect of normal GABA release. Reduces glutamate-mediated excitation	Cholestasis, hepatitis, hypotension, respiratory depression, behavioural disturbances, nystagmus	Enzyme inducer. Tolerance occurs
Benzodiazepines	Status epilepticus	Potentiate the effects of GABA binding	Sedation, hypotension, apnoea	

Epilepsy and driving

First fit/solitary fit:

- 1 year off driving (fit free) with medical review before restarting. If another fit occurs during this time, the patient must wait 1 year from that fit before review.

Loss of consciousness without known cause:

- As above.

Seizures during sleep:

- After one seizure, regulations as above. If all attacks for at least 3 years have been during sleep, and the patient has never had an awake attack, driving is allowed.

Withdrawal of antiepileptic medication:

- Advise not to drive (but not a legal obligation on the patient's part) for 6 months from time of withdrawal. If further seizures occur the above regulations apply.

Status epilepticus

This is a medical emergency. Always consider whether the patient is pregnant, as it may be an eclamptic fit, which will only be cured by delivery of the baby. Otherwise, correct reversible causes (give a glucose infusion, and replace fluids). The initial treatment is with benzodiazepines (lorazepam or diazepam) ± phenytoin. If these therapies do not stop seizure activity, an anaesthetist is required to supervise the administration of a barbiturate such as phenobarbital.

NEOPLASMS OF THE CENTRAL NERVOUS SYSTEM

Primary brain tumours

The annual incidence of primary brain tumours in adults is 7 per 100 000, accounting for about 5% of all neoplasms in the body. However, brain tumours are the most common solid tumours that occur in children. The prevalence of the different tumour types and their anatomical location varies with age:

- Adults: gliomas, metastases and meningiomas:
  - 80–85% supratentorial compartment
  - 15–20% infratentorial compartment.
- Children: medulloblastomas and cerebellar astrocytomas:
  - 40% supratentorial compartment
  - 60% infratentorial compartment.

Clinical features depend on site of the tumour and speed of growth and can be divided into three main categories:

- Features of raised intracranial pressure (headache, vomiting and papilloedema)
- Focal symptoms and signs, the nature of which depends on the anatomical site of the tumour and whether the tumour effect is irritative or destructive
- False localizing signs due to raised intracranial pressure (e.g. VIth nerve palsy).

Neuroepithelial tumours

Astrocytomas

Astrocytomas are the commonest primary tumours of the brain. They occur at any age, but most commonly between 40 and 60 years. Male:female is 2:1. Astrocytomas occur with equal incidence throughout the frontal, temporal and parietal lobes, but are uncommon in the occipital lobe. There are four pathological grades (Kernohan I–IV):

- Low-grade astrocytoma (grades I and II) - commonly seen in children/young adults
- Malignant astrocytoma (grade III)
- Glioblastoma multiformis (grade IV).

Malignant astrocytomas are far more common than benign ones.

Oligodendroglioma

Oligodendroglioma is a slow-growing tumour with low malignancy grade. It affects a younger age-group (30–50 years) and is most common in the frontal lobe. Imaging reveals a well-demarcated tumour, frequently with areas of calcification.

Medulloblastoma

Medulloblastoma is the commonest malignant solid tumour of childhood (4–8 years). It arises from embryonic tissue in the cerebellar vermis and may seed through the cerebrospinal fluid pathways to other parts of the cranium or the spinal cord.

Ependymoma

Ependymoma is the second most common tumour of childhood, although it is also found in individuals in their early 20s. It occurs throughout the ventricular system or the spinal canal but is particularly common in the fourth ventricle and in the caudal part of the spinal cord. It frequently infiltrates surrounding tissues. Fourth ventricle ependymomas usually present with symptoms of intermittent hydrocephalus, ataxia, vertigo and vomiting.

Meninges

Meningioma

Meningioma is a benign tumour arising from the dura. It generally compresses (rather than invades) neural tissues, although malignant forms may invade underlying brain. Incidence peaks between 40 and 60 years of age. It is most common in the sylvian region, the parasagittal surface of the parietal and frontal lobes, the olfactory grooves, the lesser wings of the sphenoid, the tuberculum sellae, the cerebellopontine angle and the thoracic spinal cord. Imaging reveals a well-circumscribed lesion with occasional calcification. Surgery is the mainstay of treatment.

HINTS AND TIPS

Some meningiomas contain oestrogen receptors and may enlarge markedly in pregnancy.

Nerve sheath tumour

Primary nerve sheath tumours include neurofibromas (which enlarge the nerve from within) and schwannomas (which grow at the periphery of the nerve stretching the nerve over the surface of the tumour). Schwannoma is a benign, slow-growing tumour that commonly develops in cranial nerve VIII (often called an acoustic neuroma/vestibular schwannoma). It tends to present in mid-life and is more common in females. Neurofibromas are common in neurofibromatosis syndrome (most commonly type 1), and there is a higher incidence of malignant transformation when compared to sporadic neurofibroma.

Primary central nervous system lymphoma

This tumour type is becoming more common with increasing numbers of immunosuppressed patients. Primary central nervous system lymphoma (PCNSL) are often periventricular and may be multiple. They are aggressive tumours, and account for up to 10% of CNS complications in AIDS patients.

Pituitary adenoma

Pituitary adenoma is a benign tumour that presents with neurological or endocrinological symptoms. Large tumours usually present with headache, bitemporal hemianopia (from upward pressure on the optic chiasm), and occasionally hypopituitarism. Smaller tumours present with hyperprolactinaemia and less commonly with acromegaly/gigantism, Cushing's syndrome and thyrotoxicosis.

Other tissues

- Germ cells - germinoma, teratoma
- Tumours of maldevelopment - craniopharyngioma, epidermoid/dermoid cyst, colloid cyst
- Local extension from adjacent tumours - chordoma, glomus jugulare tumour.

Metastatic brain tumours

Metastatic brain tumours are around eight times more common than primary brain malignancies. Approximately 20% of patients dying of other tumours will have intracranial metastases, 25% of which are asymptomatic. The primary tumours are predominantly bronchus, breast, bowel and melanoma.

Presenting features are similar to those of primary brain tumours but the lesions are often multiple. On CT and MRI they have a round and well-circumscribed appearance, often with surrounding oedema.

Effects of systemic cancer on the central nervous system

- Direct invasion from adjacent structures
- Metastatic disease
- Non-metastatic 'remote effect' (paraneoplastic syndromes):
    - Immunologically mediated – cerebellar dysfunction, visual dysfunction, sensory neuropathy, opsoclonus
    - Lambertz–Eaton myasthenic syndrome
    - Limbic encephalitis.
- Others (opportunistic infections, dermatomyositis, inappropriate antidiuretic hormone secretion).

INFECTIONS OF THE CENTRAL NERVOUS SYSTEM

Meningitis

Acute bacterial meningitis and aseptic meningitis are covered in Chapter 1.

Intracranial abscess

Intracranial abscesses are rare in developed countries.

Brain abscess

The routes of bacterial invasion are:

- Direct extension from middle ear, sinus or tooth infections
- Haematogenous spread: subacute bacterial endocarditis, right-to-left heart shunts, bronchiectasis
- Skull fracture/penetrating trauma to the skull.

Common causative organisms are:

- Streptococci (*Streptococcus milleri* commonly from sinus infections)
- *Bacillus fragilis* (from ear infections)
- Anaerobic bacteria from the oropharynx.

Clinical features

- Febrile illness
- Seizures
- Focal neurological signs
- Altered consciousness
- Signs of raised intracranial pressure.

Investigations

- Brain abscesses are readily evident on CT or magnetic resonance imaging. A characteristic ring enhancement is usually seen
- Evidence of systemic infection (raised white cell count, positive blood cultures)
- Look for the underlying cause (consider echocardiography, chest X-ray)
- Note that lumbar puncture is contraindicated and may be fatal.

Treatment

- Urgent surgical aspiration or excision
- Antibiotic therapy (broad spectrum with good CNS penetration)
- Lower intracranial pressure (mannitol, hyperventilation, bed tilted to 'head up' position)
- Mortality is high (10–15%).

Extradural (epidural) abscess

Extradural (epidural) abscesses usually result from osteomyelitis of the cranial bone or extension of infection from the frontal or mastoid sinuses. They cause intense local pain and oedema of the scalp.

Subdural abscess

Subdural abscess is a serious complication of paranasal sinus infection or cerebral abscess. It results in cortical vein thrombosis with a widespread neurological deficit. Seizures are common. The prognosis is poor.

Spinal abscess

Spinal abscesses are epidural in two-thirds of cases. Half of cases result from haematogenous spread of skin or urinary tract infections, and the remainder from direct spread of vertebral osteomyelitis. *Staphylococcus* is the commonest causative organism followed by *Escherichia coli* and *Proteus*. Clinical features are:

- Severe localized spinal pain
- Fever
- Signs of spinal cord compression.

MRI is the investigation of choice for spinal imaging. Spinal abscesses should be treated with immediate surgical decompression and antibiotics.

Chronic meningoencephalitis

Tuberculous meningitis

Tuberculous meningitis is uncommon in developed countries. It is more common in socially and economically deprived communities. Clinical features include:

- Prolonged prodromal illness followed by slowly evolving meningeal symptoms

- Adhesive arachnoiditis causing cranial nerve palsies and hydrocephalus
- Localized vasculitis and caseation causing focal neurological signs and seizures.

Investigations

- A head CT scan should be performed in patients with focal neurological signs or depressed consciousness.
- CSF examination shows raised lymphocyte count, high protein and low glucose.
- Ziehl–Nielsen staining occasionally reveals the presence of acid–fast bacilli, which will be confirmed by culture.

Treatment

- A combination of isoniazid, rifampicin and pyrazinamide
- Pyridoxine is given to prevent isoniazid-induced neuropathy
- Corticosteroids may also be given initially to reduce the host inflammatory response.

Mortality is high, reaching 20–30% in treated patients. Many survivors are left disabled.

Neurosyphilis

Treponema pallidum (a spirochaete) invades the CNS within 3–24 months of the primary infection in 25% of untreated cases. Although the incidence of neurosyphilis has declined, it is important to maintain a high index of suspicion since it can mimic other neurological disorders. Clinical features include:

- Asymptomatic meningeal neurosyphilis
- Meningovascular syphilis – acute hemiplegia and sudden individual cranial nerve palsies
- Tabes dorsalis – proprioceptive sensory loss, with unsteady, wide-based gait
- General paralysis (of the insane) – dementia and upper motor neuron paralysis of the limbs
- Intracranial neurosyphilitic gummata (rubbery granulomata) may cause seizures and focal neurology
- Abnormal pupils (Argyll Robertson) should be looked for, along with absent knee or ankle jerks and positive Babinski's sign.

Lyme disease

Lyme disease is a spirochaetal infection caused by *Borrelia burgdorferi*, classically after an Ixodes tick bite. It presents initially with a characteristic skin rash (erythema chronicum migrans). Fifteen per cent of patients develop neuroborreliosis, which may mimic other common neurological disorders such as:

- Chronic meningitis
- Encephalitis
- Cranial nerve palsies (particularly facial)
- Painful radiculopathy
- Peripheral neuropathy
- Mononeuritis multiplex.

Treatment is with a cephalosporin with good CNS penetration (e.g. ceftriaxone).

Viral encephalitis

Viral encephalitis is an acute febrile encephalitic illness that is often associated with a meningeal component. It can be caused by many viruses, including mumps, herpes simplex and zoster, coxsackie virus and echoviruses. Worldwide problems include HIV encephalitis which can be associated with AIDS-related dementia, rabies, West Nile fever and Japanese encephalitis. Herpes simplex encephalitis (HSE) is particularly important because it is treatable. Clinical features include:

- Headache, fever, altered consciousness
- Occasionally, acute psychiatric symptoms (delusions, hallucination), seizures or focal neurological signs
- Hemispheric signs (e.g. dysphasia, hemiparesis) are more likely in herpes simplex infection.

Investigations

- A head CT scan or MRI excludes space-occupying lesions and may show focal abnormalities in the affected lobes (particularly the temporal lobe in HSE).
- Cerebrospinal fluid examination shows a raised lymphocyte count, with slightly raised protein and normal glucose, but may be entirely normal.
- Electroencephalogram (EEG) shows diffuse slow activity (delta waves), with focal periodic complexes (in HSE).
- Blood and cerebrospinal fluid may show rising viral antibody titres.
- Viruses may be identified in the cerebrospinal fluid.

Prognosis varies according to the causative virus. Aciclovir is effective in HSE and is relatively non-toxic. It should be used whenever this diagnosis is suspected. If untreated, the overall mortality of HSE is approximately 70%, which can be reduced to 20% with aciclovir.

Other virus-induced neurological diseases

For clinical purposes, viral illnesses are best considered by the clinical syndrome they produce (Fig. 14.9).

Fungal infections

Fungi are frequently the cause of opportunistic infections in immunocompromised patients, particularly in those with HIV infection. The commonest fungi

Fig. 14.9 Other virus-induced neurological diseases

Virus	Neurological syndrome	Principal symptoms
Varicella zoster	Shingles	Painful vesicular eruption in dermatomal distribution
Retroviruses HTLV1, HIV	Tropical spastic paraparesis, AIDS	Spastic paraparesis, meningitis, myelopathy, neuropathy, dementia
Measles	Acute: meningoencephalitis; chronic: subacute sclerosing, panencephalitis (SSPE)	Deteriorating intellect, seizures, pyramidal signs
Rabies	Rabies	Psychiatric symptoms, (affective disorders), hydrophobia/aerophobia, hyper-reflexia and spasticity or ascending paralysis mimicking Guillan–Barré syndrome
Papoviruses (JC, SV40)	Progressive multifocal leukodystrophy	Dementia in an immunocompromized patient
Arboviruses	Post-encephalitic parkinsonism	Parkinsonian with dystonic movement disorders
Rubella	Progresses rubella encephalitis	Mental retardation, seizures, optic atrophy, cerebellar and pyramidal signs
Poliovirus	Poliomyelitis	Meningeal irritation, asymmetrical paralysis without sensory involvement

associated with CNS infection in the UK are *Cryptococcus, Nocardia, Candida* and *Aspergillus*. Fungal infection commonly presents with subacute meningitis complicated by cortical thrombophlebitis and cerebral abscesses. Cerebrospinal fluid examination shows moderate polymorphonuclear leucocytosis, increased protein and low glucose. The causative fungi can be demonstrated on Gram or Indian-ink staining, or by using special culture techniques.

Treatment is with antifungal agents, but mortality and morbidity are high.

Protozoan infection

Toxoplasma

Toxoplasma gondii is an intracellular protozoan parasite. Humans are occasionally infected through the ingestion of raw uncooked meat or cat faeces, or by the transplacental route. Congenital toxoplasmosis (caused by transplacental transmission) presents with hydrocephalus, hepatosplenomegaly, retino-choroiditis and thrombocytopenia.

Acquired toxoplasmosis occurs in immunocompromised patients (particularly in AIDS), with features of meningoencephalitis, seizures, focal neurological signs and depressed consciousness. Head CT scanning in acquired toxoplasmosis shows characteristic contrast-enhancing lesions.

Toxoplasma immunoglobulin G antibodies are found in most patients. Brain biopsy is diagnostic. Mortality is very high (70%).

Malaria

Cerebral malaria, resulting in a haemorrhagic encephalitis, is caused by *Plasmodium falciparum*. The main clinical features consist of fever and malaise, followed 2–3 weeks after initial infection by severe headache, delirium, seizures, progressive stupor leading to coma and, occasionally, focal neurological signs. The diagnosis is established by seeing malarial parasites in erythrocytes on a thick and thin blood film. The brain is swollen and there is widespread petechial haemorrhages. Treatment is with intravenous quinine. Mortality is high (22%).

METABOLIC DISORDERS AND TOXINS

Vitamin deficiencies

Nutritional vitamin deficiencies are rare in developed countries, although they can occur in chronic alcoholics or socially isolated people (the elderly or mentally ill). Vitamin deficiency can also result from disease

Fig. 14.10 Clinical features and common causes of vitamin deficiency

Vitamin	Function	Cause	Neurological sequelae
A	Essential for normal retinal and epithelial cell function	Malnutrition	Adults and children: blindness; infants: mental retardation and hydrocephalus
B_1 (thiamine)	Pyruvate metabolism	Malnutrition, alcoholism	Wernicke's encephalopathy, Korsakoff's psychosis, neuropathy
B_3 (nicotinic acid)	NAD, NADP coenzyme component	Malnutrition	Encephalopathy, neuropathy
B_6 (pyridioxine)	Cofactor in protein metabolism	Malnutrition, isoniazid treatment	Neuropathy, seizures (infants)
B_{12} (cobalamine)	Purine synthesis	Autoimmunity, ileal disease, gastrectomy, malnutrition	Dementia, myelopathy (subacute combined degeneration), neuropathy
Folic acid	Purine synthesis	Malabsorption, malnutrition	Myelopathy, neuropathy, neural tube defect
D	Calcium metabolism	Malabsorption, malnutrition, chronic renal failure	Myopathy
E	Antioxidant	Malabsorption	Cerebellar ataxia

(malabsorption, autoimmunity) or drugs (e.g. isoniazid), and is usually not limited to a single vitamin. Some common features and causes of vitamin deficiencies are shown in Figure 14.10.

Rarely, vitamin overdose (vitamin A) results in neurological complications (headache, papilloedema).

Toxins

Methanol

Poisoning with methanol causes headache, photophobia and, in severe cases, papilloedema, optic atrophy and blindness. Ethanol infusion (ethanol competes with methanol) and haemodialysis are the mainstays of treatment.

Alcohol

Neurological complications of alcoholism include:

- Acute intoxication. The effect of acute alcohol administration depends on the amount of alcohol consumed and on whether the subject is a naïve or chronic alcohol user. Symptoms range in severity from euphoria and mild incoordination to ataxia, dysarthria and confusion, to deep anaesthesia and respiratory suppression. Secondary effects of intoxication include head injury, hypoglycaemia and hyponatraemia.
- Alcohol withdrawal syndrome (tremors, hallucinations, seizures and delirium tremens). Action tremor usually reaches a peak 24–36 hours after the cessation of drinking and is promptly aborted by further alcohol intake. Hallucinations may be visual, auditory or tactile (often of spiders crawling up the wall/over the patient). Seizures occur 24–48 hours after the cessation of drinking. Delirium tremens combines the three previous features with severe autonomic overactivity (dilated pupils, pyrexia, tachycardia and sweating).
- Nutritional complications such as Wernicke–Korsakoff syndrome (caused by thiamine/vitamin B_1 deficiency) and neuropathy. Early clinical features are ataxia, oculomotor disturbances (oculomotor palsies and nystagmus) and confusion which, left untreated, can progress to coma and death. As confusion improves following treatment, the amnesic component of the syndrome emerges in which confabulation is a prominent feature. Neuropathy is a symmetrical sensorimotor axonal type.
- **Demyelination may be seen in the form of central pontine myelinolysis and Marchiafava–Bignami disease.**
- Hepatic complications (acute hepatic encephalopathy and chronic portosystemic encephalopathy).
- Other syndromes – dementia/brain atrophy; alcoholic cerebellar degeneration (characterized by gait and truncal ataxia); alcoholic myopathy (acute painful proximal myopathy); central pontine myelinolysis (acute syndrome of quadriparesis, pseudobulbar palsy occasionally associated with abnormal eye movements and 'locked-in' syndrome).

HINTS AND TIPS

In the Western world alcoholism is the major cause of nutritional polyneuropathy. Classically, this causes a 'stocking and glove' distribution of sensory loss. Weakness is more marked distally than proximally. Autonomic involvement results in postural blood pressure drop and sweating soles of feet.

Carbon monoxide poisoning

The high affinity of haemoglobin to carbon monoxide results in severe tissue hypoxia. Acute intoxication leads to acute encephalopathy with visual field defects, papilloedema and retinal haemorrhage. Many patients are left with chronic encephalopathy and parkinsonism. Hyperbaric oxygen may help to prevent this, even hours after exposure.

Heavy metals

Lead

Acute encephalopathy is seen largely in children. Chronic motor neuropathy typically presents with wrist drop.

Mercury

Mercury causes chronic encephalopathy with ataxia, dysarthria and tremor.

Manganese

Manganese poisoning causes chronic encephalopathy and parkinsonism.

Iatrogenic

Drugs

Drug-induced neurological disorders include:

- Encephalopathy (e.g. hypnotics, sedatives, antidepressants in large doses)
- Neuropathy (e.g. isoniazid, vincristine)
- Neuromuscular transmission blockade (e.g. penicillamine)
- Myopathy (e.g. steroids)
- Extrapyramidal syndrome (e.g. antipsychotic medications and antiemetics)
- Psychiatric symptoms (e.g. antiparkinsonian medications).

Radiotherapy

Neurological complications are related to the total radiation dose and the period over which it is given. Early features are related to localized oedema. Delayed features are related to necrosis, which often simulates tumour recurrence.

Neurogenetics 15

Objectives

In this chapter you will learn about:
- The genetic mechanisms responsible for inherited neurological diseases.
- The contribution of neurogenetics to multifactorial neurological disease.

INTRODUCTION

In addition to acquired diseases, there are also many inherited conditions of the nervous system. There are several reasons why the nervous system is particularly susceptible to genetic disease:

- An extremely large number of genes are expressed in the nervous system (40% of the body's 30 000 genes).
- The brain undergoes more postnatal maturation than any other organ, requiring the expression of new genes.
- Most cells in the central nervous system (CNS) do not divide. As a consequence, abnormal protein products of mutant genes are able to accumulate and cause progressive neurodegeneration.

TRINUCLEOTIDE REPEAT DISORDERS

The major genetic defect causing several neurological disorders (Fig. 15.1) is a large and abnormal expansion of three bases in the genome (a trinucleotide repeat). The mutation resides in a stretch of repetitive DNA sequence in which the number of repeat units is altered, rather than the sequence itself. Repeat sequences are found throughout the human genome in normal individuals. Disease occurs only if they alter the sequence of a mature peptide (e.g. expansion of the CAG codon for glutamine, or when repeats expand in non-coding regions and disturb DNA replication or mRNA stability).

Trinucleotide repeat disorders exhibit genetic anticipation; the disease demonstrates increasing severity (earlier age of onset, increasing morbidity) from one generation to the next. The anticipation phenomenon occurs because the replication machinery tends to increase the number of repeats in offspring. Alleles inherited from a father expand further.

Huntington's disease

Huntington's disease causes progressive, localized neuronal cell death associated with choreic movements and dementia. It is inherited as an autosomal dominant disease and is associated with increases in the CAG trinucleotide repeat sequence in the *huntingtin* gene. The prevalence is 4–7/100 000. Onset is usually in middle age and is insidious.

The pathology is covered in more detail in Chapter 6 but essentially there is neuronal loss in the caudate nucleus with a decrease in projections to other basal ganglia structures. Corticostriatal projections are also lost. Neurochemically, it involves a shortage of GABA and acetylcholine.

The clinical diagnosis is confirmed by genetic studies (to identify the CAG repeat). Magnetic resonance imaging (MRI) shows an increase in T2 signal in the caudate nucleus and positron emission tomography (PET) illustrates loss of glucose uptake in the caudate nuclei.

This is a relentless neurodegenerative disorder in which choreic movements and dementia become progressively severe. Phenothiazines or haloperidol may help control chorea in the early stages. Most patients die from an inter-current illness (e.g. respiratory tract infection secondary to aspiration) 10–20 years after diagnosis. Genetic counselling of affected families is important.

DISORDERS INVOLVING GENE MUTATIONS

Duchenne's and Becker's muscular dystrophy

Duchenne's muscular dystrophy (DMD) and Becker's muscular dystrophy (BMD) are two inherited muscle-wasting diseases (see Ch. 6) caused by mutations in the same gene on the X chromosome. DMD is the most

Fig. 15.1 Examples of neurological diseases associated with trinucleotide repeat sequences

	Repeat sequence	Normal number of repeats	Mutant number of repeats	Gene	Gene location	Inheritance
Coding repeat expansion						
Huntington's disease	CAG	6–34	> 35	*Huntingtin*	4p16	autosomal dominant
Spinocerebellar ataxia (type 1)	CAG	6–39	> 40	*Ataxin*	6p22–23	autosomal dominant
Non-coding repeat expansion						
Myotonic dystrophy	CTG	5–37	> 50	*DMPK*	19q13	autosomal dominant
Friedrich's ataxia	GAA	7–22	> 200	*Frataxin*	9q13	autosomal dominant
Fragile X mental retardation	CGG	5–52	> 200	*FMR1*	Xq27	X-linked dominant

common and most severe (lethal) muscular dystrophy. BMD is a similar but less aggressive form with milder symptoms and a later age of onset. DMD and BMD are caused by mutations that disrupt the genetic locus Xp21.2, the site of the *dystrophin* gene. The *dystrophin* gene codes for dystrophin, a structural protein found mostly in skeletal muscle. In DMD no functional dystrophin is produced whereas in BMD the mutation causes partial loss of function of dystrophin.

Evaluation for dystrophin mutations can be carried out on DNA (usually obtained from peripheral blood cells) or alternatively dystrophin may be examined directly (in muscle biopsies) by western blotting or immunostaining of muscle sections. This allows presymptomatic diagnosis in suspected cases and confirmation of diagnosis if the family history is non-corroborative. Prenatal diagnosis of at risk pregnancies is also possible.

Gene therapy offers the best hope for effective future intervention.

HINTS AND TIPS

Duchenne muscular dystrophy is characterized by delayed early motor development (between 1 and 3 years of age) followed by contractures, scoliosis, and eventual loss of ambulation (at approximately 12 years). Pseudohypertrophy of muscle (particularly the calf) occurs in 80%. The child is unable to climb stairs and when trying to rise from a crawling position will 'climb up himself (Gower's sign, indicative of pelvic weakness).

HINTS AND TIPS

Gene therapy involves the insertion of genes into an individual's cells in order to treat a disease. Typically, gene therapy aims to supplement a defective mutant allele with a functional one. This technology is young and has been used with only limited success. In DMD methods involve the use of viral vectors for *in vivo* gene transfer of *dystrophin* to dystrophic muscle.

Neurofibromatosis

Neurofibromatosis is a common neurological condition inherited in a autosomal dominant fashion (incidence 1:3000). It is part of a group of disorders called neurocutaneous syndromes in which tumours and hamartomas develop in the skin, retina and nervous system. There are two types; type I (von Recklinghausen's neurofibromatosis) (NF I) and type II (NF II).

In NF1, multiple neurofibromas develop from the neurolemmal sheaths of peripheral and cranial nerves. It has a relatively high prevalence (1 in 4000). Mutations causing NF1 occur in the gene for the protein neurofibromin, located on chromosome 17q. At least one functioning copy of the gene is required by cells in order to inhibit spontaneous tumour formation. Affected offspring inherit a mutation in the *neurofibromin* gene. Loss of function of the normal *neurofibromin* gene (inherited from an unaffected parent) is believed to cause the clinical manifestations of the disease.

NF1 mutations tend not to occur in a small enough number of gene locations to allow effective screening. Consequently, diagnosis relies almost exclusively on clinical criteria.

Clinical diagnosis requires two or more of the following:

- Six or more café-au-lait spots > 5 mm diameter (prepubertal) (> 15 mm after puberty)
- Two or more neurofibromas or one plexiform neurofibroma
- Axillary or inguinal freckles
- Optic glioma
- Two or more Lisch nodules (hamartomas of the iris)
- Osseous lesion
- First-degree relative affected by the above criteria.

Potential future therapies for NF1 may involve inhibiting neoplastic transformation or pharmacological compensation for the deficiency of *neurofibromin*.

NF II is caused by mutations on chromosome 22q. Diagnosis requires:

- Bilateral vestibular schwannomas (acoustic neuromas) on imaging
- A first-degree relative with NF II and a unilateral VIII nerve mass
- A first-degree relative with NF II and two of the following:
  - Neurofibroma
  - Meningioma
  - Glioma
  - Schwannoma
  - Posterior capsular lenticular opacity.

von Hippel–Lindau syndrome

von Hippel–Lindau (VHL) syndrome is a dominantly inherited multisystem family cancer syndrome associated with mutations of the VHL tumour suppressor gene on chromosome 3p25.

Features include:

- Cerebellar haemangioblastomas - associated with polycythaemia
- Retinal angiomas
- Phaeochromocytoma
- Renal, adrenal and pancreatic tumours
- Other vascular tumours of the central nervous system.

Studies have revealed significant heterogeneity in the type and the location of mutations within the VHL gene. Calculation of tumour risks for different types of VHL mutation have provided significant prognostic information, particularly with respect to the likelihood of phaeochromocytoma.

Morbidity and mortality from VHL syndrome can be reduced by identification and surveillance of affected and at-risk individuals so that complications are diagnosed early at a presymptomatic stage.

Channelopathies

Mutations in proteins associated with voltage-gated ion channels (sodium, potassium, calcium and chloride ion channels) and ligand-gated ion channels (GABA, glycine) have been described involving the nervous system. The disorders described include:

- Skeletal muscle - congenital myotonia and periodic paralysis
- Epilepsy syndromes
- Familial hemiplegic migraine
- Episodic ataxia.

Inherited spongiform encephalopathies

Familial forms of Creutzfeldt–Jakob disease (CJD) and all known cases of Gerstmann–Straüssler–Schenker disease (GSS) and fatal familial insomnia (both inherited spongiform encephalopathies) are linked to germline mutations in the coding region of the *PRNP* gene on chromosome 20. To date, no pathogenic mutations have been found in sporadic or infectious forms of CJD. However, there are features of genetic predisposition in iatrogenic CJD and kuru (a spongiform encephalopathy found only in members of a cannibalistic New Guinea tribe).

DISORDERS INVOLVING GENE DELETIONS OR DUPLICATIONS

Some disorders of the nervous system are caused by a total or partial loss of a single gene. Hereditary neuropathy with liability to pressure palsies (HNPP) is caused by a large deletion on chromosome 17 which includes the gene coding for peripheral myelin protein 22 (*PMP22*). This results in a tendency to develop recurrent focal entrapment neuropathies.

Hereditary motor and sensory neuropathy type 1 (HMSN 1) is the most common inherited peripheral neuropathy. HMSN 1 shows autosomal dominant inheritance and has an incidence of approximately 1 in 2500; 70% of affected patients have a tandem duplication of a 1.5 Mb region on chromosome 17. This region includes the *PMP22* gene.

DISORDERS OF THE MITOCHONDRIAL GENOME

Mitochondria contain their own distinct genome. They are the only organelle other than the nucleus with their own DNA (mtDNA). During fertilization mitochondria in sperm are excluded from the zygote leaving mitochondria that come only from the oocyte. Consequently, mitochondrial DNA is inherited exclusively through the maternal lineage without any recombination of genetic material. The proteins required for mitochondrial function are, however, encoded partly by mtDNA and partly by nuclear DNA. Therefore, mitochondrial disorders may be due to mutations in either mitochondrial or nuclear DNA.

Mutation rates in the mitochondrial genome are 10–100 times higher than in nuclear DNA. Reasons for this are the rapid rate of replication of mtDNA, the lack of a proofreading mechanism and the absence of an adequate mtDNA repair mechanism. mtDNA has no introns (non-coding regions of the genome) and therefore a random mutation will usually strike a coding mtDNA sequence.

A given cell can contain both mutant and normal mtDNA, a situation known as heteroplasmy. The percentage of mutant mtDNA must exceed a threshold in order to produce clinical manifestations. This threshold varies according to the tissue oxidative requirements of cells. Therefore, disease signs manifest especially in tissues with high energy expenditure (brain, heart and muscle).

There are numerous different clinical disorders associated with defects in the mitochondrial genome. Two of the commoner examples are:

- MELAS – Myopathy, Encephalopathy, Lactic Acidosis and Stroke-like episodes
- MERRF – Myoclonic Epilepsy with Ragged Red Fibres.

DISORDERS INVOLVING GENOMIC IMPRINTING

Genomic imprinting

Genomic imprinting is the phenomenon in which a specific subset of genes in the genome is expressed differently according to their parent of origin. Certain imprinted genes are expressed from a paternally inherited chromosome and silenced on the maternal chromosome. Other imprinted genes show the opposite pattern of expression and are only expressed from a maternally inherited chromosome.

Prader–Willi syndrome and Angelman's syndrome

Both Prader–Willi and Angelman's syndrome involve genes that are located in the same region of chromosome 15 and are characterized by genetic imprinting. Both conditions occur due to inactivation of one copy of the genes relevant to each disorder. Normally, the maternally derived copy of genes for Prader–Willi syndrome at the 15q11-13 locus is silent. Similarly, a paternally derived copy of one gene for Angelman syndrome at 15q11-13 is normally silent. In both cases, when the normally active copy of the gene(s) is absent, abnormality results. The region implicated in inactivating the genes involved in imprinting is located in close proximity to the genes for both disorders. As a consequence, both syndromes can result from the same chromosomal deletion. The parent from whom the chromosome 15 that gets deleted has come, determines which of the two disorders results:

- Prader–Willi syndrome (mental retardation with obesity, short stature and hypogenitalism) results from loss of imprinted genomic material in the paternal 15q11–13 locus.
- Angelman's syndrome (severe mental retardation, cerebellar ataxia, craniofacial abnormalities and epilepsy) results from loss of maternal genomic material at 15q11–13.

DISORDERS OF MULTIFACTORIAL AETIOLOGY WITH A GENETIC COMPONENT

There is continuing neurogenetic research into diseases that are generally not considered to be inherited disorders. The clinical similarity between some inherited and sporadic disorders suggests that they may also have features of disease pathogenesis in common; an understanding of the inherited form may help to determine the cause of the sporadic form.

Alzheimer's disease

Alzheimer's disease (AD) (Ch. 14) is the most common cause of dementia in elderly people. The underlying aetiology of AD is unknown but it is generally accepted to be the result of multiple factors, some being environmentally derived and others genetically inherited (Fig. 15.2).

One significant risk factor for developing AD is a positive family history. However, the typically late onset of the disease complicates attempts to identify an inherited component because affected family members often die from unrelated causes before developing signs of dementia. Despite this limitation, familial AD with autosomal dominant inheritance has been identified in a subset of Alzheimer's patients. These cases primarily involve the early-onset type.

Deposition of neuritic plaques is central to AD pathogenesis. Amyloid precursor protein (APP) is the precursor of ß-amyloid, which forms the central core of

Fig. 15.2 Factors thought to influence the development of Alzheimer's disease
Familial or genetic factors
Family history of Down's syndrome
Head trauma
Smoking
Aluminium
Mercury
Hormone replacement therapy (protective)
Anti-inflammatory drugs (protective)
Education (protective)

neuritic plaques. A mutation in the gene coding for APP (found on chromosome 21) is associated with early onset familial AD. Two other genes are linked to AD, one (on chromosome 14) encodes the protein presenilin 1 and the other (on chromosome 1) encodes presenilin 2, both of which are enzymes involved in the cleavage of APP. Mutation in these genes most likely accounts for approximately 50% of cases of early onset AD, probably by increasing the production of APP.

HINTS AND TIPS

Almost all individuals with Down's syndrome have an extra copy of chromosome 21 (trisomy 21). If they live into their 40s, nearly all show neuropathological changes similar to those seen in Alzheimer's disease. This is attributed to excess production of ß-amyloid protein as a result of over-expression of the *APP* gene.

A genetic link is also seen in development of late-onset AD. Apolipoprotein E (ApoE) is a protein found in the blood and brain that occurs in three isoforms: ApoE2, ApoE3 and ApoE4. Inheriting a copy of the *APOE4* allele is associated with a four-fold increase in risk of developing AD, apparently by contributing to amyloid deposition. Those who inherit two copies of the *APOE4* gene have a 16-fold increased risk. The *APOE2* form is protective with those who inherit two copies of *APOE2* being at low risk of developing AD. Unlike familial causes of AD, the *APOE4* gene is only a susceptibility factor in that it increases the risk of AD, but does not make it certain. Other, as yet unidentified factors, probably environmental, must also contribute.

Parkinson's disease

Idiopathic Parkinson's disease (PD) is an age-related neurodegenerative disorder (Ch. 6). It is associated with a combination of asymmetrical bradykinesia, hypokinesia and rigidity (sometimes in combination with postural changes and rest tremor). Loss of dopaminergic cells in the pars compacta of the substantia nigra is the central pathological event. The aetiology of PD is unknown (Fig. 15.3) and the conditions we label as PD may actually represent different diseases with a common final pathway.

Accumulating evidence suggests a significant genetic component for susceptibility to idiopathic PD. Epidemiological studies show that the risk of PD is at least doubled in first-degree relatives with lifetime risk in first-degree relatives of sporadic PD cases estimated at 17%. A number of gene mutations for PD have been characterized including:

- Single amino acid substitution in the *α-synuclein* gene. α-synuclein is one of a family of small proteins of unknown function. It is found at high levels in Lewy body neuronal inclusions (a pathological hallmark of PD).
- Deletions in the *parkin* gene. The *parkin* gene is involved in early onset parkinsonism responsive to levodopa. Patients have slowly progressive parkinsonism caused by homozygous deletions in the *parkin* gene.
- Missense mutations in the gene for UCH-L1 (a de-ubiquinating gene).

Motor neuron disease

Motor neuron disease (MND) causes progressive injury and cell death of lower motor neuron groups in the spinal cord and brainstem and frequently of upper motor neurons in the motor cortex (Ch. 6). The causes of the neurodegenerative processes remain uncertain (Fig. 15.4) but neurogenetics plays a role. Over 60 different mutations have been described in approximately

Fig. 15.3 Factors thought to influence the development of Parkinson's disease
Genetic factors (*parkin*, α-synuclein, UCH-L1)
Administration of MPTP (a substance derived during illicit heroin production)
Consumption of an excitotoxic amino acid found in high concentrations in the cycad bean
Manganese poisoning
Exposure to herbicides/pesticides
Living in a rural environment
Smoking (? protective)

Fig. 15.4 Factors implicated in the aetiology of motor neuron disease

Viruses	chronic viral infection
Toxins	certain metals (lead, selenium, mercury, manganese)
Minerals	chronic calcium deficiency
Genetics	mutation in the *SOD1* gene, amongst others

Irrespective of what triggers the process, the final common pathway of anterior horn cell death is a complex interaction of genetic factors, glutamate excess and oxidative stress.

250 pedigrees of familial MND. It has been shown that mutations in the gene encoding the enzyme SOD1 (Cu/Zn superoxide dismutase) on chromosome 21 underlie 20% of familial cases and 2% of all cases of MND. Motor neurons have a high expression of SOD1 compared with other cells in the nervous system. It is thought that the mutant enzyme exerts its deleterious effects through a toxic gain of function (perhaps resulting in increased formation of highly damaging hydroxyl radicals).

The genetic changes responsible for the remaining 80% of familial cases of MND are still largely unknown. Linkage analysis indicates that chromosome 2q and 9q may contain genetic alterations responsible for rare forms of MND of juvenile onset.

Pharmacology of the central nervous system

16

Objectives

In this chapter you will learn about:

- The main groups of drugs used to modify central nervous system (CNS) function.
- The mode of action of antiemetics.
- The mode of action of general anaesthetics.
- Addiction.

ANXIOLYTICS AND HYPNOTICS

Anxiety is an exaggeration of a normal state with a cognitive component (unpleasant feelings of fear and restlessness) and an autonomic component (tachycardia, gastrointestinal upset, sweating). Anxiolytics reduce the symptoms of anxiety, whereas hypnotics enable people to sleep. This distinction is not clearcut, particularly if anxiety is the main impediment to normal sleep.

The two main classes of drugs used for anxiolysis and hypnosis are:

- Benzodiazepines
- 5-hydroxytryptamine (5-HT) modulators.

The pharmacology of these and other drugs is summarized in Figure 16.1.

Figure 16.2 shows the mechanism and site of action of benzodiazepines. Dependence occurs after 4–6 weeks and is both psychological and physical. The withdrawal syndrome (in 30% of patients) comprises rebound anxiety and insomnia, tremors and twitching. Withdrawal is more severe after taking a short-acting benzodiazepine. Figure 16.3 outlines the differences between the benzodiazepines. Half-life times are important clinical considerations, particularly in elderly people, as a prolonged sedated state could result.

DRUGS USED IN AFFECTIVE DISORDERS

Affective disorders involve a disturbance of mood and are thought of as pathological extremes along a normal continuum of mood change. They are classified according to which extremes they encompass and the type of symptoms that patients report:

- Unipolar affective disorders present either with mania (euphoria, increased motor activity, flight of ideas and grandiose delusions) or depression (misery, malaise and despair).
- Bipolar affective disorder involves swings between episodes of depression and mania.

Depression can be divided into two broad categories:

- 'Reactive' depression, where there is a clear psychological cause, involving less severe symptoms and less likelihood of biological disturbance. This might happen, for example, in response to a bereavement.
- 'Endogenous' depression, where there is no clear cause. More severe symptoms (e.g. suicidal thoughts) are seen and there is a greater likelihood of biological disturbance (e.g. sleep disturbance, anorexia, weight loss or gain). Depression with some of these features tends to respond better to drug therapy.

Monoamine theory of depression

For many years, it was thought that depression was due to reduced activity of monoamines (dopamine, noradrenaline (norepinephrine)). These observations explain why:

- Monoamine oxidase inhibitors can improve mood by reducing the catabolism of monoamines.
- Tricyclic antidepressants can improve mood by blocking the uptake of noradrenaline from the synaptic cleft.
- Reserpine produces a depression-like syndrome in animal models by causing a depletion of amines.
- Methyldopa produces depression by inhibiting noradrenaline synthesis.

However, the monoaminergic theory cannot explain why:

- Amfetamine, cocaine and L-dopa, which all affect monoamine systems, do not elevate the mood of depressed patients.

Fig. 16.1 Drugs used in the treatment of mood disorders

Class	Drug	Mechanism of action	Clinical effects	Indications	Side effects	Overdose
Anxiolytics and sedation	Benzodiazepines (e.g. lorazepam, diazepam)	Binds to $GABA_A$-receptors to increase GABA affinity which hyperpolarizes the cell	Sedation and sleep, anxiolytic, anticonvulsant, reduces voluntary muscle tone	Anxiety states, preoperative sedation, status epilepticus, acute alcohol withdrawal, sedation during endoscopy	Psychomotor impairment and drowsiness; incoordination, weakness, diplopia; amnesia; disinhibition (leading to inappropriate behaviours, including aggression); dependence	Alone benzodiazepines produce a long sleep; in combination with alcohol, the central nervous system (CNS) depressant effects are potentiated resulting in fatal respiratory depression; treatment is with a benzodiazepine antagonist, flumazenil
	5-HT modulators (e.g. busipirone)	Binds to presynaptic 5-HT receptors to decrease endogenous 5-HT release	Similar to benzodiazepines	Anxiety	Less pronounced than benzodiazepines; dizziness, nervousness and excitement	
Antidepressants	Tricyclic antidepressants (e.g. amitriptyline)	Reduce noradrenaline and 5-HT from the synaptic cleft	Elevates mood in part through increasing monoamine levels	Endogenous depression, phobic disorders, obsessive–compulsive disorder and panic disorder	Muscarinic: dry mouth, blurred vision, constipation; adrenergic: postural hypotension, arrhythmia; central effects: sedation, convulsions, mania, weight gain; interactions with alcohol and antihypertensive drugs; avoid if patient suicidal	Potentially fatal: presents with confusion mania and dysrhythmias (potentiated NAergic transmission)

	Monoamine oxidase (MAO) inhibitors (e.g. phenelzine and moclobemide)	Reduce the activity of MAO, reducing monoamine (e.g. 5-HT, NA) breakdown therefore increasing available monoamines in the synaptic cleft. MAO_A inhibition correlates best with antidepressant efficacy	As for tricyclics	Endogenous depression	Interactions with tyramine in food (cheese, wine) resulting in noradrenaline release causing large blood pressure increases and cerebrovascular accidents; sympathetic: hypotension; muscarinic: dry mouth, blurred vision, constipation; phenelzine can be hepatotoxic	Presents with convulsions
	Selective serotonin reuptake inhibitors (SSRIs; e.g. fluoxetine, paroxetine)	Selectively blocks 5-HT reuptake	Reduce depressive symptoms	Usually first-line treatment for depression	No amine, anticholinergic and adrenergic actions; non-fatal in overdose; nausea and headache common but subside; insomnia; rare serotonin syndrome when used with MAOIs (hyperthermia and cardiovascular collapse)	Safe in overdose; now the most widely prescribed class of antidepressants
Mood stabilizer	Lithium (e.g. lithium carbonate)	Modulation of second-messenger pathways of cAMP and inositol triphosphate (IP_3)	Stabilizes mood, probably through 5-HT mechanisms	Bipolar disease, refractory depression	Narrow therapeutic window; monitor plasma lithium levels; CNS: tremor, weakness, headache, nausea and vomiting; kidney: diabetes insipidus, which may lead to nephrotoxicity; never prescribe with diuretics; hypothyroidism; oedema and weight gain	Presents with vomiting, diarrhoea; tremor, ataxia and coma; potentially fatal

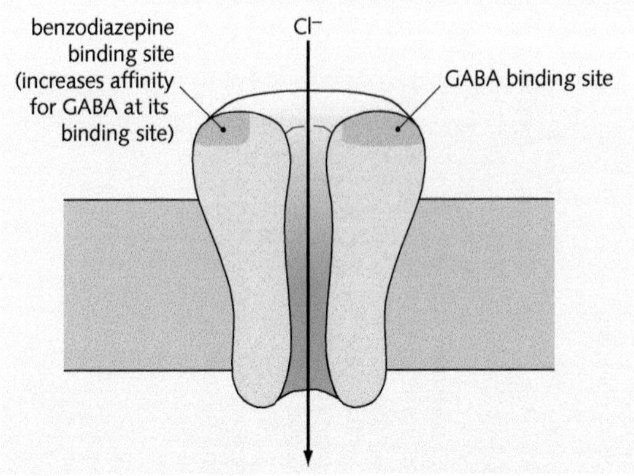

Fig. 16.2 Mechanism and site of action of benzodiazepines.

- Atypical antidepressants (e.g. iprindole) work without manipulating monoaminergic systems.
- There is a 'therapeutic' delay of 2 weeks between the full neurochemical effects of antidepressants and the start of their therapeutic effect.
- It is unlikely that monoamine mechanisms alone are responsible for the symptoms of depression.

Figure 16.1 shows the main classes of antidepressants used in clinical practice.

An overview of the pharmacological actions of antidepressant drugs is given in Figure 16.4.

HINTS AND TIPS

Outside the central nervous system (CNS), 5-HT is found most abundantly in control of the gastric system. Stimulation of this system with serotonin selective reuptake inhibitors (SSRIs) produces a surge in signalling resulting in the feeling of nausea. This is temporary and goes away in 1–2 weeks, but patients must be told to expect this so they do not stop their medication.

ANTIPSYCHOTICS (NEUROLEPTICS)

Antipsychotic drugs are used in the treatment of schizophrenia, which can be thought of as a collection of disordered thoughts, perceptions and behaviours. Some symptoms tend to occur together and different types of schizophrenia can be described according to this grouping:

- Positive symptoms (pathological by their presence; delusions, hallucinations, impaired reasoning)
- Negative symptoms (pathological by the absence of normal functioning; social withdrawal, lack of drive, behavioural disorders).

Theories of the cause of schizophrenia

Theories as to the cause of schizophrenia must allow for genetic factors (monozygotic twins have 50% concordance, 17% in dizygotic twins) and environmental factors (stressful events often precede onset and influence the course of the illness).

The dopamine theory (increased dopamine transmission):

- Evidence for this is that the clinical dose of an antipsychotic is proportional to its ability to block the D_2 receptor. Positron emission tomography (PET) ligand scans have shown that there are increased D_2 receptors in the nucleus accumbens. Psychiatric side effects are seen with drugs that increase dopaminergic transmission (L-dopa, amfetamine, bromocriptine).
- Evidence against this is that the level of dopamine metabolites in the cerebrospinal fluid (CSF) of patients is normal or low. This suggests that dopamine is not the only factor causing symptoms, but likely influences the activity of other neurotransmitter systems (e.g. acetylcholine).

Fig. 16.3 Properties of benzodiazepines

Drug (half-life)	Metabolite (half-life)	Duration of action (h)	Clinical use
Lorazepam (1–12 h)	None	12–18	Anxiolysis, hypnosis, anticonvulsant
Temazepam (8–12 h)	None	12–18	Anxiolysis, hypnosis
Diazepam (20–40 h)	Nordiazepam (60 h)	24–48	Anxiolysis, anticonvulsant
Clonazepam (50 h)	None	24–48	Anxiolysis, anticonvulsant (absence seizures)

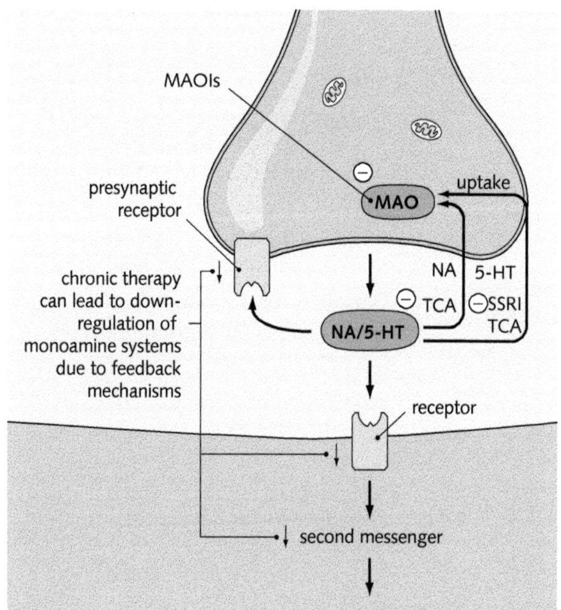

Fig. 16.4 Mechanism of action of antidepressants.

The developmental theory (disordered development):

- Evidence for this is that schizophrenic patients show reduced temporal lobe size compared with controls. Those born in winter months are more likely to develop schizophrenia, possibly because of viral infection in the mother before birth.
- Evidence against is that not all studies agree on these findings and the theory does not explain the efficacy of neuroleptic drugs.

Neuroleptic side effects: dopamine pathways

There are three main dopamine pathways in the brain:

1. Mesolimbic dopamine, running from the midbrain to the nucleus accumbens and amygdala, affecting thought and motivation
2. Nigrostriatal dopamine, running from the midbrain to the caudate nuclei, affecting motor control (see Ch. 6)
3. Tubero-infundibular dopamine, running from the hypothalamus to the pituitary gland, regulating prolactin secretion.

The side effect profile of neuroleptics is explained by:

- Disruption of the dopamine pathways
- Blockade of muscarinic receptors
- Blockade of α1-receptors.

Figure 16.5 summarizes the main antipsychotics used in medical practice and their side effects. A summary of the pharmacological effects is given in Figure 16.6.

HINTS AND TIPS

The naming of the pharmacological differences between typical and atypical antipsychotics is a common and popular exam question, but the differences are easily learnt!

NAUSEA AND VOMITING

The vomiting response consists of:

- Reverse peristalsis, where the contents of the duodenum and jejunum are propelled back into the stomach
- Closure of the glottis
- Relaxation of the lower oesophageal sphincter
- Contraction of the muscles of the abdominal wall.

These events, together with the sensation of nausea, are coordinated by an area in the medulla. This is known as the vomiting centre, which sends outputs to the dorsal motor nucleus of cranial nerve X and to the spinal motor neurons innervating the abdominal musculature. The types of stimulus that produce a vomiting response are explained by the inputs to the vomiting centre.

The chemoreceptor trigger zone in the area postrema in the medulla senses information about circulating compounds as it is not protected by the blood–brain barrier. Its neural circuits have many receptors (e.g. D_2, 5-HT_3, opioid) that allow pharmacological intervention to reduce information flow about chemical triggers. Drugs inducing nausea include L-dopa, opioids, anticancer agents (e.g. cisplatin), digitalis and anaesthetics.

The vestibular system sends balance information to the vomiting centre. In motion sickness (pallor, sweating, nausea and vomiting), there is a conflict between the visual and vestibular systems. This can be treated behaviourally or with drugs that reduce vestibular input. Vestibular disease presents with vertigo (false sense of rotary movement), particularly in:

- Labyrinthitis (seen acutely in viral infection, with symptoms of vertigo, nausea and vomiting)
- Ménière's disease (vertigo, nausea, vomiting, tinnitus and deafness) caused by increased endolymphatic pressure.

The solitary nucleus sends viscerosensory information about chemicals in the gut collected by cranial nerve X. The enteroendocrine system in the gut wall responds to gut contents and by 5-HT mechanisms can affect the firing of cranial nerve X afferent neurons:

- The spinal cord sends information about trauma: nausea can accompany physical injury

Fig. 16.5 Antipsychotic drugs			
Class	**Compound**	**Mechanism of action**	**Side effects**
Typical	Phenothiazine with aliphatic side-chain (e.g. chlorpromazine)	D_2 receptor blockade in the mesolimbic dopaminergic pathway	Strong sedation, moderate autonomic side effects and moderate extrapyramidal motor disturbance; corneal and lens deposits seen
	Phenothiazine with a piperidine side chain (e.g. thioridazine)	D_2 receptor blockade in the mesolimbic dopaminergic pathway	Moderate sedation, strong autonomic side effects and mild extrapyramidal motor disturbance; corneal and lens deposits seen
	Phenothiazine with a piperazine side chain (e.g. fluphenazine)	D_2 receptor blockade in the mesolimbic dopaminergic pathway	Low sedation, mild autonomic effects and strong extrapyramidal motor disturbance
	Thioxanthene (e.g. flupenthixol); similar to piperazine phenothiazines	D_2 receptor blockade in the mesolimbic dopaminergic pathway	Low sedation, mild autonomic effects and strong motor disturbance
	Butyrophenone (e.g. haloperidol); similar to piperazine phenothiazines	D_2 receptor blockade in the mesolimbic dopaminergic pathway	Low sedation, mild autonomic effects and strong motor disturbance
Atypical	Clozapine	Blocks 5-HT_{2A} receptors as well as α-adrenergic and histamine receptors; minimal anti-dopaminergic action	Sedation (via histamine blockade), hypotension, hypothermia; main concern is with agranulocytosis (reduced granule inflammatory cells from toxic bone marrow suppression, e.g. neutrophils); patients must be monitored. Rarely cholestatic jaundice and skin rashes
	Risperidone, olanzapine, quetiapine, amisulpiride	Blocks 5-HT and DA transmission although exact mechanism unclear	Favourable side effect profile, but risks of hyperglycaemia, cerebrovascular accidents, akathisia, constipation, dizziness, drowsiness, insomnia, dry mouth, tremor and weight gain

- The limbic cortex sends information from the special senses: certain odours and sights can cause nausea.

Figure 16.7 summarizes the connections of the medullary vomiting centre and the sites of drug action.

Antiemetics

Figure 16.8 shows the action, uses and side effects of some antiemetic drugs.

GENERAL ANAESTHESIA

All general anaesthetics produce:

- Loss of consciousness, of reflex responses to noxious stimuli, of spatial orientation, of volitional control and of memory, and reductions in respiratory rate and blood pressure.
- Death at high doses, caused by respiratory depression and cardiovascular depression by actions on the medulla; in addition, cardiac depression may be brought about by direct effects on the myocardium.

Anaesthesia used to be characterized by an initial excitatory phase (modern anaesthetics act very quickly so that this phase is no longer prolonged or troublesome) followed by a dose-dependent increase in anaesthetic depth. This was seen with agents such as ether. Single anaesthetic agents are rarely used in modern practice, as their complementary effects allow lower doses to be employed. This leads to fewer side effects. Often a combination of intravenous and inhalational agents is used to exploit their different kinetic properties.

The principles of surgical anaesthesia are to produce:

- Loss of consciousness
- Analgesia
- Muscle relaxation.

There is no obvious pharmacological structure–activity relationship for anaesthetic agents; their mechanisms of action are complex, either by affecting the reticular formation (most anaesthetics) or by a direct depression of cortical activity (e.g. propofol).

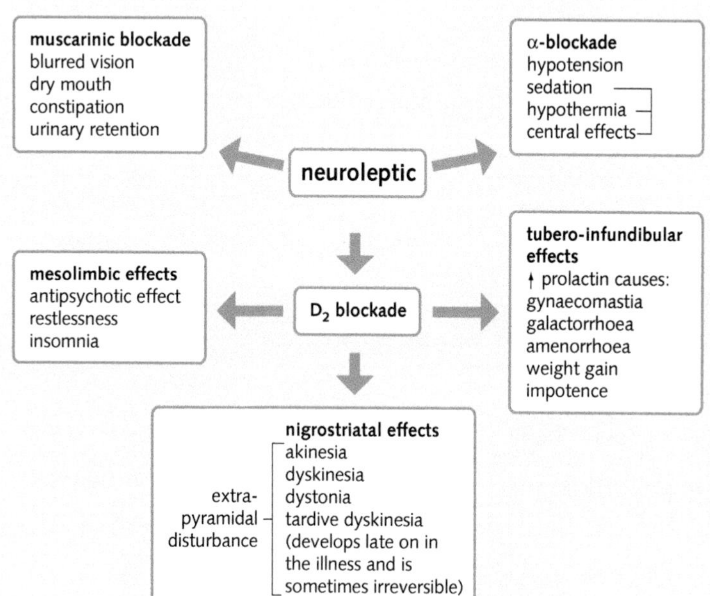

Fig. 16.6 Pharmacological effects of neuroleptic medication.

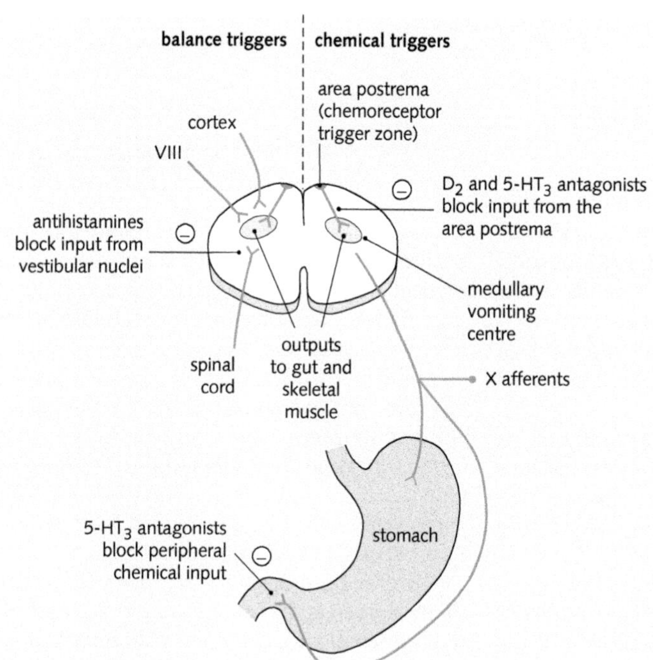

Fig. 16.7 Sites of action of antiemetics.

The potency of any anaesthetic is directly related to its hydrophobic nature, generally measured as its lipid solubility as the oil:gas (for gases and vapours) and oil:water (for aqueous agents) partition coefficient. One possible mechanism of action is that anaesthetics interact with a hydrophobic region (either lipid, protein or lipoprotein) of the neuronal membrane, causing membrane expansion and consequent malfunction. Evidence for this is that anaesthesia in mammals may be reversed by high ambient pressure (in excess of 100 atm; 10.1 MPa).

Fig. 16.8 Antiemetic drugs

Class	Drug	Site of action	Uses	Side effects
Antimuscarinic	Hyoscine	Vomiting centre, antagonizing vestibular input	Motion sickness	Drowsiness, dry mouth, blurred vision, impaired short-term memory
Antihistamine	Cinnarizine and cyclizine	Vomiting centre, antagonizing vestibular input	Motion sickness, vestibular disease	Less than antimuscarinics
Histamine analogue	Betahistine	Reduces endolymphatic pressure in the membranous labyrinths	Ménière's disease	
D_2 antagonists	Metoclopramide and domperidone	Chemoreceptor trigger zone reducing sensitivity to chemical triggers in the blood	Reduces drug-induced nausea and vomiting; combination with paracetamol to treat migraine	Drowsiness, fatigue, motor restlessness
5-HT_3 antagonist	Ondansetron and granisetron	Chemoreceptor trigger zone and peripherally in the gut reducing transmission from 5-HTergic enteroendocrine cells in response to chemical triggers in the gut	Reduces drug-induced nausea and vomiting. Addition of dexamethasone (steroid) increases efficacy in chemotherapy patients requiring high doses	Headache, gastrointestinal upset

Induction and recovery

Induction and recovery describe how quickly anaesthesia occurs after administration and how quickly the body recovers from anaesthesia. The speed of induction with, and recovery from, an anaesthetic depends on the physical properties of the anaesthetic and how quickly it can equilibrate between the lungs, blood and CNS for inhalants and gaseous agents, or from blood and CNS for aqueous agents.

Intravenous agents (e.g. propofol) are often used for the induction of anaesthesia as they can produce unconsciousness in approximately 20 seconds. This is generally preferable for patients, as many find face masks can make them feel claustrophobic.

Inhalational anaesthetics (e.g. isoflurane) are more commonly used for the maintenance of anaesthesia. This is because they give a more rapid control of the level of consciousness.

After equilibration, 95% of the administered anaesthetic is in the body fat. Fat has a low blood flow and so it takes a long time for anaesthetics to enter and leave the body fat. A fat-soluble anaesthetic can build up gradually in adipose tissue, and then be released back into the circulation over a long period of time.

The most common general anaesthetics are compared in Figure 16.9.

ADDICTION

The neural systems that mediate reward and pleasure use a variety of neurotransmitter agents, and dopamine in particular has been implicated. Dopaminergic pathways important for reinforcement are recruited by some commonly misused drugs that are reinforcing (Fig. 16.10).

Addictive drugs such as cocaine, amphetamine, opiates and nicotine act like positive reinforcers. Animals will readily press a lever to give themselves an intravenous infusion of amphetamine. Drugs of abuse potentiate the reinforcing effects of electrical brain stimultion, reducing the frequency of pulses needed to produce a behavioural response.

Reinforcing drugs also increase the levels of dopamine released at the terminals of projections of the ventral tegmental area. Cocaine and amphetamine raise the level of dopamine in the nucleus accumbens by blocking the dopamine transporter thereby prolonging the time dopamine remains in the synaptic cleft. The nucleus accumbens has strong connections to the limbic system and hypothalamus. Nicotine is possibly the most addictive, most widely abused drug. It increases the level of dopamine in the mesocorticolimbic pathway, enhancing the release of dopamine by acting on presynaptic cholenergic receptors.

Fig. 16.9 Anaesthetic drugs

Route	Drug	Potency (oil: gas)	Induction/ recovery	Notes and side effects
Inhaled	N_2O	Low (1.4)	Fast	Only analgesic by itself. Used 60% O_2/40% N_2O as carrier for other agents
	Halothane	High (220)	Medium	Depresses myocardium, baroreceptor reflex, sympathetic system producing hypotension. 20% metabolized and may cause hepatic damage
	Enflurane	Medium (98)	Medium	Depresses myocardium producing hypotension. 2% metabolized so no hepatic damage. May cause seizures
	Isoflurane	Medium (91)	Medium	Causes vasodilatation producing hypotension. Only 0.2% metabolized. Less epileptogenic than enflurane but may cause myocardial ischaemia
Injected	Thiopental	High	Fast	Depresses myocardium and respiratory centre. No analgesic effect. Duration or unconsciousness 5–10 minutes due to liver, kidneys, etc., and then to muscle. Eventual redistribution to body fat so almost total
	Propofol		Fast	Cardiovascular and respiratory depression. Rapidly metabolized and suitable for total intravenous anaesthesia

Fig. 16.10 Drugs of misuse

Class	Drug	Action	Effects	Side effects	Tolerance	Dependence
Psychomotor stimulants	Amfetamine	Causes release of NA and DA from terminals	Central DA effects: euphoria, excitement, locomotor stimulation with repetitive behaviour (stereotypies), anorexia	Insomnia, irritability, headache, psychosis, tremor	Develops as amfetamine depletes terminals of transmitter	Increases activity in dopamine reward system (VTA to nucleus acumbens), producing psychological dependence
	Cocaine	Blocks NA and DA uptake (uptake 1)	Peripheral noradrenergic effects: increased blood pressure, decreased gastrointestinal mobility	Cardiac dysrhythmias, convulsions, respiratory and vasomotor depression		
Hallucinogens	Lysergic acid diethylamide (LSD)	5-HT_2 partial agonist	Altered perception, thoughts, feelings	Persistent effects lasting several weeks, flashbacks to previous 'trips'	Quickly develops	None
	MDMA (Ectasy)	Amfetamine-like and LSD-like	Euphoria, altered thoughts	Idiosyncratic responses – coma, convulsions, hyperpyrexia, rhabdomyolysis	Cross-tolerance with LSD	None

VTA, ventral tegmental area

In addition to the positive reinforcement of the drug, two other features characterize addiction:

- *Tolerance* refers to progressive adaptation to the dosage that produces euphoria. In other words, higher and higher doses are needed to achieve the same effect.
- Dependence refers to the negative visceral consequences of withdrawal of the drug, e.g. nausea.

Therefore, drug misuse is driven by the avoidance of the adverse effects of withdrawl as well as the rewarding effects of the drug.

Clinical assessment of the nervous system

Objectives

In this chapter you will learn about:

- How to take a structured and comprehensive neurological history.
- How to develop an awareness of the communication skills that are particularly relevant to neurology.
- How to perform a structured and comprehensive neurological examination.
- How to use the information elicited from the neurological history and examination to answer the question 'Where is the lesion?'.
- Neurophysiological investigations.
- Routine investigations (blood tests, etc.) and how they relate to neurological problems.
- Imaging of the nervous system.

BEGINNING THE INTERVIEW

Taking a good history is the most important skill in medicine. As well as providing the foundation for a good doctor–patient relationship, the history enables formulation of a differential diagnosis and a focus for the clinical examination.

Observation of the patient as they walk into the examination room or as you approach the bed is vital:

- Do they appear unwell?
- Do they have an abnormal gait (shuffling, high-stepping) or use walking aids (sticks, crutches, frame, wheelchair, callipers)?
- Do they appear to be independent or clearly need help from others?
- Are there any obvious morphological abnormalities (e.g. weakness on one side, drooping of the face, wasting of the muscles)?

Begin the interview by:

- Introducing yourself
- Explaining who you are
- Asking if you may talk to and examine them
- Asking their age and occupation
- Asking whether they are right- or left-handed.

Observe the patient's environment:

- Notice the oxygen, fluids, intravenous infusions, medicines, warfarin card and sputum pot.
- Cards and flowers from friends and relatives may indicate a supportive home network.

You will observe important points regarding their neurological status immediately:

- Do they respond appropriately (indicating probable preservation of important higher mental functioning)?
- Do they appear to be depressed (which may be part of their neurological condition or may indicate a reaction to it)?
- Do they appear to be elated (again, a feature of some neurological illnesses such as multiple sclerosis)?
- Is their speech normal?
- You may notice additional features such as tremor, agitation, twitches and abnormal movements.

THE STRUCTURE OF THE HISTORY

The presenting complaint

From the patient's point of view. Ask:

- 'What is the main problem?'
- 'What was it that caused you to go to your doctor/come to the hospital?'
- When presenting the history to others, use the patient's own words (e.g. 'This woman complains of seeing double' rather than 'This woman has horizontal diplopia').

The history of the presenting complaint:

- When did the patient first note it?
- Has it worsened, improved or stayed the same since?
- What is its nature (e.g. headache may be sharp, dull, an ache, a throb, etc.)?
- Is there anything that makes it better (e.g. medicines, sleep, exercise) or worse (e.g. time of day, posture, exercise)?
- Have any other symptoms developed since this first complaint was noticed (e.g. main complaint may be weakness of the hand, but a numb patch may have developed more recently)?

- Have any tests already been performed, and if so where and by whom?
- Has the patient ever had other neurological symptoms in the past (these may be related, e.g. an episode of transient visual loss 5 years previously in a young woman now complaining of difficulty in walking)?
- Run through a checklist of neurological symptoms.

Neurological symptoms

Remember these by working from the 'head down':

- Headache
- Fits, faints and funny turns
- Memory problems
- Visual disturbance
- Hearing disturbance
- Speech difficulty
- Dizziness
- Swallowing difficulty
- Weakness
- Numbness
- Bladder or bowel disturbance
- Walking difficulty.

Systemic enquiry

Do not underestimate the importance of going through these categories (if only briefly). Co-existent disease may have a huge impact on disability, and may be linked to the presenting complaint (e.g. weight loss and back pain may be indicative of a tumour, which may be related to new-onset neurological symptoms). Things to ask about include:

- General – fatigue, anorexia, weight change, itch, rashes, low mood, fevers/nights sweats
- Gastrointestinal – swallowing difficulty, nausea and vomiting, haematemesis, heartburn, indigestion, abdominal pain, change in bowel habit, blood or mucus per rectum
- Cardiorespiratory – chest pain, breathlessness, orthopnoea, palpitations, cough, sputum, wheeze, haemoptysis
- Genitourinary – dysuria, frequency, nocturia, change in appearance/smell of urine, prostatic symptoms, incontinence, sexual function
- Musculoskeletal – joint pain, stiffness, swelling, loss of joint function, immobility.

Past medical history

Any serious illnesses in the past or now? It is useful to write an abbreviated list of important negatives in your clerking, to show that these have been checked. The mnemonic 'MJTHREADS' is commonly used as a reminder: myocardial infarction, jaundice, tuberculosis, hypertension, rheumatic fever, epilepsy, asthma, diabetes, stroke.

Drug history

- Is the patient taking any medicines now, or have any been taken for some time in the past?
- Are there any known drug allergies?

Family history

Are there any 'family illnesses'? Are parents, siblings, and children alive and well, and if not, what did they die from and at what age? Draw a family tree (Fig. 17.1) if appropriate.

Social history

- Home circumstances – own home, stairs, social-services help, family support, responsibilities for children/disabled relatives, etc.
- Smoking (ever)?
- Alcohol (ever heavy consumption)?
- Drug misuse?
- Diet (are they likely to have a vitamin deficiency? Ask about supplementation)?
- Heterosexual or homosexual (use your judgement as to whether this is an appropriate question – in a 90-year-old lady with dementia, it is likely to cause eyebrows to be raised!)?

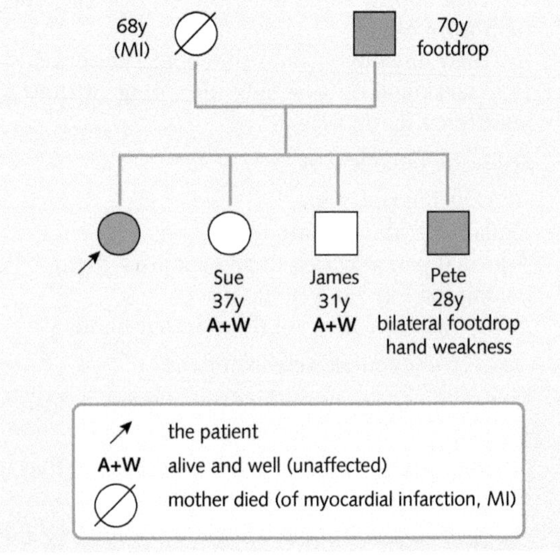

Fig. 17.1 The Lane family tree: an example of autosomal dominant inheritance. In this case, hereditary motor and sensory neuropathy (HMSN).

Summary

When presenting the history, run through the categories described above, always starting with the same pattern (e.g. 'Miss Randolph is a 40-year-old right-handed secretary who presents with numbness of both feet'):

- Describe the history of the presenting complaint, past medical history and review of systems. You do not have to mention specifically all negative points, but it is worth pointing out those that are important (e.g. 'she has no history of diabetes').
- List any medication currently taken by the patient.
- Describe the family history, if relevant; if not, say that 'there is no relevant family history'.
- Describe important social points (e.g. 'she drinks only moderate alcohol and has never smoked').

Then move on to your examination findings.

When presenting the history, always start with the same sequence:
- Name
- Age
- Handedness
- Occupation
- Complaint (in the patient's words).

COMMUNICATION SKILLS

Patients with neurological problems often present particular problems with communication. This can make them daunting to approach, as we feel embarrassed about our fumblings. Remember that these people have to deal with discrimination and ignorance all the time. The most important thing you can do is to respect them.

Approaching the patient

Make sure that you look respectable. Introduce yourself to the patient and ask their permission to talk to them. Always speak to the patient first, rather than any relatives who may be around, even if they appear to be unconscious or incapable of responding. Many older people like to shake their doctor's hand, but do be aware of cultural differences (see later). Ensure that the patient is comfortable and that you are too. Ask the patient's permission to sit on a chair. Preferably, you should be at eye level with them, or slightly lower. Eye contact is important in building trust with a patient, which you will need when embarking on the examination. It is worth making sure you are in a comfortable position to write.

Beginning the conversation

If possible, leave your note taking until later – perhaps just jotting down important dates of operations, etc., that you might otherwise forget. Start by checking the patient's name, age, occupation and handedness. This is a good opportunity to build a relationship with them – show interest in their occupation or where they live.

Begin your history taking with open questions such as 'Tell me what led you to come to hospital' or 'Tell me what has been happening with your health lately'.

Particular issues in neurological patients

Be sensitive to any disability that the patient has. If they are deaf, make sure you enunciate your words very clearly and raise your voice if appropriate. Remember that neurological conditions often leave cognitive functions unaffected, so do not speak to any adult patient as if they were a child. Give patients plenty of time and try not to interrupt. If a patient finds speaking difficult and slow, they probably find it much more frustrating than you do!

THE NEUROLOGICAL EXAMINATION

Speech

This will probably be one of the first things you assess, albeit unconsciously, during the history.

Speech production is organized at three levels: phonation, articulation and language production.

Phonation

Phonation is the production of sounds as the air passes through the vocal cords. A disorder of this process is called dysphonia.

Assessment

In dysphonia, the speech volume is reduced and the voice sounds rather husky. Dysphonia is usually due to lesions of the recurrent laryngeal nerves, or to respiratory muscle weakness (e.g. Guillain–Barré syndrome).

Articulation

Articulation is the manipulation of sound as it passes through the upper airways by the palate, the tongue and the lips to produce phonemes. A disorder of this process is called dysarthria.

Assessment

To assess articulation, ask the patient to repeat 'British Constitution', 'baby hippopotamus', and 'West Register Street'. If the speech articulation is abnormal, this could be caused by:

- Cerebellar dysarthria – speech is slurred or 'staccato'
- Extrapyramidal dysarthria – speech is soft and monotonous
- Pseudobulbar dysarthria – speech is high pitched with a 'strangulated' quality ('Donald Duck' speech)
- Bulbar dysarthria – speech has a nasal quality that may worsen as the patient continues to speak (suggesting myasthenia gravis).

Language production

Language production is the organization of phonemes into words and sentences, and is controlled by the speech centres in the dominant hemisphere. A disorder of this process is called dysphasia.

Assessment

To assess language production:

- Establish the patient's handedness. Dysphasia is a feature of dominant hemisphere dysfunction.
- Listen to the patient's spontaneous speech, assessing its fluency and contents.
- Assess the patient's comprehension by observing his or her response to simple commands: 'Open your mouth, look up to the ceiling'.
- Assess the patient's ability to name objects. Use your wrist-watch (face, hands, strap, buckle).
- Assess the patient's ability to repeat sentences: 'No ifs, ands or buts'.

If any of these features is abnormal, the patient may be dysphasic (but they must be distinguished from a patient who is depressed and has psychomotor retardation, or severe dysarthria).

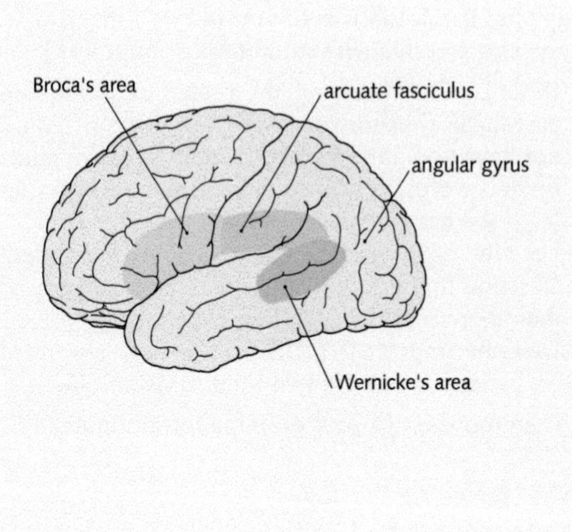

Fig. 17.2 Broca's and Wernicke's areas and their connecting arcuate fasciculus.

Cerebrovascular disease and brain tumours are the commonest causes of dysphasia. Dysphasia is classified according to speech fluency and content, comprehension and anatomical location of the lesions (Figs. 17.2 and 17.3).

Mental state and higher functions

Consciousness

Consciousness is the state of being aware of self and the environment. It has two components:

- The level of arousal
- The content of consciousness.

Fig. 17.3 Classification of dysphasia

Type	Lesion	Speech fluency	Speech content	Comprehension of speech	Association
Expressive	Broca's area	Non-fluent	Normal	Normal	Telegrammatic speech, dysarthria
Receptive	Wernicke's area	Fluent	Impaired	Impaired	Neologisms, excessive speech
Conductive	Arcuate faciculus	Fluent	Normal	Normal	Impaired function in repetitive tasks
Global	Parietal lobe/ dominant hemisphere	Non-fluent	Impaired	Impaired	Contralateral visual/sensory inattention, defects in written language, variable extent of other disabilities according to size of lesion

The level of arousal

A number of ill-defined terms are used to describe the different levels of arousal:

- Full wakefulness and responsiveness – normal arousal status
- Obtundation – patient is drowsy and not fully responsive
- Stupor – patient appears to be asleep, with little or no spontaneous activity; however, he or she is rousable when stimulated
- Coma – patient is unresponsive and unrousable.

This aspect of consciousness is conventionally assessed using the Glasgow Coma Scale (see below).

The content of consciousness

The content of consciousness is dependent on the patient's level of cognitive functioning. The content of consciousness can be assessed only when a reasonable degree of arousal is present. This aspect of consciousness is conventionally assessed with the Mini-Mental State Examination (see below).

Appearance and behaviour

Assessment of the patient's mental state begins as soon as you meet them. The physical appearance can be helpful. Demented patients may look bewildered but unconcerned, or apathetic and withdrawn. Look for evidence of self-neglect, which is often concealed by relatives. Observe the patient's response to your questions during the history taking, assessing their comprehension and whether they retain insight into their problem.

Affect

Ask the patient if he or she has been feeling anxious, depressed or irritable, and decide if his or her mood is appropriate. Euphoric and manic patients look inappropriately cheerful and energetic, and tend to ignore or play down their problems and disabilities. Patients with emotional lability have sudden unprovoked outbursts of laughing or crying, which can be very distressing to them.

In cognitive impairment, patients' emotional reactions vary according to the severity of their illness:

- In the early stages, anxiety and depression might result from preserved insight into the increasing intellectual difficulties.
- In advanced stages, a flattening of the affect becomes apparent, and may lead to the patient being apparently totally unresponsive.

Attention and orientation

Attention

Ensure that the patient's comprehension is normal. Formal assessment of attention is carried out using serial reversals:

- 'Can you spell "world" backwards for me, please?'
- 'Can you name the months of the year backwards, starting with December?'
- 'Can you count backwards from 20?'

Orientation

Assess the patient's orientation in time, place, and person. To test the patient's orientation in time, ask:

- 'What day of the week is it today?'
- 'What month are we in?'
- 'What time of day is it?' – this is a very sensitive marker for dementia.

To test the patient's orientation in place, ask:

- 'Can you tell me where you are now?'
- 'What city are we in?'

To test the patient's orientation in person, ask:

- 'Who is this person?' (point to a family member, a nurse or a doctor).

Memory

Immediate memory (recall)

Establish that the patient's comprehension and attention are normal. Immediate recall is tested with digit span: 'Can you repeat these numbers after me, please?'. Start with two or three figures, avoiding recognizable sequences. A normal individual can repeat a five- to seven-digit sequence.

Recent memory

Ask the patient about recent political, social or sporting events, taking into account his or her premorbid intelligence and socioeconomic status.

Ask the patient to memorize a short address (try '23 West Register Street'). Ask him or her to repeat the address after you to ensure that it has been registered. Distract the patient for the next 10 minutes (by continuing your assessment of his or her mental status), then ask him or her to repeat the address. Most normal individuals will be able to recall all the data.

Visual memory can be tested by displaying a drawing for 5 seconds and asking the patient to redraw the design 10 seconds later (Fig. 17.4). Patients with visuospatial disorders will have difficulty with the task, even if their visual memory is intact.

Remote memory

Ask the patient about childhood, schooling, work history or marriage. A relative should verify the accuracy of his or her answers. If no relative is available, ask a question about a time period relevant to the patient.

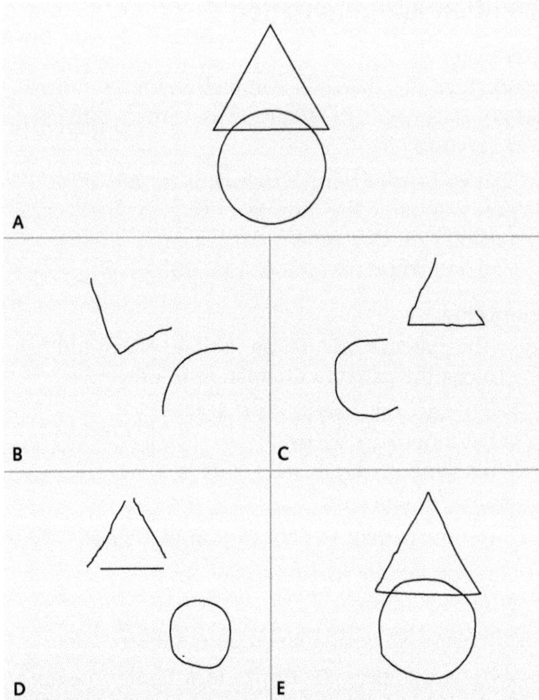

Fig. 17.4 Visual memory test showing the standard design (A) and reproductions scored from 0 to 3 (B–E).

In elderly people, this might be 'In what year did World War 1 start?' or, in younger patients 'In what year did England win the football World Cup?'. These questions should again be adjusted for premorbid intelligence and socioeconomic status. Immediate and recent memory is usually affected early in dementia. However, remote memory is relatively spared in patients with minor degrees of brain damage, but is always affected in those with advanced dementia.

Calculation

This should be tested in the light of the patient's education. Give the patient simple addition or subtraction sums. Serial sevens or threes (subtracting sevens or threes serially from 100) is a useful test.

Dyscalculia is a prominent feature of Gerstmann's syndrome (dyscalculia, right–left disorientation and finger agnosia), caused by dominant parietal lobe lesions.

Abstract thinking

This is tested by asking the patient to interpret *common* proverbs:

- 'A bird in the hand is worth two in the bush.'
- 'People in glasshouses should not throw stones.'

Abstract thinking can also be tested by assessing the patient's ability to identify the similarities between pairs of objects: 'Cow and dog, air and water'.

Constructional ability and neglect

Constructional ability and neglect are tested by asking the patient to construct simple designs (triangle, square) using match-sticks, and to draw or copy designs of increasing complexity (Fig. 17.5):

- 'Please draw a clock, put the hours on it, and set the time at 3 o'clock.'

Patients with non-dominant parietal lesions have poor constructional ability (which is often associated with neglect to the contralateral side of the body, including the visual fields). This is often reflected in the patient's drawings (they copy only the right side of the design, or they draw the clock and put all the numbers on the one side, usually the right side).

Right–left disorientation

Establish that the patient's comprehension is normal. Right–left disorientation is assessed by giving the patient simple commands of increasing complexity:

- 'Show me your right hand.'
- 'Put your left hand on your right ear.'

Right–left disorientation is seen in patients with dominant parietal lobe lesions.

Dyspraxia

Dyspraxia is the inability to perform a skilled movement in the absence of weakness, incoordination, sensory loss or abnormal comprehension. Dyspraxia can be confined to the limbs, the trunk or the buccofacial musculature.

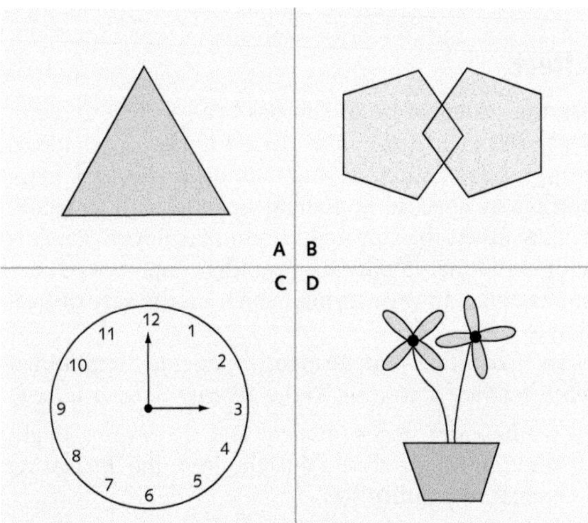

Fig. 17.5 Constructional tests: drawings of increasing complexity to be reproduced by the patient.

Dyspraxia is tested by asking the patient to carry out particular tasks of increasing complexity:

- 'Stick out your tongue.'
- 'Pretend to whistle.'
- 'Show me how to use a toothbrush.'
- 'Show me how to take the cap off a toothpaste tube and squeeze the toothpaste onto a brush.'

There are some special forms of dyspraxia:

- Dressing dyspraxia
- Constructional dyspraxia
- Gait dyspraxia.

Agnosia

Agnosia is the inability to recognize a sensory input in the absence of primary sensory pathway dysfunction. It can affect a certain sensory modality in a global fashion (visual agnosia, auditory agnosia), or can affect a specific class of stimuli (colour agnosia).

Agnosia is tested by showing the patient a few objects and asking him or her to name each one. Allow the patient to manipulate the objects, which might improve recognition (by allowing him or her to use a different sensory input). Assess other sensory modalities:

- Auditory agnosia (inability to recognize sounds)
- Tactile agnosia (inability to recognize objects placed in the hand: astereognosis)
- Finger agnosia (inability to name fingers)
- Topographic agnosia (inability to comprehend three-dimensional sense).

Mini-Mental State Examination

It is often difficult to perform an extensive testing of higher cortical functions in every patient. The Mini-Mental State Examination (Fig. 17.6) allows a rapid assessment:

- The maximum score is 30
- Scores 28–30 do not support the diagnosis of dementia
- Scores 25–27 are borderline
- Scores <25 are suggestive of dementia (if acute confusional state and depression are unlikely).

Cortical and subcortical dementia

Learn to differentiate between the features of cortical and subcortical dementia (Fig. 17.7). Patients with cortical dementia retain the ability to answer questions at a

Fig. 17.6 The Mini-Mental State Examination

Orientation

1. What is the year, season, date, month, day? (One point for each correct answer.)
2. Where are we? Country, county, town, hospital, floor? (One point for each answer.)

Registration

3. Name three objects, taking 1 second to say each. Then ask the patient all three once you have said them. (One point for each correct answer.)

Repeat the questions until the patient learns all three.

Attention and calculation

4. Serial sevens. Stop after five answers. (One point for each correct answer.)

Alternative: spell 'world' backwards.

Recall

5. Ask for names of three objects asked in question 3. (One point for each correct answer.)

Language

6. Point to a pencil and a watch. Ask the patient to name them for you. (One point for each correct answer.)
7. Ask the patient to repeat 'No ifs, ands, or buts'. (One point if done correctly.)
8. Ask the patient to follow a three-stage command: 'Take the paper in your right hand, fold the paper in half, put the paper on the floor.' (Three points if done correctly.)
9. Ask the patient to read and obey the following: CLOSE YOUR EYES. (Write this in large letters). (One point if done correctly.)
10. Ask the patient to write a sentence of his or her own choice. (The sentence must contain a subject and an object and make sense.) Ignore spelling errors when scoring. (One point if done correctly.)
11. Ask the patient to copy two intersecting pentagons with equal sides (Fig. 17.5B). (Give one point if all the sides and angles are preserved, and if the intersecting sides form a quadrangle.)

Maximum score = 30 points

Fig. 17.7 Features of cortical and subcortical dementia							
	Example	**Cognition**	**Insight**	**Memory**	**Response time**	**Personality**	**Mood**
Cortical dementia	Alzheimer's disease Pick's disease	Severely disturbed	Absent	Difficulty learning new information	Normal	Unconcerned	May be depressed
Subcortical dementia	Parkinson's disease Huntington's chorea	Impaired problem solving	Partially retained	Difficulty retrieving learned information	Slow	Apathetic	Often depressed

relatively normal speed. However, their answers are irrelevant and 'hopeless'.

Q: How many arms do you have?
A: Oh, not many!

Patients with subcortical dementia have difficulty in retrieving memories and their response time is therefore long. They are not totally 'hopeless' and often find the right answer with some help.

Q: Who is the monarch on the throne in England now?
A: Erm . . . I don't know.
Q: Is it George, Victoria or Elizabeth?
A: Queen Elizabeth.

Clinical syndromes associated with specific focal hemispheric dysfunction

Frontal lobe

Conditions associated with frontal lobe dysfunction are:

- Altered personality, altered mood, loss of interest, loss of initiative
- Expressive dysphasia (dominant hemisphere) and dyspraxia
- Hemiparesis and primitive reflexes
- Sphincter incontinence (bifrontal lesions).

Parietal lobe

Conditions associated with parietal lobe dysfunction on the dominant side are:

- Dysphasia, dyslexia, dysgraphia
- Dyscalculia
- Right–left disorientation
- Finger agnosia.

Conditions associated with dysfunction of the non-dominant side are:

- Neglect to the contralateral side of the body
- Constructional and dressing dyspraxia
- Topographic agnosia.

Conditions associated with dysfunction of the non-dominant or dominant side are:

- Hemisensory disturbance or inattention
- Lower quadrant homonymous field defect.

Temporal lobe

Conditions associated with temporal lobe dysfunction are:

- Amnesic syndromes
- Dysphasia (dominant lobe)
- Upper quadrant homonymous field defect.

Occipital lobe

Conditions associated with occipital lobe dysfunction are:

- Visual field defects
- Distortion of vision
- Impaired visual recognition (visual agnosia).

Gait

In normal gait, the erect moving body is supported by one leg at a time while the other swings forward in preparation for the next support move. The normal gait sequence consists of three components – heel strike, stance and toe off. Only one foot will be on the floor at any time, although both the heel of the anterior foot and the toes of the posterior foot will be on the ground momentarily when the body weight is transferred from one leg to the other. Normal gait requires input from the motor, sensory, cerebellar and vestibular systems.

Assessment

The gait of a patient is assessed as follows:

- Ask the patient to walk up and down the examination room in his or her usual fashion, with his or her arms loose by his or her side.
- Observe the patient's posture, the pattern of his or her arm and leg movements and the control of his or her trunk.
- If gait appears normal, ask the patient to heel-toe walk ('I would like you to walk heel to toe as if you are walking on a tightrope'). Walk alongside

the patient to support him or her if he or she appears unsteady.

- If gait appears abnormal, classify it into one of the following patterns.

Hemiplegic gait

Hemiplegic gait (Fig. 17.8A) is caused by unilateral upper motor neuron leg weakness. The ipsilateral arm is held flexed and adducted while the ipsilateral leg is extended (pyramidal pattern of weakness). To move the affected leg, patients tilt their pelvis to be able to swing the affected leg forward in a 'circumduction' manner.

Spastic gait

Spastic gait is caused by bilateral upper motor neuron leg weakness. Both legs are spastic and patients walk in small steps with their toes pressing firmly on the floor as if they are walking in mud. The legs are held in adduction with the knees touching each other, giving the gait a 'scissored' quality.

Cerebellar ataxic gait

Cerebellar ataxic gait (Fig. 17.8B) is caused by cerebellar (and occasionally vestibular) lesions. Patients walk on a wide base and appear unsteady, with erratic body movements. They stagger to the affected side in unilateral lesions (backwards if the lesion is in the cerebellar vermis). The condition may be embarrassing for the patient as people assume that they are drunk. Mild cases can be detected only by asking patients to walk on a narrow base (heel-toe walking).

Sensory ataxic gait

Sensory ataxic gait (Fig. 17.8C) is caused by proprioceptive and somatosensory loss. The gait is rather unsteady but patients are able to compensate to some extent using their visual input. Patients tend to stamp their feet down against the floor, owing to the loss of all sensory input. Patients become very ataxic in the dark or if the eyes are closed (see Romberg's test below).

Footdrop gait

Footdrop gait (Fig. 17.8D) is caused by common peroneal nerve lesion (if unilateral), or peripheral neuropathy (if bilateral). Patients over-flex the hip and the knee to be able to lift their toes off the floor, giving the gait a high-stepping quality.

Parkinsonian gait

Parkinsonian gait (Fig. 17.8E) is slow and shuffling with small stride length, flexed posture and reduced arm swinging. Patients often have problems in starting to walk and in turning while walking, which is achieved by using an exaggerated number of steps. This gait should be differentiated from the less common *marche à petit pas* seen in bilateral frontal lobe lesions, in which gait is shuffling but the arms and the trunk are not affected.

Waddling gait

Waddling gait is caused by proximal myopathy. Patients have exaggerated lumbar lordosis. They bend their pelvis forward and walk with a waddle, tilting from one side to the other.

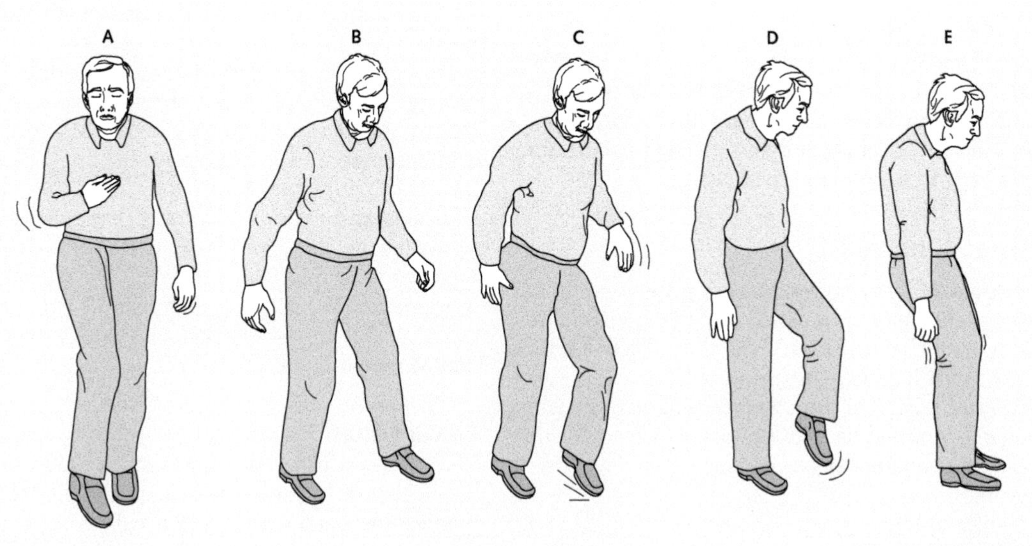

Fig. 17.8 Gait disorders. Hemiplegic (A), cerebellar ataxic (B), sensory ataxic (C), unilateral footdrop (D) and parkinsonian (E).

Antalgic gait

Antalgic gait is caused by painful musculoskeletal conditions. Patients walk with a 'limp' in an attempt to minimize the use of the painful leg.

Apraxic gait

Apraxic gait is caused by parietal lobe lesions. Patients have no difficulty in manipulating their limbs when sitting or lying, but when attempting to walk they experience great difficulty in organizing their gait and placing their feet in the right positions. Gait appears to have an odd and bizarre character. Patients are liable to 'freeze' to the ground, unable to initiate movements.

Hysterical gait

Hysterical gait is erratic and unpredictable. Patients stagger widely with exaggerated arm movements. Falls and injuries are unusual but their presence does not exclude this diagnosis.

Fig. 17.9 Causes of olfactory symptoms
Anosmia (loss of smell)
Congenital Nasal sinuses infections/tumours Head injury/cranial surgery Frontal lobe tumours Subfrontal meningiomas
Parosmia (persistent unpleasant smell)
Nasal infections/tumours Head injury Depression
Olfactory hallucination
Temporal lobe epileptic seizures
Paroxysmal unpleasant smell (burning rubber, smell of gas psychosis)

Romberg's test

To perform Romberg's test, ask the patient to stand with his or her feet together and assess his or her stability. Next, ask the patient to close his or her eyes, making sure that you will be able to support him or her if he or she falls.

Patients with cerebellar or vestibular lesions are usually ataxic on a narrow base with their eyes open. Their ataxia might get marginally worse when the eyes are closed. Patients with proprioceptive sensory loss might be slightly ataxic on a narrow base with their eyes open, but they fall when they close their eyes (positive Romberg's test).

The cranial nerves

Examination of the cranial nerves is a key part of the central nervous system assessment. It provides a number of neurological signs that aid lesion localization, particularly in unconscious patients.

Olfactory nerve (I)

To test the olfactory nerves, first ask patients about any recent change in their sense of smell (anosmia, parosmia, olfactory hallucination) (Fig. 17.9). Then, test their ability to smell coffee, cinnamon or tobacco, by examining each nostril in turn. Avoid using very irritating odours (e.g. ammonia or camphor), which could stimulate the trigeminal nerve endings, even in anosmic patients.

Unilateral loss of smell is usually asymptomatic. Bilateral loss of smell is usually associated with an altered sense of taste (loss of the ability to appreciate aromas). Remember to examine the olfactory nerve in all patients presenting with personality changes, disinhibition or dementia (frontal lobe tumours), and in all cases of head injury.

The eye (II and III)

Visual acuity

Visual acuity is tested using a Snellen chart in a well-lit room. Seat or stand the patient 6 m from the chart. Small, hand-held Snellen charts can be read at a distance of 2 m. Near visual acuity is tested using reading charts but this does not necessarily correlate well with distance acuity.

Correct the patient's refractive errors with glasses or a pinhole. Ask the patient to cover each eye in turn with his or her palm, and find which line of print he or she can read comfortably. Visual acuity is expressed as the ratio of the distance between the patient and the chart to the number of the smallest visible line on the chart (normally 6/6) (Fig. 17.10).

If the patient is unable to read characters of line 60 (visual acuity less than 6/60), assess his or her ability to count your fingers at 1 m (VA: CF), see your hand movements (VA: HM), or perceive a torch light (VA LP). If unable to perceive light (VA: NLP), then the patient is medically blind.

Colour vision

Colour vision is tested using Ishihara plates in a daylight-lit room. Test each eye separately. If 13/15 plates or more are read correctly, colour vision can be regarded as normal. This test is designed principally to detect congenital colour vision defects, but is sensitive in detecting mild degrees of optic nerve dysfunction.

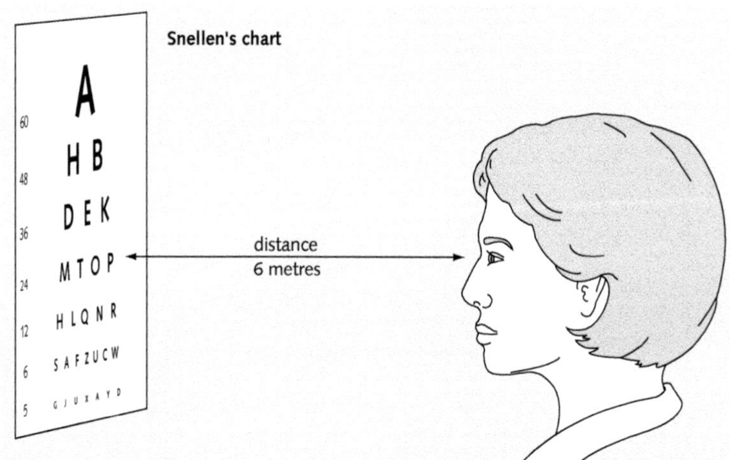

Fig. 17.10 Visual acuity. The patient is able to read line number 24, but not number 12. Visual acuity is 6/24.

Visual fields

Sit about 1 m from the patient with your eyes at the same horizontal level. Start by testing for visual inattention. Ask the patient to look at your eyes and hold your hands outstretched halfway between you and the patient. Stimulate the patient's visual fields by moving each hand separately and then both hands together, and ask the patient to indicate which of your hands has moved each time.

In patients with parietal lobe lesions, a visual stimulus presented in isolation to the contralateral field is perceived, but it is missed when a comparable stimulus is presented simultaneously to the ipsilateral field (neglect).

Visual fields are examined by confrontation, during which you compare your own visual fields with the patient's (provided that yours are normal). The patient's visual field will match yours only if your head positions are exactly comparable and if your hand is exactly halfway between you and the patient; this is seldom the case.

Visual fields in poorly cooperative patients are assessed by using visual threat (sudden, unexpected hand movement into the patient's visual field).

Peripheral fields

Examine each eye in turn. To test the patient's right visual field, ask him or her to cover his or her left eye with his or her left palm and to look at your left eye throughout the examination.

Cover your own right eye with your right hand, and test the patient's peripheral field by bringing the moving fingers of your left hand into the upper and then the lower quadrants of the patient's temporal fields. Ask the patient to inform you as soon as he or she sees your fingers.

Now cover your own right eye with your left hand and examine the patient's nasal fields with your right hand using the same method.

Blind spot

The blind spot is tested using a 10 mm red hat pin. Ask the patient to cover his or her left eye and focus on looking at your nose. Move the pin from the central into the temporal field along the horizontal meridian, having explained to him or her that the pin will disappear briefly and then reappear again, and that he or she should indicate when this happens. Once you have found the patient's blind spot, you can map its shape and compare its size with yours.

Central field

The central field is tested by moving a red hat pin along the central visual field (fixation area) in the horizontal meridian. Ask the patient to indicate if the pin disappears (absolute central scotoma) or if the colour appears diminished (relative scotoma). A central scotoma extends temporally from the fixation area into the blind spot.

Visual field defects

Bedside testing of visual fields can detect only large scotomas. Different patterns of visual field defects can be recognized clinically (Fig. 17.11).

Eyelids and pupils

Inspection

Note the position of the eyelids. If there is a ptosis, decide whether it is partial or complete; assess its fatigability by asking the patient to sustain upward gaze for

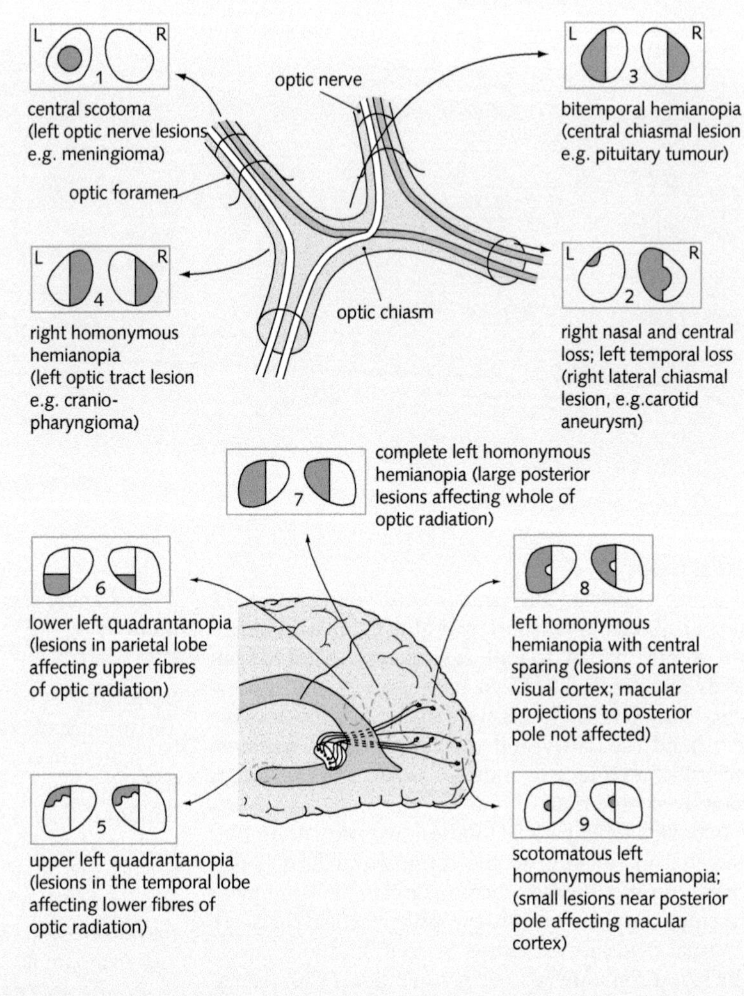

Fig. 17.11 Visual field defects (courtesy of Dr Ross, St Thomas's Hospital, London).

at least 1 minute. Next, assess the size and shape of the pupils. They should be circular and symmetrical (Fig. 17.12).

Light response

Light responses should be assessed using a bright torch light. Ask the patient to fixate on a distant target and shine the light in each eye in turn from the lateral side. Observe the direct (ipsilateral) and the consensual (contralateral) responses. Assess the presence of an afferent pupillary defect by swinging the light from one eye to the other, dwelling 3 seconds on each. As you swing the light from, say, the right eye to the left, the pupil of the latter (which has just started to dilate because of loss of its consensual reaction) should immediately constrict. A delayed constriction indicates loss of sensitivity of the afferent pathways (optic nerve damage).

Accommodation

Hold your finger 50–60 cm from the patient and ask him or her to fixate on it. Bring your finger towards the patient's eyes. Observe the normal reaction of bilateral pupillary constriction and convergence (adduction).

Fundoscopy

This is often the most feared part of the neurological examination. The key to picking up signs is simply a matter of practice – try to look at the fundi of every patient you clerk.

Ask the patient to fixate on a distant target, avoiding bright lights. Using an ophthalmoscope, examine the patient's right eye using your right eye, and the patient's left eye using your left eye. Warn the patient that you will have to get close to them to do this, and try to keep breathing!

unilateral		reaction to light	associated signs
third nerve palsy		negative	ptosis (partial or complete) external ophthalmoplegia
Horner's syndrome		poor reaction to shade	ptosis (always partial) anhydrosis endophthalmus
Holmes–Adie syndrome		slow reaction	constriction to pilocarpine (0.1%) lower limb areflexia
bilateral			
Argyll Robertson		negative	depigmented iris normal accommodation neurosyphilis
midbrain compression		negative	coma lateralizing signs
pontine stroke		negative	coma hyperventilation hyperpyrexia

Fig. 17.12 Pupillary abnormalities.

Adjust the ophthalmoscope lens until the retinal vessels are in focus and trace them back to the optic disc. Assess the optic disc shape, colour and clarity of its margins. The temporal disc margins are normally slightly paler than the nasal margins. The physiological cupping varies in size but does not extend to the disc margins.

Next, assess the retinal vessels. The arteries are narrower than the veins and brighter in colour. The vessels should not be obscured as they cross the disc margins. Look for retinal vein pulsation, which is present in about 80% of normal individuals and is an index of normal intracranial pressure. This is seen best at the disc margins where the veins cross over the arteries. Note the width of the blood vessels and look for arteriovenous nipping at the crossover points.

Assess the rest of the retina, noting any evidence of discoloration, haemorrhages or white patches of exudate. Ask the patient to look at the light of the ophthalmoscope, which brings the macula into view. Classify funduscopic abnormalities into those affecting the optic disc, retinal vessels or the retina (Fig. 17.13).

Patients with acute optic neuritis might have funduscopic abnormalities similar to papilloedema. However, in optic neuritis, eye movements can be painful and visual acuity is substantially reduced.

Eye movements (III, IV and VI)

Inspect the eyes and note the position of the eyelids and the presence of any strabismus (squint). Concomitant strabismus remains constant throughout the range of eye movements and is usually asymptomatic. Incomitant (paralytic) strabismus varies during the range of eye movements.

If the patient is capable of voluntary eye movements, the pursuit and saccadic systems should be tested to assess whether eye movements are conjugate, and to detect the presence of diplopia and nystagmus:

- Isolated painful third nerve palsy is suggestive of a posterior communicating artery aneurysm.
- Pupil-sparing third nerve palsy is suggestive of vascular aetiology, particularly diabetes.
- Monocular diplopia is suggestive of either refractive defects (cornea or lens) or hysteria.
- Very complicated and variable diplopia is suggestive of myasthenia gravis. Look for orbicularis oculi weakness in these cases.

Pursuit eye movements

Steady the patient's head with one hand and hold the index finger of your other hand 40–50 cm in front of his or her eyes. Ask the patient to follow your slowly moving finger throughout the range of binocular vision in both the horizontal and the vertical planes in a letter 'H' pattern.

Assess the smoothness, speed and magnitude of the movements. Look for nystagmus and ask the patient to report any diplopia. In the presence of diplopia, identify the direction of the maximum separation of images and the two muscles responsible for moving the eyes in this direction (Fig. 17.14). Identify the source of the outer image, which comes from the defective eye, by covering each eye in turn. This will allow you to name the muscle(s) and the nerve(s) involved.

Saccadic eye movements

Ask the patient to keep his or her head still, and to look left, right, up and down as quickly as possible. Assess the velocity and the accuracy of the movements. Look for slow or absent adduction (internuclear ophthalmoplegia) (Fig. 17.15).

Fig. 17.13 Common fundoscopic abnormalities

Structure	Abnormality	Pathology
Optic nerve	Papilloedema	Raised intracranial pressure, venous obstruction (e.g. cavernous sinus thrombosis, orbital tumour), high cerebrospinal fluid (CSF) protein (e.g. Guillain–Barré syndrome, spinal cord tumours), malignant hypertension, hypercapnia
	Optic atrophy	Optic neuritis (e.g. multiple sclerosis, Devic's disease), optic nerve/ chiasmal compression (e.g. meningioma, optic nerve gliomas, pituitary tumours, Paget's disease of the skull, arachnoiditis), toxic/ metabolic (e.g. methyl alcohol, B_{12} deficiency), long-standing raised intracranial pressure), infections (e.g. neurosyphilis), hereditary (e.g. Leber's optic atrophy)
Retinal arteries	Silver-wiring, increased tortuosity, arteriovenous nipping	Hypertension
	Gross narrowing with retinal pallor and reddened fovea	Central retinal artery occlusion
	Cholesterol or platelet emboli	Cerebrovascular disease
Retinal veins	Venous engorgement	Papilloedema (see above), central retinal vein occlusion
Retina	Haemorrhages	Superficial flamed-shaped (hypertension) and deep dot-shaped (diabetes), subhyaloid between the retina and the vitreous (subarachnoid haemorrhage)
	Exudates Pigmentation	Soft cotton-wool and hard exudates (diabetes) Retinitis pigmentosa (e.g. hereditary, Refsum's disease, Kearns–Sayre syndrome), choroidoretinitis (e.g. toxoplasmosis, sarcoidosis, syphilis), post-laser treatment (diabetes)

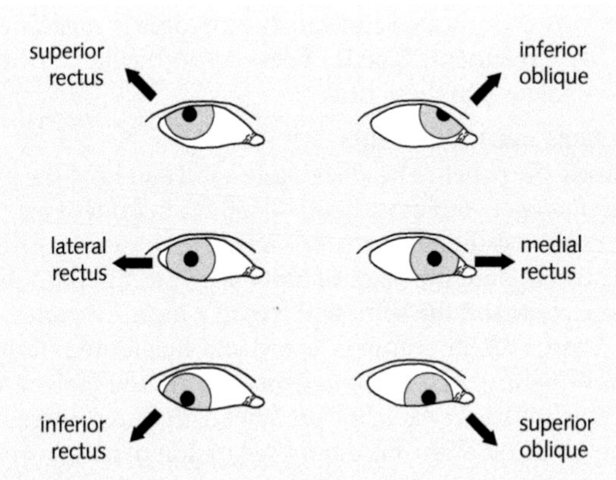

Fig. 17.14 Muscles responsible for eye movements in particular directions.

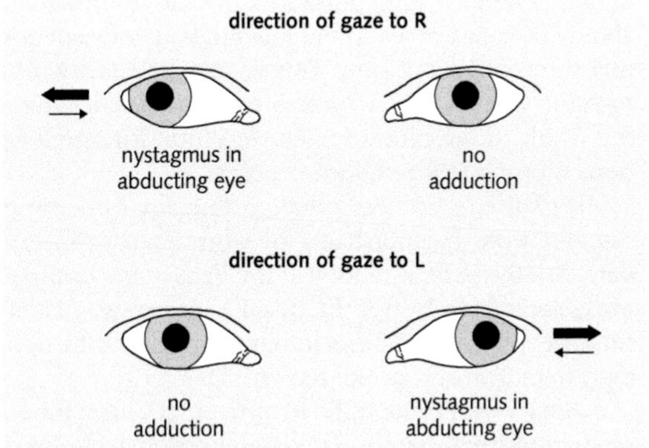

Fig. 17.15 Bilateral internuclear ophthalmoplegia.

If pursuit or saccadic eye movements are absent, oculocephalic reflex (doll's eye movements) will differentiate between supranuclear and nuclear ocular paralysis. Ask the patient to fixate on your eyes while you rotate his or her head in the horizontal and the vertical planes. In supranuclear lesions the reflex is intact, allowing the patient's eyes to remain fixated on yours.

Ocular nerve paresis

Clinical signs of ocular nerve paresis are given in Figure 17.16. Causes of ocular paresis are given in Figure 17.17.

Nystagmus

Nystagmus is an involuntary rhythmic oscillation of the eyes caused by lesions affecting brainstem vertical and horizontal gaze centres and their vestibular and

Fig. 17.16 Clinical signs of ocular nerve paresis

Nerve	Signs
Iii	Ptosis, eye is deviated laterally and slightly downwards (divergent strabismus), pupil may be dilated and unresponsive (pupil sparing in diabetes and vascular causes)
Iv	Impaired depression (and intortion) of the fully adducted eye, head might be tilted to the opposite side to avoid diplopia when reading or looking down
Vi	Impaired abduction (convergent strabismus)

Fig. 17.17 Causes of ocular paresis

Type		Pathology
Supranuclear gaze paresis	Horizontal	Frontal lobe lesions, eyes deviated to the side of the lesion. Common with massive stroke, head injury. Paralysis and voluntary conjugate gaze, with preserved brainstem reflexes (e.g. to coloric stimulation), brainstem pretectal lesions: eyes deviated to opposite side
	Vertical	Brainstem pretectal region: Parinaud's syndrome (vertical gaze paralysis, pupillary dilation, absent accommodation reflex) Extrapyramidal diseases (e.g. Parkinson's disease, progressive supranuclear palsy): impaired vertical gaze (initially upward)
Nuclear and nerve (III, IV, VI) palsies	Brainstem	Vascular lesions, tumours, demyelination, Wernicke's encephalopathy
	Peripheral	Raised intracranial pressure (VI as a false localizing sign, III caused by tentorial herniation) Vascular lesions (e.g.atheroma, diabetes, temporal arteritis, syphilis) aneurysms (posterior communicating artery: III, cavernous sinus: III, IV, VI) Meningeal inflammation and malignant infiltration, skull base tumours (nasopharyngeal carcinoma, chordoma) Cranial polyneuropathy (Guillain–Barré syndrome, sarcoidosis) Orbital tumours and granulomas, sinus disease
Muscle disease		Myasthenia gravis, thyroid eye disease, mitochondrial cytopathy

cerebellar connections. It is usually asymptomatic, except for oscillopsia when patients experience movements of their visual fields.

Nystagmus must be differentiated from normal endpoint nystagmoid jerks seen at extreme deviation of gaze, and from the voluntary rapid oscillation of eyes. Both are brief and unsustained.

Testing

Note the presence of nystagmus in the primary position of gaze (when looking forward), and while examining eye movements, and decide whether it is pendular or jerky, and whether the movements are horizontal, vertical, rotatory or of mixed nature.

Record its amplitude (fine, medium, coarse), persistence and the direction of gaze in which it occurs (the direction of nystagmus is, by convention, the direction of the fast component). Causes of nystagmus are given in Figure 17.18.

The face (V and VII)

Trigeminal nerve (V)

Sensory

Sensory testing is performed using the same techniques as for the rest of the body (described later). Test light touch, pin prick, and temperature over the forehead, the medial aspects of the cheeks and the chin, which correspond to the ophthalmic, maxillary and mandibular branches of the trigeminal nerve, respectively (Fig. 17.19). A partial loss can be detected by comparing the response to the same stimulus on the other sites on the face.

Corneal response is elicited by lightly touching the cornea (not the conjunctiva) with a wisp of cotton wool. Synchronous blinking of both eyes occurs. An afferent defect (Vth cranial nerve lesion) results in depression or absence of the direct and consensual reflex. An efferent defect (VIIth cranial nerve lesion) results in an impairment or absence of the reflex on the side of the

Fig. 17.18 Causes of nystagmus

Type	Description	Pathology
Pendular	Oscillations of equal velocity	Long-standing impaired macular vision (since early childhood), miner's nystagmus
Jerky	Fast phase towards the side of the lesion	Unilateral cerebellar lesions
	Fast phase to the opposite side of the lesion	Unilateral vestibular lesions
	Direction of nystagmus varies with the direction of gaze	Brainstem pathology
	Upbeat nystagmus Downbeat nystagmus	Lesions at or around the superior colliculi Lesions at or around the foramen magnum
Rotatory	Specific to one head position, and fatigues with repeated testing	Unilateral labyrinthine pathology
Rotatory or mixed	All other types	Brainstem pathology

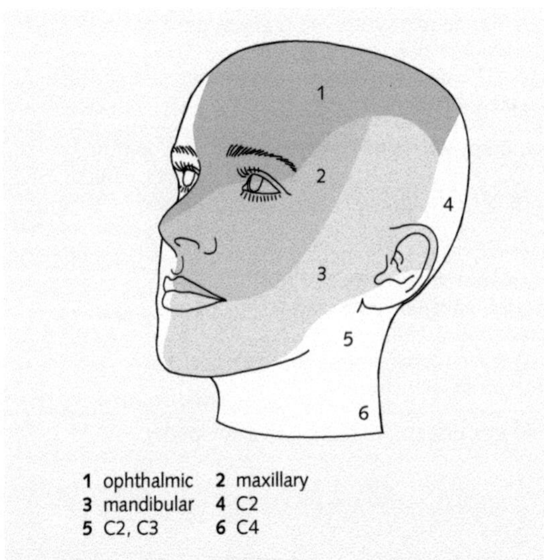

Fig. 17.19 Trigeminal sensory innervation to the face.

facial weakness. The clinical pattern of sensory loss depends on the anatomical site of the lesion (Fig. 17.20).

Motor

Inspect for wasting of the temporalis muscles, which produces hollowing above the zygoma. Ask the patient to clench his or her teeth together and palpate the masseters, noting any wasting. The pterygoid muscles are assessed by resisting the patient's attempts to open his or her mouth. In unilateral trigeminal lesions, the lower jaw deviates to the paralytic side as the mouth is opened.

Jaw jerk

Jaw jerk is a brainstem stretch reflex. Ask the patient to open his or her mouth slightly. Rest your index finger on the apex of the jaw and tap it with the patella hammer. The response, mouth opening, is due to a contraction of the pterygoid muscles. An absent reflex is not significant, but the reflex could be brisk in pseudobulbar palsy (see later).

Facial nerve (VII)

Motor response

Inspect the patient's face, looking for asymmetry of the nasolabial folds and the position of the two angles of the mouth. Assess the movements of the upper part of the face by asking the patient to elevate his or her eyebrows, close his or her eyes tightly and resist your attempt to open them. Movements of the lower side of the face are assessed by asking the patient to blow out his or her cheeks with air, purse his or her lips tightly together and resist your attempt to open them, show his or her teeth, or whistle. Finally, ask the patient to smile, and observe any facial asymmetry.

If you detect any weakness or asymmetry, decide if the weakness is confined to the lower part of the face (upper motor neuron lesion) or both the upper and the lower parts of the face (lower motor neuron lesion) (Figs. 17.21 & 17.22). Do not miss bilateral facial weakness. In this case, the face appears to sag, with lack of facial expression.

Look for Bell's phenomenon (eyeball rotates upwards and outwards on attempting to close the eye). The lack of this sign may indicate that the patient is not attempting to close his or her eye, raising the suspicion of a psychological reason for their symptoms.

Taste

Formal assessment of taste is rarely of practical benefit. Taste is examined by applying a solution of salt, sweet (sugar) or sour (vinegar) to the anterior two-thirds of the tongue and comparing the response on the two

Fig. 17.20 Clinical syndromes of the trigeminal nerve

Site of lesion	Signs	Pathology
Dorsal pons	Altered light touch, with preserved pain and temperature	Vascular, tumour
High central	'Onion-skin' circumoral analgesia which advances outwards	Syringobulbia
Low central medulla or high intrinsic cervical lesion above C2	'Onion-skin' analgesia which starts at the peripheral parts of the face and advances towards the nose and the mouth	Syringomyelia
Lateral medulla	Ipsilateral loss of pain and temperature	Lateral medullary syndrome
Upper cervical cord, foramen magnum	Generalized sensory loss which starts first in ophthalmic division and advances downwards	Cervical spondylosis, meningiomas
Sensory root or ganglia	Generalized sensory loss of all modalities	Acoustic neuroma, meningioma, angioma
Peripheral branch	Selective sensory loss of all modalities	Orbital tumours, neuromas

Fig. 17.21 Clinical syndromes of facial weakness

Site of lesion	Signs	Pathology
Supranuclear	Contralateral (or ipsilateral) UMN weakness	Vascular, tumour
Brainstem	Ipsilateral LMN weakness	Vascular, tumours, syrinx, demyelination
Cerebellopontine angle	Ipsilateral LMN weakness	Acoustic neuromas, meningiomas, angioma
Basal meninges	Often bilateral LMN weakness	Sarcoidosis, malignant meningitis
Petrous bone	Ipsilateral LMN weakness	Middle ear infections, Bell's palsy, geniculate herpetic zoster
Face	Ipsilateral LMN weakness	Parotid tumours, trauma
Muscle disease	Usually bilateral LMN weakness	Myasthenia gravis, myotonic dystrophy, muscular dystrophy
Others	Usually bilateral LMN weakness	Guillain–Barré syndrome

LMN, lower motor neuron; UMN, upper motor neuron

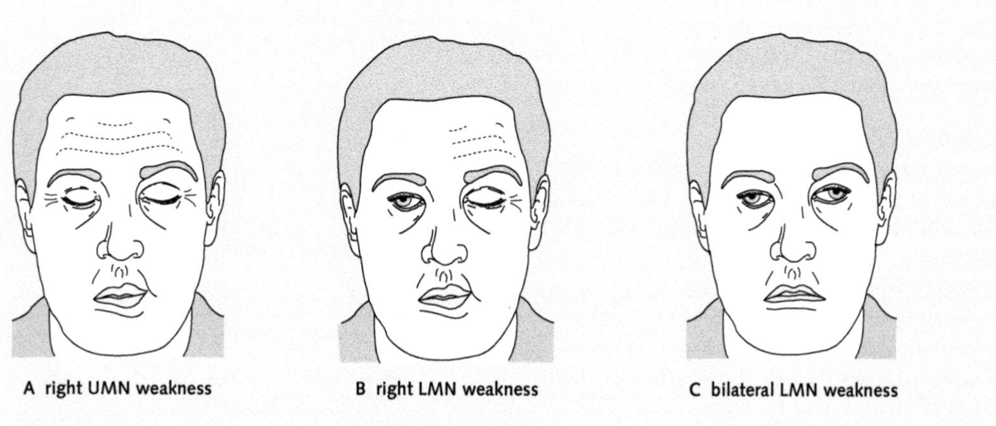

Fig. 17.22 Facial weakness. The patient is asked to close his or her eyes and purse his or her lips. Note the defective eye closure and Bell's phenomenon in B and C. LMN, lower motor neuron; UMN, upper motor neuron.

sides. The mouth should be rinsed with water between testing. Cranial nerve VIII lesions proximal to the middle ear will cause loss of taste.

Hyperacusis

Hyperacusis (undue sensitivity to noise) is suggestive of a lesion proximal to the middle ear, affecting the nerve to the stapedius.

Auditory nerve (VIII)

Hearing

Clinical bedside assessment of hearing is not sensitive and can detect only gross hearing loss. Audiometry is usually required for detailed assessment. Assess each ear separately while masking the hearing in the other ear by occluding the external meatus with your index finger. Test the patient's hearing sensitivity by whispering numbers into his or her ear and asking him or her to repeat them.

If hearing is impaired, examine the external auditory meatus and the tympanic membrane with an auriscope to exclude infections or wax. Determine if the hearing loss is conductive (middle ear pathology) or perceptive (inner ear pathology) by performing Rinne's and Weber's tests.

Rinne's test

Place a vibrating 512 Hz tuning fork on the mastoid process (bone conduction) and then hold it close to the ear (air conduction). Ask the patient to determine which sound is loudest. Normally, air conduction is louder than bone conduction (positive Rinne). In sensorineural deafness, this will be the same. In conductive deafness, bone conduction will be louder.

Weber's test

Place a vibrating 512 Hz tuning fork at the midline over the vertex and ask the patient to determine whether the sound is perceived equally loudly in both ears (normal status), or in one ear more than the other. Sound is heard louder in the affected ear in conductive deafness, and in the unaffected ear in perceptive deafness.

Vestibular functions

Sensory information from the vestibular system is important in the control of posture and eye movements. The vestibular functions are assessed by examining these two areas:

- Posture: patients with vestibular lesions complain of vertigo and are mildly ataxic but usually able to compensate, using their visual input. However, patients with acute vestibular lesions can be markedly ataxic, with a tendency to fall towards the affected side.
- Nystagmus: unilateral vestibular dysfunction causes jerky/rotatory nystagmus with the fast phase towards the unaffected side (see nystagmus).

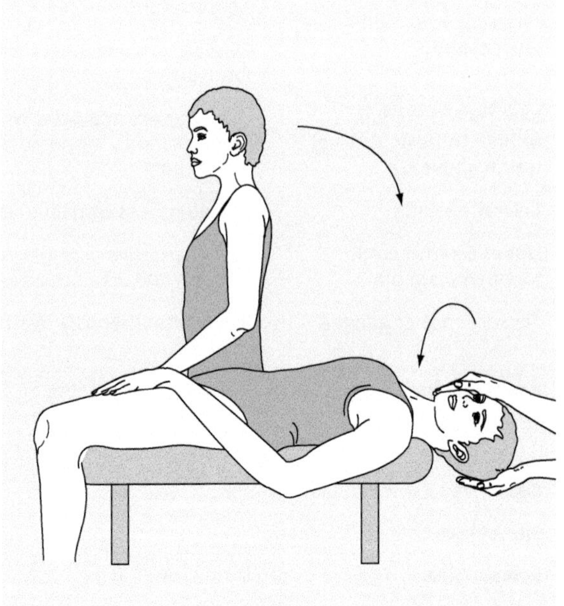

Fig. 17.23 Technique for exhibiting positional nystagmus (Hallpike's manoeuvre).

Hallpike's manoeuvre

Hallpike's manoeuvre should be performed in all patients with positional vertigo (vertigo precipitated by a particular head position).

Sit the patient at the side of a couch facing away from the edge. Pull the patient quickly backwards and to one side so that the head hangs about 30–45° below the horizontal plane rotated to one side (Fig. 17.23). Ask the patient to keep his or her eyes open and to report any vertigo and look for nystagmus. Sit the patient up and observe any nystagmus. Repeat the manoeuvre to the other side. If positive, repeat the manoeuvre to the same side and determine if the pathology is central or peripheral (not always easy) (Fig. 17.24).

Fig. 17.24 Features of peripheral and central positional nystagmus

	Peripheral	Central
Site of pathology	Semicircular canals	Brainstem
Vertigo	Always present	May be absent
Nystagmus	Rotatory	Horizontal/rotatory
Onset	Delayed by 3–10 seconds	Immediate
Repeated testing	Response fatigues	Usually does not fatigue

Caloric testing
This test is not routinely done in all neurological examinations.

Establish that the patient's tympanic membranes are intact. With the patient lying supine with the head elevated at 30°, flush 250 mL of cold water (30°C) into the external auditory meatus. After a delay of 20 seconds, this produces a tonic deviation of the eyes to the same side with compensatory nystagmus to the opposite side lasting for more than 1 minute. Unconscious patients with intact vestibular function will have the tonic deviation only.

The test is repeated 5 minutes later with hot water (44°C), which induces tonic deviation of the eyes to the opposite side and compensatory nystagmus to the side of the irrigated ear.

Labyrinthine or vestibular nerve lesions cause depression of both the 'hot' and the 'cold' responses from the affected side (canal paresis), whereas central lesions cause an enhancement of nystagmus in one of the directions, whether triggered by hot or cold water (directional preponderance).

Clinical patterns of cranial nerve VIII lesions are shown in Figure 17.25.

The mouth (IX, X and XII)

Mouth and tongue

Inspect the tongue as it lies in the floor of the mouth for evidence of wasting (unilateral or bilateral), fasciculations (shimmering movements at the surface of the tongue) or other involuntary movements (Huntington's chorea, orofacial dyskinesia). Ask the patient to protrude his or her tongue, and then move it rapidly from side to side.

Fig. 17.25 Clinical patterns of VIIIth cranial nerve lesions

Site of lesions	Clinical features	Pathology
Peripheral	Auditory and/or vestibular symptomatology	Cranial trauma Barotrauma Infections Occlusion of the internal auditory artery Ménière's disease Toxins and drugs
Central	Auditory or vestibular symptomatology, often with other cranial nerve involvement (V, VII) and long tract signs	Cerebrovascular disease, multiple sclerosis, cerebellopontine angle tumours, brainstem tumours, syringobulbia

Fig. 17.26 Clinical patterns of tongue weakness

Lower motor neuron lesions	Unilateral	Focal atrophy, fasciculations and deviation to the ipsilateral (paralysed) side
	Bilateral	See bulbar palsy (Fig. 17.27)
Upper motor neuron lesions	Unilateral	Deviation to the paralysed side
	Bilateral	See pseudobulbar palsy (Fig. 17.27)

Abnormalities can be caused by unilateral or bilateral upper motor neuron or lower motor neuron lesions (Fig. 17.26).

Pharynx and gag reflex

With the patient's mouth wide open, inspect the soft palate, the uvula, and the posterior pharyngeal wall at rest and during phonation (by asking the patient to say 'aah').

If you suspect a positive finding, press the end of an orange stick into the posterior pharyngeal wall, first on one side then the other. Assess the afferent pathway of the gag reflex (IXth cranial nerve) by asking the patient if the sensation is comparable on the two sides, and the efferent pathway (Xth cranial nerve) by inspecting the normal response of a symmetrical rise of the soft palate in the midline. This is a very unpleasant sensation for the patient and should be carried out with care.

The upper motor neuron innervation of the palatal and pharyngeal muscles is bilateral and unilateral lesions cause no significant dysfunction. In unilateral lower motor neuron lesions, the palate lies slightly lower on the affected side and deviates to the intact side during phonation or while testing the gag reflex.

Minor and inconsistent deviations of the uvula should be ignored.

The larynx

Formal assessment of the vocal cords is usually performed by indirect laryngoscopy, which is not part of the clinical examination. Bedside evaluation is confined to the assessment of phonation and cough.

Unilateral lesions of the recurrent laryngeal nerve cause partial upper airway obstruction with stridor, hoarseness of voice and 'bovine' cough. Bilateral lesions cause severe stridor and aphonia.

The accessory nerve (XI)

The function of the trapezius muscles is assessed by asking the patient to shrug their shoulders, first without, and then against, resistance. The bulk and the strength of the sternocleidomastoid muscle is assessed by asking the patient to rotate their head to the contralateral side against the resistance of your hand.

Bulbar and pseudobulbar palsies (IX, X, XII)

These syndromes describe bilateral weakness of the bulbar muscles of either an upper or a lower motor neuron type (Fig. 17.27).

Multiple cranial nerve palsies

Patchy loss of function

These palsies are usually caused by:

- Malignant meningitis (due to carcinoma, lymphoma or leukaemia)
- Granulomatous meningitis (due to sarcoidosis, tuberculosis or syphilis)
- Bone disease (due to metastasis or Paget's disease).

Diffuse loss of function

These palsies are usually caused by:

- Guillain–Barré syndrome
- Motor neuron disease
- Myasthenia gravis
- Polymyositis.

The motor system

In most cases, the cardinal sign of motor impairment is weakness. Remember that other findings (signs) will vary with the sites of pathology (Fig. 17.28).

Acute upper motor neuron lesions cause decreased tone (flaccid paralysis) and absent reflexes, although Babinski's response (see below) will be extensor. Whenever possible, begin with an inspection of the patient's gait. While the patient is standing:

- Can the patient stand on his or her toes and heels without support?
- Can the patient hop? Most patients with significant leg weakness cannot hop.

Fig. 17.27 Clinical features and causes of pseudobulbar and bulbar palsies

	Clinical features	Cause	Pathology
Pseudobulbar palsy	Dysarthria (spastic), choking attacks, emotional lability; the tongue is stiff, spastic, slow but not wasted; jaw jerk and gag reflexes are brisk	Bilateral upper motor neuron lesions of IX, X and XII (supranuclear)	Bilateral cerebrovascular disease, motor neuron disease, multiple sclerosis, supranuclear palsy, Creutzfeldt–Jakob disease
Bulbar palsy	Dysarthria (nasal), dysphagia and nasal regurgitation; the tongue appears wasted, flaccid and fasciculating, and the gag reflex is absent	Bilateral lower motor neuron lesions	• Nuclear: medullary infarction, tumour, syrinx, encephalitis • Peripheral nerve: cranial polyneuropathy (e.g. Guillian–Barré syndrome, sarcoidosis, diphtheria), neoplasms (e.g. meningeal infiltration, metastasis), skull base lesions (e.g. metastasis, chordoma, glomus tumour), skull base anomaly (e.g. Chiari malformation) • Disorders of neuromuscular transmission: myasthenia gravis • Primary muscle disease: polymyositis, muscular dystrophy

Fig. 17.28 Variation in examination findings with site of pathology

Site of lesion	Wasting	Tone	Power	Reflexes
Upper motor neuron	None	Increased	Decreased	Increased
Lower motor neuron	Wasted	Decreased	Decreased	Decreased
Neuromuscular junction	Rarely	Usually normal, decreased	Decreased (fatigable)	Usually normal
Muscle	Sometimes	Normal	Decreased	Decreased

Not every patient will have every feature and occasionally patients may diverge from these features, but this remains a useful guide.

Following this, ask the patient to lie on the bed, and make sure his or her arms and legs are exposed.

An examination of the motor system should include the following four features:

- Tone
- Power
- Coordination
- Reflexes.

Inspection

Look for:

- Wasting – a reduction of muscle bulk in certain muscles compared with others. Wasted muscles are usually weak, and wasting is characteristic of lower motor neuron (i.e. anterior horn cell, nerve root and nerve) dysfunction.
- Scars – indicating previous injury or surgery, which may have damaged a nerve
- Fasciculations – seen as rippling or twitching of a muscle at rest, a feature of lower motor neuron problems (especially, but not exclusively, motor neuron disease)
- Involuntary movements such as tremor may be obvious.

Tone

'Tone' means how floppy (decreased tone) or stiff (increased tone) a limb feels. Some patients with increased tone in the legs may complain that their legs 'jump', especially in bed. Other patients have difficulty relaxing during an examination, which can artificially increase stiffness in their limbs. You must, therefore, do your upmost to put them at ease.

Arms

To examine tone, relax the patient and ask them to make themselves 'go floppy'. Take his or her arm and slowly flex and extend the elbow, then hold his or her hand (with elbow flexed) and pronate/supinate the forearm. Try to make your movements as unpredictable as possible, as cooperative patients may unconsciously try to 'help' you move their arms. If tone is increased, you may feel a 'supinator catch' – an interruption of the smooth movement on supination. Other signs in the arm include 'cog-wheel' rigidity, typically seen in Parkinson's disease.

Legs

There are several ways to examine tone in the legs:

- Rock each leg from side to side on the bed, holding it at the knee. Normally, the foot lags behind the leg. If tone is increased, the foot and leg move stiffly, as one unit. If tone is decreased, the foot flops from side to side.
- Flex and extend the knee, supporting both the upper leg and the foot.
- Place your hand under the patient's knee and quickly lift the knee about 15 cm; normally the foot will stay on the bed; if tone is increased, it may jump up with the lower leg.

Clonus describes the rhythmic contractions evoked by a sudden passive stretch of a muscle, elicited most easily at the ankle. A few beats may be normal in anxious patients, but 'sustained clonus' is characteristic of an upper motor neuron lesion.

Increased tone occurs in two main forms:

- Spasticity (derived from the Greek word *spastikos*, to tug or draw) is associated with upper motor neuron lesions, characterized by resistance to the first few degrees of movement, then a sudden lessening of resistance with a 'give way' (so-called clasp-knife) effect.
- Rigidity is characteristic of extrapyramidal disorders such as Parkinson's disease, distinguished clinically from spasticity by constant resistance to passive movement at a joint (lead-pipe rigidity). If tremor is superimposed on rigidity, the resistance is jerky or of 'cog-wheel' type.

Power

Power needs to be tested in each of the main muscle groups. Power in each muscle is given a grade defined by the Medical Research Council scale (Fig. 17.29), which can initially seem complicated, but is very useful for assessing changes.

The scheme illustrated in Figure 17.30 and Figure 17.31 allows testing of the main muscle groups of the arms. The scheme illustrated in Figure 17.32 and Figure 17.33 allows testing of the main muscle groups of the legs.

Fig. 17.29 The Medical Research Council (MRC) scale for muscle weakness

Grade	Response
0	No movement
1	Flicker of muscle when patient tries to move
2	Moves, but not against gravity
3	Moves against gravity but not against resistance
4	Moves against resistance but not to full strength
5	Full strength (you cannot overcome the movement with your equivalent muscle group)

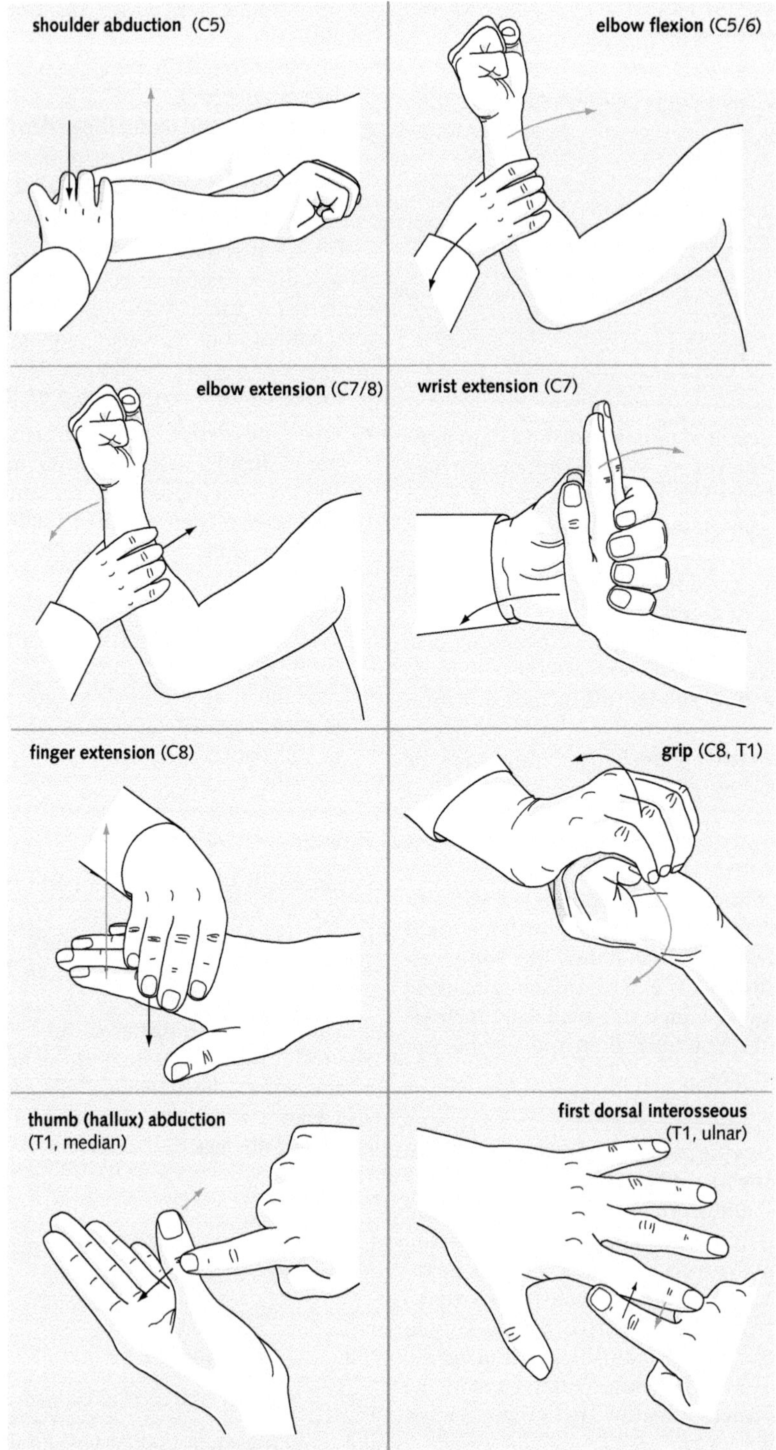

Fig. 17.30 Testing muscle groups of the upper limb. The blue arrow indicates the direction of movement of the patient, and the black arrow the direction of movement of the examiner. Each muscle group should be given a grade as defined by the MRC scale (see Fig. 17.29).

Fig. 17.31 Scheme for examination of power in the upper limbs

Movement	Instruction	Muscle/myotome
Shoulder abduction	Bend your elbow and hold your arms up and out to the side Don't let me push them down	Deltoid/C5
Elbow flexion	Bend your elbow and don't let me straighten it	Biceps/C5, C6
Elbow extension	Now straighten your elbow and don't let me bend it	Triceps/C7, C8
Wrist extension	Push your hands up like this and don't let me stop you	Wrist extensors/C7
Finger extension	Straighten your fingers out and don't let me push them down	Finger extensors/C8
Grip	Grip my fingers	Finger flexors/C8, T1
Thumb abduction	[With palms flat] point your thumb to the ceiling and don't let me push it down	Abductor pollicis brevis/C8, T1, median nerve
Index finger abduction	Spread your fingers wide and don't let me push them together	Abductors (dorsal interossei)/T1, ulnar nerve

It is useful to get into the habit of giving the same instruction to each patient you examine.

Fig. 17.32 Scheme for examination of power in the lower limbs

Movement	Instruction	Muscle/myotome
Hip flexion	Lift your leg straight off the bed, keep it up	Iliopsoas/L1, L2
Hip extension	Straighten your knee and don't let me bend your leg	Quadriceps/L3, L4
Hip adduction	Keep your knees together and don't let me pull them apart	Hip adductors/L2, L3
Knee flexion	Bend your knee and keep it bent	Hamstrings/L5, S1
Ankle dorsiflexion	Pull your foot up towards your nose, don't let me push it down	Tibialis anterior and long extensors/L4, L5
Plantiflexion (towards the floor)	Point your foot down to the bed, keep it there	Gastrocnemius/S1
Knee extension	Press your legs flat against the bed and don't let me pull them up	Gluteal muscles/L5, S1

Reflexes

Tendon reflexes are most easily determined by stretching the tendon with a tendon hammer. Tap either onto the tendon directly or onto a finger placed over the tendon (biceps and supinator) (Fig. 17.34A). You should examine the tendon reflexes in the leg, as shown in Figure 17.34B. These may be:

- Increased
- Decreased
- Absent.

If absent, this should be confirmed by reinforcement (Fig. 17.34C shows this for the legs). There are two methods:

- Ask the patient to clench their teeth tightly just before you tap the reflex.
- Ask the patient to grip their hands and pull sideways (hard!) just before you tap the reflex.

The latter is obviously not appropriate when testing arm reflexes.

Tendon reflexes are conventionally notated as shown in Figure 17.35. Abdominal reflexes can be tested as shown in Figure 17.34D. The plantar response is elicited by scratching of the sole (Fig. 17.34E).

Coordination

Whether a patient can perform smooth and accurate movements is dependent partly on power in the muscles, lack of which may cause clumsiness, but more importantly on the cerebellar system. Assess:

- Gait – a wide-based, sometimes lurching gait is seen in cerebellar disease. Unsteadiness is made more obvious if the patient is asked to walk 'heel to toe'.
- Arms – the finger–nose test: ask the patient to touch your finger, held about 50 cm in front of the patient,

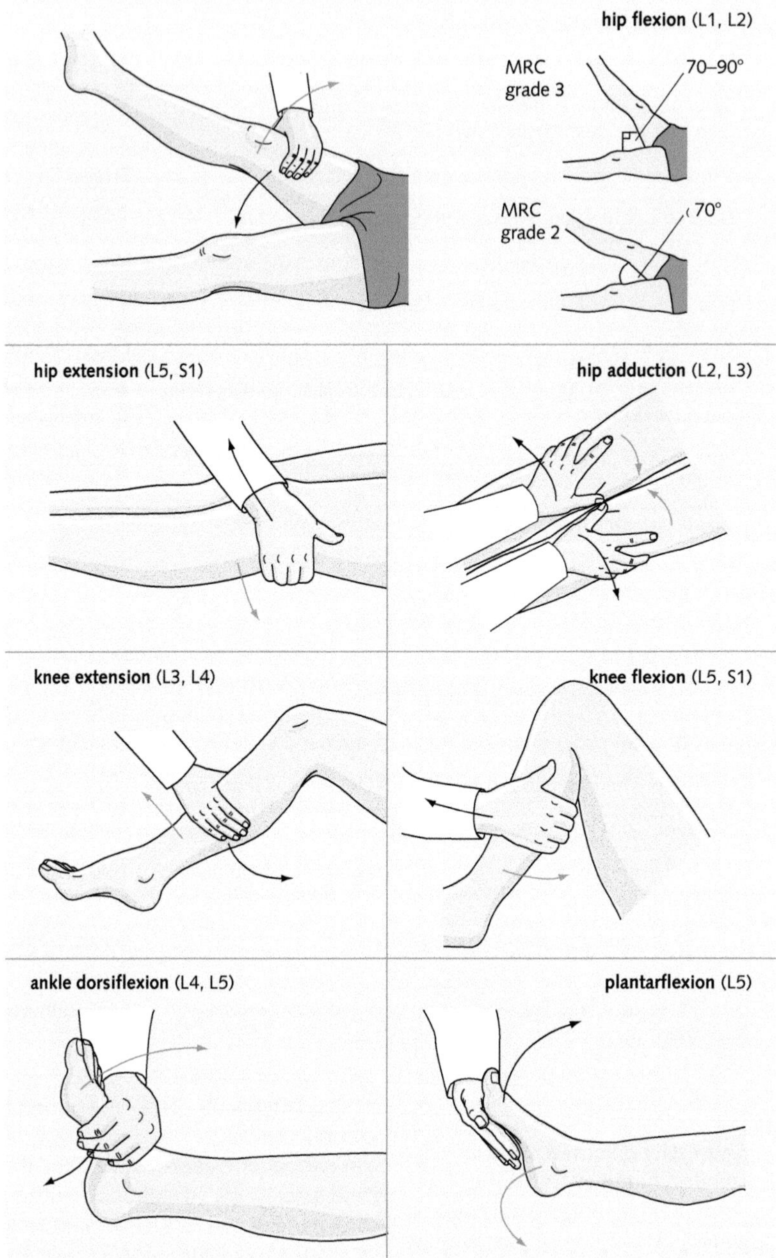

Fig. 17.33 Testing muscle groups of the lower limb. The blue arrow indicates the direction of movement of the patient, and the black arrow the direction of movement of the examiner. Each muscle group should be given a grade as defined by the MRC scale (see Fig. 17.29).

with his or her index finger and then to touch his or her nose, then move back and forth. You may have to move the patient's finger for him or her on the first attempt. Cerebellar lesions may cause 'overshooting' of the target, missing your finger (past-pointing) or tremor (intention tremor). Dysdiadochokinesis describes the impairment of rapid alternating movements seen in such patients, and is tested by asking them to slap their palm while alternately pronating and supinating their other arm.

- Legs – the heel–shin test. Ask the patient to place one heel on the other knee and slowly slide the heel

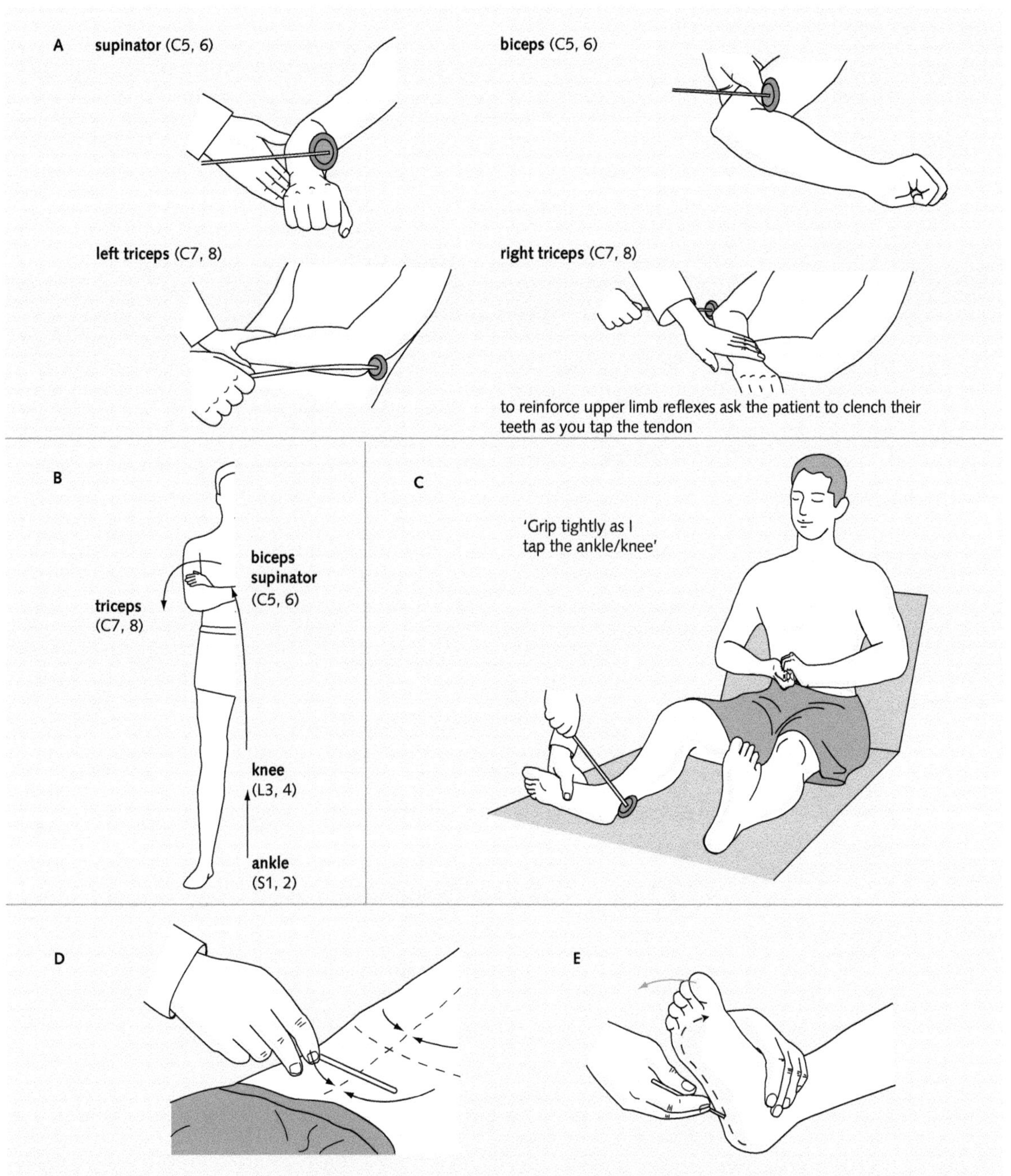

Fig. 17.34 Eliciting reflexes. A, Upper limb tendon reflexes. B, A simple way to remember root values of reflexes. C, Testing ankle jerk with reinforcement. D, Abdominal reflexes: test in four quadrants shown. E, The normal response is a downgoing hallux. In an upper motor neuron lesion, the hallux dorsiflexes and the other toes fan out (the Babinski response).

down the lower leg, then up again. Intention tremor may be seen.

Note that the presence of inaccuracy is the most important sign. These movements must be tested on each side in turn.

Abnormality of these movements in a patient with a cerebellar problem is described as ataxia, and may be associated with other signs of cerebellar disease:

- Nystagmus
- Dysarthria.

Fig. 17.35 Annotation of tendon reflexes	
Normal	+
Brisk	++
Very brisk, with associated clonus	+++
Absent	0
Present with reinforcement only (decreased)	±

Fine movements

Early stages of an upper motor neuron or extrapyramidal disorder may be picked up by noting impairment of fine finger movements: ask the patient to pretend to play a piano and to touch the thumb with each finger of the same hand in turn.

Abnormal movements (dyskinesias)

Abnormal movements include:

- Decreased movement (e.g. the bradykinesia of Parkinson's disease)
- Increased movement.

The main types of increased movement you will encounter are shown in Figure 17.36, and may involve the limbs (more usually the arms) and face. All are involuntary.

The most important aspect of examination of dyskinesias is inspection, and most of the features described in Figure 17.36 can be elicited by this alone. In addition:

- Tremor at rest – ask the patient to sit with his or her hands overhanging his or her lap, close his or her eyes and count backwards from 100 to 'bring out' resting tremor.
- Tremor with different actions – the patient will complain if anything in particular makes his or her tremor worse (e.g. holding a cup), so examine those actions in particular. The same applies to myoclonus and dystonias.
- Walking may exaggerate certain movement disorders (e.g. dystonias), so examine this too.

The akinetic rigid syndromes are characterized by abnormal movement:

Fig. 17.36 Types of abnormal movement (dyskinesia)		
Tremor	**Action**	
	Physiological	Normal, low amplitude, in outstretched hands
	Drug induced	Exaggerated of normal (e.g. sympathomimetics, lithium)
	Essential	Coarser, especially when assuming a posture (e.g. holding a glass), usually autosomal dominant; especially in upper limbs; may involve the head (titubation)
	Resting	Ask the patient to sit with his hands in his lap, most common in Parkinson's disease
	Intention	Cerebellar, as above
Jerks	**Tic**	Abrupt, repetitive, stereotyped jerk-like movements; especially facial; no cause is often found; can be suppresed
	Chorea	Fleeting, irregular, semi-purposeful, disorderly movements affecting any body part; caused by, e.g., Huntington's disease, stroke involving the subthalamic nucleus (causing ipsilateral chorea, or hemiballismus), drugs (e.g. neuroleptics), or systemic lupus erythematosus
	Athetosis	Slow, writhing movements, often with chorea
	Myoclonus	Brief shock-like muscle contractions
	Focal	Of one body part (e.g. palatal myoclonus)
	Segmental	Caused by focal disease of the spinal cord or brainstem and involving body segments supplied by this region (e.g. arm)
	Generalized	A large number of causes including liver and renal failure, Creutzfeldt–Jakob disease, anoxia, and myoclonic epilepsy
		May also be *at rest*, with *action* (e.g. postanoxia), or *stimulus sensitive* (e.g. postencephalitis)
Dystonia	**Focal**	Sustained muscle contraction causing unusual postures, may be painful
	Segmental	Involving one body part (e.g. writers' cramp, torticollis)
	Axial	Affecting adjacent body segments
	Hemidystonia	Involving neck and back
	Generalized	On one side of the body (e.g. cerebral palsy)
		All limbs and axial muscles involved (e.g. metabolic disorders – Wilson's disease, Parkinson's disease)
		Drug-induced dystonia may be acute (e.g. metoclopramide, neuroleptics), or chronic (e.g. L-dopa, phenytoin)

- Parkinson's disease
- Steele–Richardson syndrome (with vertical eye movement disturbance and mild dementia)
- Multiple system atrophy (MSA):
  - MSA- P (Parkinsonism) +/- autonomic failure
  - MSA- C (cerebellar) +/- autonomic failure.

When examining a patient with Parkinson's disease, the most commonly encountered disorder of movement, look in particular for:

- Bradykinesia (slow movements) (especially obvious on fine finger movements)
- Rigidity – carefully examine tone for cog-wheeling
- Tremor – 'pill-rolling', at rest
- Festinant gait – slow, shuffling, flexed, decreased arm swing, unstable on turning, may 'freeze'. May show retropulsion (will walk backwards if stopped). Initiation of movements is affected, so watch the patient rise from a chair, or start to walk from a stationary position
- Facial akinesia – characteristic facies with poverty of movement and lack of expression. May have a 'positive glabellar tap': with the hand above the patient, repeatedly tap between the eyes. A normal person will stop blinking after a few taps, but a patient with Parkinson's disease will continue to blink. In practice, this is not particularly useful, but is a favourite with examiners. Increased salivation or drooling may also be evident
- Handwriting – small and cramped. Keep a sample of this in your examination notes.

Causes of mixed upper and lower motor neuron signs:
- Motor neurone disease
- Single spinal cord and adjacent root lesion (e.g. cervical spondylosis)
- Acquired immune deficiency syndrome (AIDS)
- Syphilis
- Chronic upper motor neuron weakness causing 'disuse atrophy'.

Sensation

Patients use various terms to describe sensory disturbance: numbness, weakness, tingling/pins and needles (paraesthesiae), odd unpleasant touch (dysaesthesia) and painful touch (hyperaesthesia).

Tell the patient that you are going to test whether he or she can feel certain sensations.

Sensory testing

Do not spend hours doing this; you will exhaust the patient and yourself. Be sensible and tailor your examination to the patient's complaint. Remember, sensation from one side of the body travels in sensory tracts to the contralateral cerebral hemisphere. If the patient complains of loss of sensation, start sensory testing in the abnormal area, and move out from there.

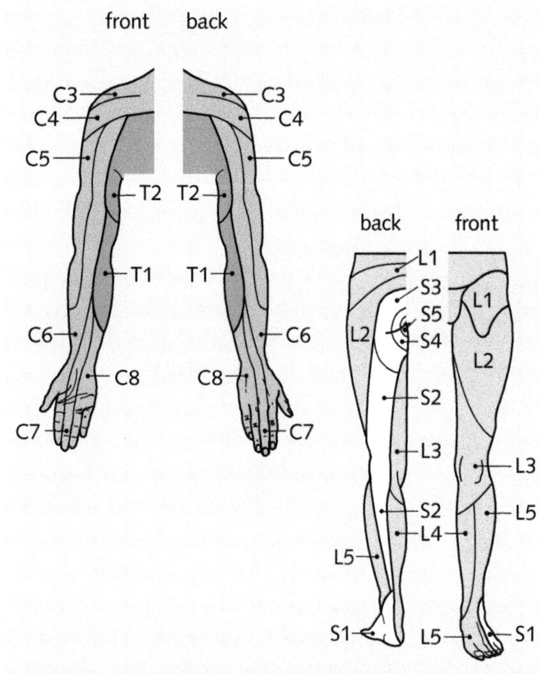

Fig. 17.37 Dermatomes of the upper and lower limbs.

The dermatomes of the upper and lower limbs are shown in Figure 17.37.

Pin prick

Use a sensory testing/needlework pin, not a needle. Test the pin on the sternum first: 'Can you feel this as sharp?' With the patient's eyes open, start at the tips of the fingers/toes and work your way proximally. If the patient does not complain of sensory disturbance, it is not necessary to traverse the entire body with the pin. Remember, this is testing pain sensation. Ask the patient 'Is it sharp or blunt?'

Light touch

Test with cotton wool and with the patient's eyes closed. Start at fingers/toes and work proximally.

Ask the patient to 'Say yes when you feel me touching you'.

Joint position sense

Move the distal interphalangeal joint of the index finger/toe up or down, holding the sides of the digit. With the patient's eyes closed, ask them 'Is your toe/finger moving up … or down?' Demonstrate what you mean by 'up' and 'down' before testing, as patients often do not understand.

Vibration sense

Use a 128 Hz tuning fork. Set it vibrating, and place it on the patient's sternum. Ask the patient 'Can you feel this vibrating?' Place the tuning fork on the distal interphalangeal joint of the great toe (hallux). Ask 'Can you feel it now?'. If not, move the turning fork to the medial malleolus, the tibial tuberosity and the greater trochanter to determine the level at which vibration sense remains intact.

Vibration sensation is often lost early in neuropathies.

Two-point discrimination

Test two-point discrimination with specific compasses and with the patient's eyes closed. While testing on the pulp of the index finger (normal 3 mm) and hallux (5 mm), ask 'Do you feel one point or two?'

Temperature

With the patient's eyes closed, touch the skin with the flat forks of a tuning fork, not vibrating. Ask 'Does this feel hot or cold?'

Lhermitte's symptom

Lhermitte's symptom is a sudden, electric-shock-like sensation travelling down the neck and back when the neck flexes. It is caused by a lesion in the spinal cord, most typically multiple sclerosis.

HINTS AND TIPS

If the patient complains of sensory disturbance, start testing that area first. If there is no complaint, start distally and move proximally. Test each sensation in turn in the arms, then each sensation in turn in the legs. Pain sensation is not agony sensation and therefore do not use a blood-taking needle!

The autonomic nervous system

The autonomic nervous system innervates the viscera and is influenced by the hypothalamus via both direct descending pathways and endocrine hormones. It is important to appreciate the anatomy and roles of the individual sympathetic and parasympathetic systems, especially in relation to the effects of drugs on each. Clinically, 'autonomic failure' usually involves both systems simultaneously, most commonly presenting with a combination of symptoms, as shown in Figure 17.38.

Thorough examination of this system is not necessary in every neurological patient unless the patient complains of symptoms of autonomic failure or the diagnosis is suspected. These tests may be performed at the bedside whilst more specialized tests may be performed by an autonomic function laboratory.

Fig. 17.38 Signs and symptoms of autonomic failure

Affected system or site	Signs and symptoms
Cardiovascular system	Postural hypotension (or, uncommonly, hypertension); impaired response of pulse to respiration, posture or Valsalva manoeuvre; resting tachycardia
Genitourinary system	Impotence, ejaculatory failure, changes in bladder function (including incontinence)
Gastrointestinal tract	Constipation or diarrhoea
Secretory systems	Inability to sweat; dry mouth and eyes
Pupils	Horner's syndrome; dilation or constriction; sluggish or absent light response

Examination of the cardiovascular system

Measure the blood pressure after the patient has been lying down for a few minutes. Then stand the patient up, wait for a minute and take the blood pressure again. The systemic blood pressure normally rises a little. A fall of > 20 mm Hg in systolic pressure is abnormal (postural hypotension).

The pulse can be monitored by a continuous electrocardiogram recording (measurement of the R–R interval is a useful way of measuring such pulse changes) in response to posture, with deep respiration (sinus arrhythmia may be lost) and with Valsalva's manoeuvre.

Valsalva's manoeuvre

Ask the patient to take a deep breath in, then to blow out through a 20 mL syringe (they will not be able to push the plunger out). Normally, a tachycardia occurs during the forced expiration, followed by a reflex bradycardia on release. The blood pressure drops initially, then is maintained throughout the expiration, before overshooting on release. This response is lost in autonomic failure.

Examination of other systems

Examination of other effects of autonomic failure includes:

- The pupils (Fig. 17.39)
- Effects of stress (such as grip, arousal, mental activity) on pulse and blood pressure
- Pharmacological tests of cardiovascular function
- Sweating responses with heat and pharmacological agents
- Skin responses to pharmacological agents
- Urodynamic tests and sphincter electromyography.

Fig. 17.39 Examination of the pupils in the presence of autonomic dysfunction

Test	Normal response	Autonomic failure
Instillation of 1:1000 adrenaline (epinephrine)	No effect	Dilation if have sympathetic post-ganglionic denervation
Instillation of 2.5% methacholine	No effect	Constriction if have parasympathetic denervation

Examination of the unconscious patient

Assessment of the patient

As with any medical emergency, resuscitation is the priority.

- An unconscious patient is a medical emergency and, as such, resuscitation takes priority (A, B, C, etc.).
- Because hypoglycaemia is easily treatable, a finger-prick glucose test should be performed immediately.
- The Glasgow Coma Scale gives an easily recognizable estimation of the level of consciousness.
- Pupils, eye movements, tone, and reflexes may be the only source of neurological localization.

A – check the airway – in danger either because protective reflexes (e.g. coughing) are suppressed or the respiratory centre is compromised. Clear debris and insert an oropharyngeal/nasopharyngeal airway or endotracheal tube if necessary.

B – breathing – early stages of respiratory centre depression cause 'periodic' (Cheyne–Stokes) breathing, with alternate hyperventilation and apnoea. Later, the patient may hyperventilate. Breathing then becomes irregular, then gasping, prior to respiratory arrest. Give oxygen and count the respiratory rate. Abnormality indicates that artificial ventilation may be necessary.

C – circulation – pulse and blood pressure. Raised intracranial pressure causes raised blood pressure and a slow pulse, and progression of this indicates increasing pressure. Drug overdoses may cause arrhythmias. Hypotension may need to be corrected. Attach an electrocardiogram monitor.

D – disability – assess the patient's general and neurological status (a rapid but careful examination of each system is mandatory). Obtain a history from a relative or friend (this is often the most helpful part of the assessment and can save a great deal of time). Look for drug bottles, prescriptions or a MedicAlert bracelet.

E – environment and exposure – the patient must be examined from head to toe, but do not forget that hypothermia is an important cause of neurological disability.

G – never forget glucose! – hypoglycaemia is a common and easily treatable cause of unconsciousness (usually caused by insulin overdose). Check blood glucose immediately in every unconscious patient and treat with intravenous glucose if low. If high, check the urine for ketones and treat as a diabetic ketoacidosis.

The Glasgow Coma Scale (Fig. 17.40) is a widely used, standard, consistent and fairly sensitive measure of the level of unconsciousness. It enables:

Fig. 17.40 The Glasgow Coma Scale. Coma score is E + M + V. The maximum (fully conscious) score is therefore 15 and the range 3–15

Eyes (E)	
Opening spontaneously (with blinking)	4
Open to command or speech	3
Open in response to pain (applied to limbs or sternum)	2
Not opening	1
Motor function (M)	
Obeys commands	6
Localizes to pain	5
Withdraws from pain	4
Flexor response to pain (decorticate)	3
Extensor response to pain (decerebrate)	2
No response to pain	1
Vocalization (V)	
Appropriate speech	5
Confused speech	4
Inappropriate words	3
Groans only	2
No speech	1

- Small changes in the patient's unconscious level to be noted quickly
- Medical staff to communicate rapidly with each other regarding the patient's condition.

You should also consider:

- Narcotics (e.g. pin-point pupils, needle tracks, slow respiratory rate); give naloxone
- Is the patient fitting? If so, give intravenous lorazepam or diazepam
- Head injury (if found, assume also has cervical spine injury until proved otherwise)
- Neck stiffness (e.g. meningitis, subarachnoid haemorrhage). If there is any suspicion of meningitis, do not delay treatment whilst a CT of the brain and lumbar puncture is performed. Take blood for culture and treat immediately with an intravenous antibiotic according to the local treatment protocol for meningitis.

Particular points to note in the neurological assessment are:

- Pupils, eye movements (Fig. 17.41) and fundi. Papilloedema is a late stage of raised intracranial pressure and this diagnosis cannot be excluded if the fundi are normal. Retinal haemorrhages may be seen with subarachnoid haemorrhage.
- Tone, power (is there any movement, spontaneously or in response to command or pain?) and reflexes can localize the cause. Brainstem lesions usually cause bilateral (symmetrical or asymmetrical) signs, sometimes just reflex changes. Supratentorial lesions usually cause asymmetrical signs (e.g. hemiparesis).

Investigations

Undertake urgent investigations (e.g. blood glucose, urea and electrolytes, liver function tests, full blood count, arterial blood gases, urine and blood drug screens, thyroid function tests, blood cultures).

Chest X-ray, skull X-ray, computed tomography brain scan, lumbar puncture and electroencephalogram may also be necessary.

Other management

The patient is likely to need urethral catheterization (also enables fluid balance to be monitored). Other aspects of longer-term care include:

- Continued monitoring of A, B, C and Glasgow Coma Scale
- Turning to prevent pressure sores
- Eye, mouth, bladder and bowel care
- Passive limb movements to prevent contractures.

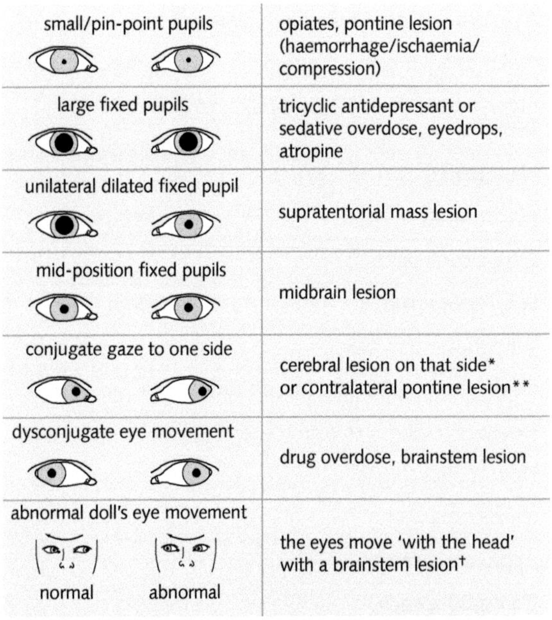

small/pin-point pupils	opiates, pontine lesion (haemorrhage/ischaemia/compression)
large fixed pupils	tricyclic antidepressant or sedative overdose, eyedrops, atropine
unilateral dilated fixed pupil	supratentorial mass lesion
mid-position fixed pupils	midbrain lesion
conjugate gaze to one side	cerebral lesion on that side* or contralateral pontine lesion**
dysconjugate eye movement	drug overdose, brainstem lesion
abnormal doll's eye movement (normal / abnormal)	the eyes move 'with the head' with a brainstem lesion†

Fig. 17.41 Pupils and eye movements in the unconscious patient. *'Looking towards the lesion'; **'Looking away from the lesion'; †Normally, if the head is held and turned quickly from side to side, the eyes swivel in the opposite direction to the head.

FURTHER INVESTIGATIONS

Neurophysiological investigations

Electroencephalography

The electroencephalography (EEG) measures electrical potentials generated by the neurons lying under an electrode on the scalp and compares these either with a reference electrode or a neighbouring electrode. The normal trace is symmetrical and, therefore, asymmetries, as well as specific abnormalities, may indicate an underlying disorder. Interpretation of EEGs is complex, and you should not worry if you cannot pick up subtle abnormalities. Before accurate brain imaging was possible, EEG was used to detect focal lesions. These are now more commonly picked up with CT or MRI, but EEG remains useful for detecting underlying abnormalities of cerebral function, and especially for:

- Epilepsy (see below)
- Diagnosis of encephalitis
- Coma
- Aid to diagnosis of Creutzfeldt–Jakob disease
- Diagnosis of subacute sclerosing panencephalitis
- Diagnosis of metabolic encephalopathies.

The main role of EEG is in the assessment of epilepsy. It can help in the following ways:

- Diagnosis of a seizure disorder
- Classification of seizure type, which may optimize therapy
- Assessment for surgical intervention
- Diagnosis of pseudoseizures (especially with simultaneous video recording – telemetry)
- 'Invasive EEG monitoring' refers to electrodes inserted directly into the brain. This is undertaken before surgery (e.g. to remove an epileptic focus).

Different normal rhythms are characteristically found over different regions of the brain (Fig. 17.42). Other than these rhythmic activities, other abnormal activity may be generated in certain conditions (Figs. 17.43 & 17.44).

Fig. 17.42 Normal electroencephalographic (EEG) rhythms

Rhythm	Characteristics	Site and comments
Alpha	8–13 Hz (normal)	Posterior; especially with eyes closed
Beta	>13 Hz (normal)	Anterior; increased with sedatives (e.g. barbiturates)
Theta	4–7 Hz (normal)	Normal in young and when drowsy
delta	<4 Hz (abnormal except in sleep)	Slow rhythm generated over a structural lesion and in sleep

Fig. 17.43 Some abnormal electroencephalographic activities

Activity	Interpretation
Generalized slow-wave activity	Metabolic encephalopathy, drug overdose, encephalitis
Focal slow-wave activity	Underlying structural lesion
Focal/generalized spikes or spike and slow wave activity	Epilepsy
Three-per-second (3/sec) bilateral, symmetrical spike-and-wave activity (Fig. 17.44)	Typical absence seizures (idiopathic generalized epilepsy)
Periodic complexes (generalized, sharp waves every 0.5–2.0 seconds)	Creutzfeldt–Jakob disease

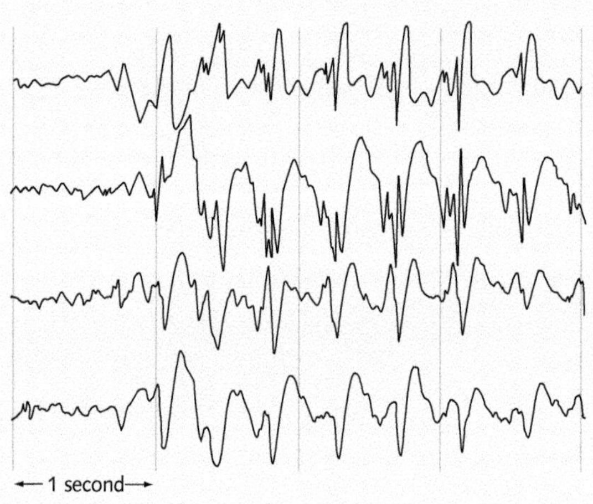

Fig. 17.44 Three-per-second (3/s) spike-and-wave activity. Characteristic of absence seizures.

HINTS AND TIPS

The EEG may be normal in patients who have clearly had seizures. There is an increased likelihood of seeing an abnormality if a recording is made under conditions of sleep deprivation, hyperventilation or photic stimulation (flashing lights).

Electromyography and nerve conduction studies

Usually performed together, these investigations examine the integrity of skeletal muscle, peripheral nerves and lower motor neurons. They are useful in:

- Determining the cause of weakness (e.g. neuropathy, myopathy, anterior horn cell disease)
- Determining the distribution of the abnormality (e.g. generalized/focal)
- Suggesting the type of myopathy (e.g. dystrophy or myositis) or neuropathy (e.g. axonal or demyelinating; motor, sensory or sensorimotor)
- Diagnosing myasthenia gravis
- Assessing baseline deficits before surgery (e.g. carpal tunnel syndrome)
- Objectively assessing the response to medical therapies, especially new treatments in trials (e.g. human immunoglobulin in Guillain–Barré syndrome).

Normal muscle at rest is electrically silent (apart from during needle insertion), unless the needle is placed in the region of a motor end-plate (when miniature end-plate potentials can be recorded). During voluntary movement, individual motor unit potentials (recordings

Fig. 17.45 Common abnormalities in electromyography (EMG) and nerve conduction

Abnormality	Change in electromyographic trace
Denervation	Increased insertional activity, large amplitude, long duration, polyphasic MUPS, fibrillations; fasciculations
Myopathy	Small, short, polyphasic MUPS
Myotonia	High-frequency bursts
Myasthenia	Abnormal decrement on repetitive stimulation; jitter with single-fibre studies (indicating variable neuromuscular transmission time)
Abnormality	**Change in nerve conduction**
Axonal neuropathy	Small action potential, normal nerve conduction velocity
Demyelinating neuropathy	Slow nerve conduction velocity; prolonged latency (time to travel from one point to the next); normal or slightly reduced action potential

MUPs, motor unit potentials

of the activity from the muscle fibres innervated by a single motor neuron) can be seen. Figure 17.45 shows common abnormalities.

Fibrillations and fasciculations

Fibrillation potentials (up to 300 mV) are due to spontaneous contractions of individual muscle fibres after denervation, probably due to hypersensitivity of the muscle membrane to acetylcholine. They cannot be seen through the skin, but may be seen in the tongue in motor neuron disease.

Fasciculation potentials (up to 5 mV, usually every 3–4 seconds) are contractions of groups of muscle fibres after denervation, visible on both electromyography and through the skin as a twitch or ripple. They may be normal, especially in calf muscles, usually at a rate of 1/s.

HINTS AND TIPS

Fasciculations are a particular feature of motor neuron disease.

Nerve conduction studies

These studies can be used to study the motor and sensory function of the large myelinated fibres of the accessible (named) nerves (e.g. the median nerve). These studies measure conduction velocity and amplitude:

- Sensory studies – involve stimulating a nerve at a given point (e.g. the index finger) and measuring at two different points proximally (the wrist (t_1) and mid-forearm (t_2)). By measuring the time difference for the action potential to appear at the two sites and measuring the distance between the two points it is possible to determine the mean conduction velocity:

$$\text{Sensory conduction velocity} = \frac{\text{distance}}{(\text{time}_2 - \text{time}_1)}$$

The amplitude of action potential can be measured on an oscilloscope screen.

- Motor studies – here there are two stimulating sites (e.g. the antecubital fossa and wrist) with one recording site (the thenar eminence). The maximal muscle response to supramaximal stimulation can be measured as an amplitude. Conduction time is measured in a similar fashion to above.

Two types of abnormality are seen on nerve conduction studies:

- A slowing of the conduction time due to demyelination (remember myelin insulates nerves, speeding transmission).
- A reduction in amplitude due to a loss of axons (remember large nerves are made up of a collection of nerve axons originating from the spinal cord or the periphery). These are both shown in Figure 17.45.

Other studies

These include:

- Evoked potentials (EPs) – this is a method of testing the integrity of sensory pathways from their end-organ receptors to the cerebral cortex. Recordings are made from a scalp EEG. When the stimulus is repeatedly delivered to the end-organ it causes a change in brain activity, which can be averaged over several trials so that any changes are due to the effects of the stimulus. These studies come in three varieties:
  1. Visual EPs – usually a patterned chequerboard
  2. Brainstem auditory EPs – usually 'clicks'
  3. Somatosensory EPs – usually via stimulation of the lower limb.
- Magnetic brain stimulation.

ROUTINE INVESTIGATIONS

You should be aware of simple tests of neurological relevance. In this section, five areas of investigation are covered:

- Haematology (Fig. 17.46)
- Biochemistry (Fig. 17.47)
- Immunology (Fig. 17.48)
- Microbiology (Fig. 17.49)
- Cerebrospinal fluid findings (Fig. 17.50).

Fig. 17.46 Possible consequences of abnormalities in blood or serum levels of haematological indices

Test	Normal range	Abnormality	Possible interpretation
Full blood count			
Haemoglobin (Hb)	13.5–18.0 g/dl male; 11.5–16.0 g/dl female	Low; anaemia High, polycythaemia	May cause non-specific neurological symptoms (e.g. dizziness, weakness, fainting); may suggest an underlying chronic illness, predispose to stroke and chorea
Mean cell volume (MCV)	79–96 fl.	High, macrocytic anaemia Low; microcytic anaemia	Vitamin B_{12} deficiency (peripheral neuropathy, SCDC, dementia) May indicate an underlying chronic illness; associated with idiopathic intracranial hypertension
White cell count (WBC)			
Neutrophils	2–7.5 × 10^9	High; neutrophilia Low; neutropenia	Meningitis or other infection Leukaemia/lymphoma (infiltrative disease, space-occupying lesions, peripheral neuropathy); multiple myeloma (neuropathy, vertebral collapse, hyperviscosity syndrome)
Lymphocytes	1.5–3.5 × 10^9	High; lymphocytosis Low; lymphopenia	Viral infection (transverse myelitis, Guillain–Barré syndrome) Leukaemia/lymphoma, as above
Eosinophils	0.04–0.44 × 10^9	High; eosinophilia	Hypereosinophilic syndrome (rare)
Platelet count	150–400 × 10^9	High; thrombo-cythaemia Low; thrombocytopenia	Predisposes to stroke, intracranial bleeding
Erythrocyte sedimentation rate (ESR)	<20 mm/h	High	Vasculitis (e.g. PAN, SLE, giant cell arteritis) may cause cerebral, cranial and peripheral nerve infarcts, confusion and fits
Coagulation tests			
Activated partial thromboplastin time (APK or PTTK)	35–45 s	High	SLE; antiphospholipid syndrome
Protein C, protein S	Varies with laboratory	Low; deficiency	Inherited predisposition to thrombosis
Factor 5 Leiden	Varies with laboratory	Present	Mutation causes a single amino acid substitution in factor 5, which results in activated protein C resistance and predisposition to thrombosis
Vitamin B_{12}	> 150 ng/L	Low; deficiency	Peripheral neuropathy, SCDC, confusion/dementia
Folate	2.1–2.8 mg/l	Low; deficiency	Peripheral neuropathy, dementia

Individual laboratories may have different normal ranges
APT, activated partial thromboplastin; PAN, polyarteritis nodosa; PTTK, partial thromboplastin time; SCDC, subacute combined degeneration of the cord; SLE, systemic lupus erythematosus

Fig. 17.47 Possible consequences of abnormalities in blood or serum levels of biochemical indices

Test	Normal range	Abnormality	Interpretation
Urea and electrolytes (U and Es)			
Sodium	135–145 mmol/l	High: hypernatraemia Low: hyponatraemia	Both may cause weakness, confusion and fits
Potassium	3.5–5.5 mmol/l	High: hyperkalaemia Low: hypokalaemia	Hyper/hypokalaemic periodic paralysis
Urea	2.5–6.7 mmol/l	High: renal failure	Confusion, peripheral neuropathy
Creatinine	< 150 mmol/l	High: renal failure	Confusion, peripheral neuropathy
Glucose (fasting)	4–6 mmol/l	High: diabetes Low: hypoglycaemia	Neuropathy, coma confusion, coma, focal signs
Calcium	2.2–2.6 mmol/l	Low: hypocalcaemia	Tetany
Liver function tests: (LFTS) bilirubin and liver enzymes	Bilirubin range 3–17 μmol/L; enzymes vary between laboratories	High	Liver disease: confusion, tremor, neuropathy
Creatine kinase	24–195 u/l	High	Muscle disease: myositis, dystrophy
Thyroid function tests: thyroid stimulating hormone (TSH)	0.5–5 mu/L	Low TSH: thyrotoxicosis High TSH: hypothyroidism	Tremor, confusion, hyperreflexia Apathy, confusion, hyporeflexia, neuropathy

Individual laboratories may have different normal ranges

Fig. 17.48 Immunology

Test	Associated disorder
Antinuclear factor (ANA)	Systemic lupus erythematosus (SLE): fits, confusion, neuropathy, aseptic meningitis. Sjögren's syndrome: gritty eyes, neuropathies, mixed connective tissue disease (MCTD)
Anti-double-stranded DNA (DSDNA) antibodies	SLE
Rheumatoid factor	Rheumatoid arthritis: cervical spine subluxation, neuropathies, vasculitis
Anti-Ro (SSA), and anti-La (SSB) antibodies	Sjögren's syndrome
Antiphospholipid antibodies (e.g. anticardiolipin)	Antiphospholipid syndrome
Anti-ribonucleoprotein (RNP) antibodies	MCTD: myositis, trigeminal nerve palsies
Jo-1 antibodies	Polymyositis
Antineutrophil cytoplasmic antibodies (ANCA)	PANCA (peripheral): polyarteritis nodosa CANCA (classic): Wegener's granulomatosis
Antiacetylcholine receptor antibodies (ACHR)	Myasthenia gravis
Anti-GM1 antibodies	Multifocal motor neuropathy, Guillain–Barré syndrome
Anti-GAD antibodies	Stiff-man syndrome

Fig. 17.49 Microbiology	
Test	**Associated disorder**
VDRL (venereal disease reference laboratory)	Primary syphilis; false positive in pregnancy, systemic lupus erythematosus, malaria
TPHA (*Treponema pallidum* haemagglutination assay)	Syphilis; false positive with non-venereal treponemes (yaws, pinta)
Hepatitis B surface antigen (HBSAG)	Some cases of polyarteritis nodosa
HIV	AIDS

Fig. 17.50 Cerebrospinal fluid findings			
Disease	**Protein (g/dL)**	**Glucose**	**Cells**
Normal	< 0.5	> 50% blood glucose	< 5/ml lymphocytes, no polymorphs
Bacterial meningitis	1.0–5.0	< 50%	> 1000/ml, polymorphs predominate
Viral meningitis	0.5–1.0	Normal	< 1000/ml, lymphocytes predominate
Tuberculous meningitis	1–10	< 50%	< 1000/ml, lymphocytes predominate

For each test, normal ranges are given, with neurological differential diagnoses for high and low values. Cerebrospinal fluid protein levels are given in g/dL and serum levels are in g/L.

IMAGING OF THE NERVOUS SYSTEM

Plain radiography

Skull radiography

Skull radiography has a limited role in current neurological practice. The main indication is head injury when more sophisticated imaging is not immediately indicated. The standard views are:

- Lateral
- Posteroanterior
- Towne's view (fronto-occipital).

Learn about the normal skull radiographic markings (Figs 17.51 and 17.52) and the main abnormalities seen on skull radiographs (Fig. 17.53).

Spinal radiography

The standard views in spinal radiography are:

- Lateral
- Posteroanterior.

Learn about the main abnormalities seen on spinal radiographs (Fig. 17.54).

Computed tomography

Using an X-ray source and a series of photon detectors housed in a gantry, CT produces a series of consecutive 2D axial brain digital images, which show the X-ray density of the brain tissue. The densities of different brain tissues vary according to their X-ray absorption properties, ranging between low (black: air, cerebrospinal fluid) to high (white: bone, fresh blood) (Figs 17.55A and 17.56A). The diagnostic yield of the CT scan is increased by injecting iodine-containing contrast agents, which enhance the distinction between the different brain tissues and outline the areas of blood–brain barrier breakdown (around tumours or infarctions). Learn about the main abnormalities seen on the CT scan (Fig. 17.57).

MRI

Nuclear magnetic resonance is the term that describes the interaction between the hydrogen protons in the different body structures and strong external magnetic fields. As the patient lies in the scanner, the naturally spinning hydrogen protons align with the strong magnetic field of the scanner. When a further external magnetic field (radiofrequency pulse) of a specific frequency is applied at a right angle, the protons 'flip' out of the main external magnetic field. As the protons

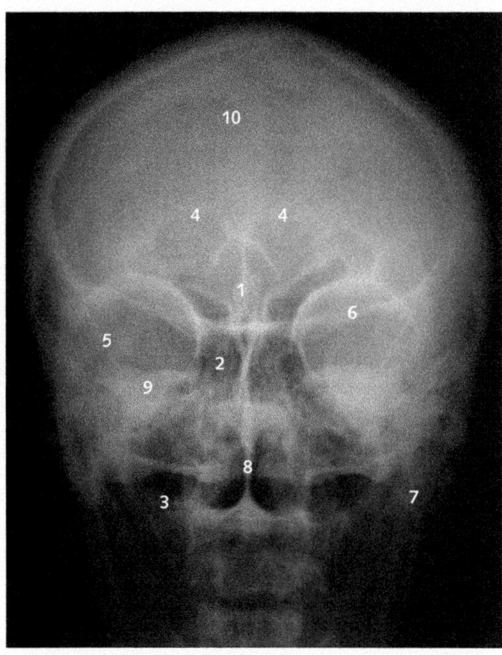

1 crista galli
2 ethmoidal air cells
3 floor of maxillary sinus (antrum)
4 frontal sinus
5 greater wing of sphenoid
6 lesser wing of sphenoid
7 mastoid process
8 nasal septum
9 petrous part of temporal bone
10 sagittal suture

Fig. 17.51 Normal posteroanterior skull radiograph (courtesy of J Weir and PH Abrahams).

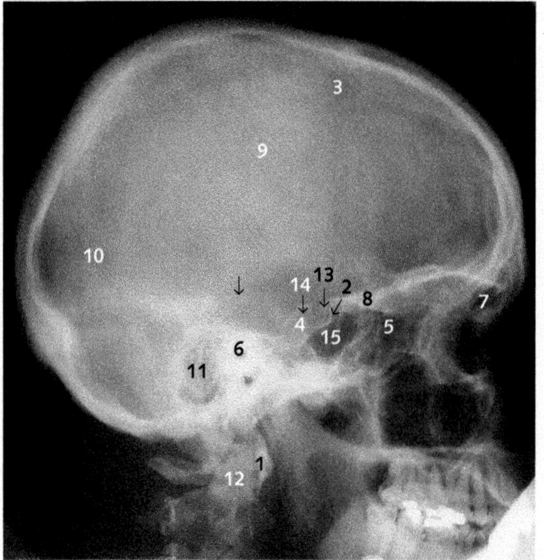

1 anterior arch of atlas (first cervical vertebral)
2 anterior clinoid process
3 coronal suture
4 dorsum sellae
5 ethmoidal air cells
6 external acoustic meatus
7 frontal sinus
8 greater wing of sphenoid
9 grooves for middle meningeal vessels
10 lambdoid suture
11 mastoid air cells
12 odontoid process (dens) of axis (second cervical vertebra)
13 pituitary fossa (sella turcica)
14 posterior clinoid process
15 sphenoidal sinus

Fig. 17.52 Normal lateral skull radiograph (courtesy of J Weir and PH Abrahams).

'relax' back to their original position, they emit a radiofrequency signal that can be digitally analysed and displayed as an image. This 'relaxation' time has two components, known as T1 and T2, which determine the magnetic resonance parameters of the different brain tissues (Figs 17.55B and 17.56B). T1 and T2 images are useful for imaging different nervous system pathologies:

Fig. 17.53 Main abnormalities seen on skull radiograph	
Pathology	**Abnormality**
Trauma	Skull fractures, intracerebral haematomas (midline shift of a calcified pineal gland)
Tumours	Bone erosions (metastasis, multiple myeloma) or hyperostosis, (meningiomas), calcifications (craniopharyngioma, glial tumours), enlargement/destruction of the pituitary fossa (pituitary tumours)
Raised intracranial pressure	Separation of the sutures (children), erosion of the posterior clinoids, thinning of the vault, and flattening of the pituitary fossa
Developmental defects	Craniostenosis, platybasia
Inflammatory processes	Opacification of the paranasal sinuses
Vascular	Calcified intracranial aneurysms and vascular malformations

Fig. 17.54 Main abnormalities seen on spinal radiograph	
Pathology	**Abnormality**
Trauma	Fractures, fracture–dislocations, subluxations
Tumours	Erosion of the pedicles (long-standing tumours), erosions of the vertebral bodies (metastatic tumours)
Degenerative disease	Narrowing of the disc spaces, calcification of the intervention discs, osteophyte formation

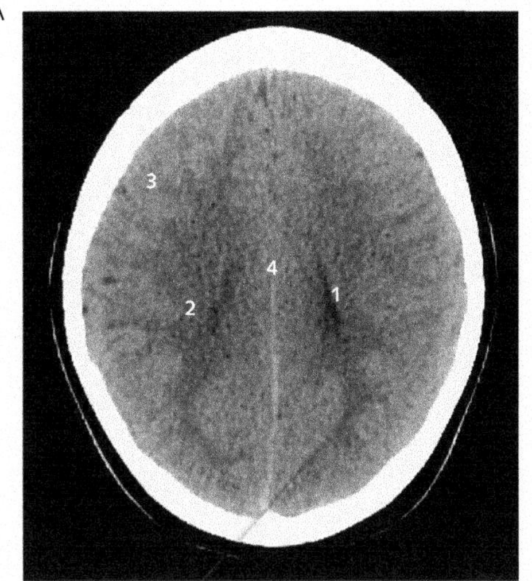

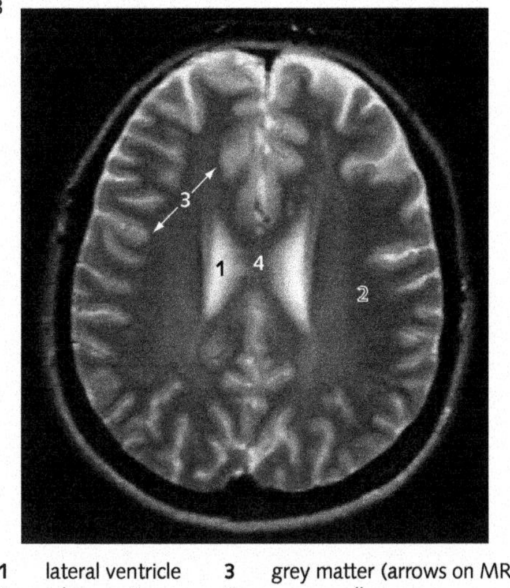

1 lateral ventricle
2 white matter
3 grey matter (arrows on MRI)
4 corpus callosum

Fig. 17.55 Computed tomography (A) and magnetic resonance imaging (B) (T2-weighted image) showing the normal structure of the brain.

A

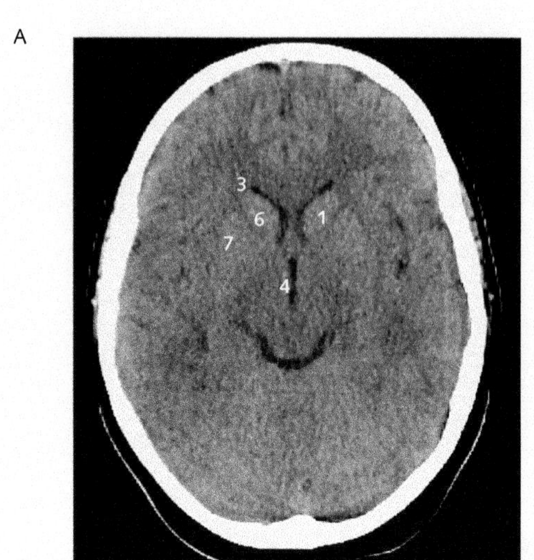

B

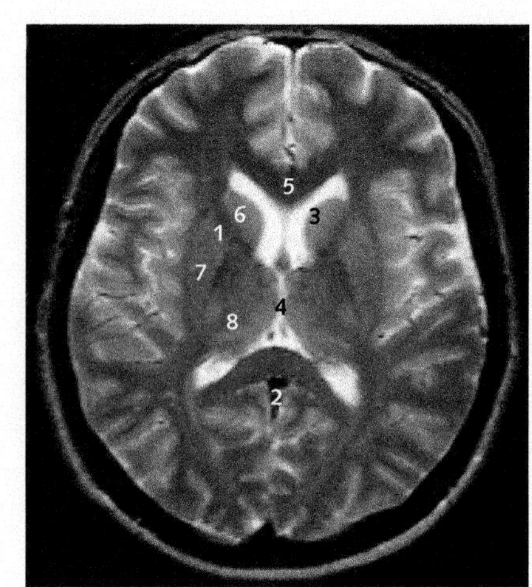

1	internal capsule	**5**	genu of corpus callosum
2	vein of Galen	**6**	head of caudate nucleus
3	frontal horn of lateral ventricle	**7**	putamen
4	third ventricle	**8**	thalamus

Fig. 17.56 Computed tomography (A) and magnetic resonance imaging (B) (T2-weighted image) showing the normal structure of the brain.

Fig. 17.57 Main abnormalities seen in computed tomography scanning

Pathology	**Abnormality**
Trauma	Extracerebral and intracerebral haematomas (HD), brain confusion (mixed HD and LD)
Vascular lesions	Infarction (LD), haemorrhage (HD), subarachnoid haemorrhage (HD) in the basal cisterns and sulci, angiomas and aneurysms (intensely enhancing lesions)
Tumours	Enhancing irregular lesions surrounded by LD (oedema)
Degeneration	Brain atrophy (ventricular enlargement, widening of sulci and flattening of the gyri)
Hydrocephalus	Ventricular enlargement with no evidence of cortical atrophy
Infections	Abscesses (ID lesions surrounded by ring enhancement), focal encephalitis (LD)
Spinal lesions	Lesions of the vertebrae, the intervertebral discs and the spinal cord

HD, high density; LD, low density

- T1 – water/CSF is dark, allowing increased anatomical resolution, thus T1 studies are good for anatomical studies
- T2 – water/CSF is bright thus pathological tissue is seen easier (they usually contain more water). Spinal pathologies usually show well-demonstrated blockages in CSF flow. T2 images have poor anatomical resolution.

The paramagnetic agent gadolinium-labelled DTPA (diethylene triamine penta-acetic acid, or pentetic acid) is used as a contrast agent. Learn about the main abnormalities seen on magnetic resonance imaging (Fig. 17.58).

Fig. 17.58 Main abnormalities seen on magnetic resonance imaging	
Pathology	**Abnormality**
Demyelinating disease	Multiple sclerosis (periventricular white matter lesions)
Tumours	Lesions in the pituitary fossa, cerebropontine angles, craniocervicial junctions and the orbits (images not affected by artefacts from the surrounding bony structures)
Vascular diseases	Large aneurysms and venous sinus thrombosis (magnetic resonance angiography)
Infections	Encephalitis, progressive multifocal leucoencephalopathy
Spinal lesions	Intramedullary lesions (syringomyelia, tumours, demyelination); extramedullary lesions (degenerative disease, tumours, abscesses)

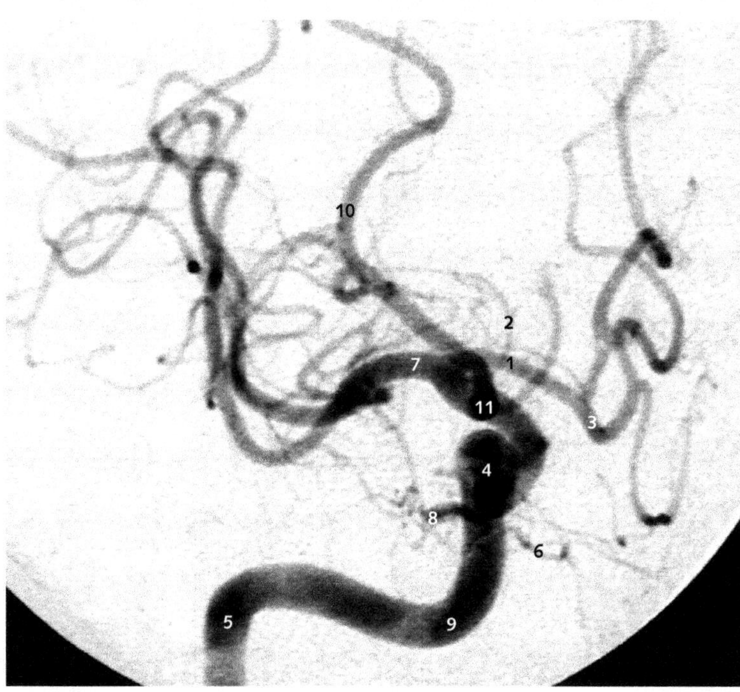

Fig. 17.59 Arterial phase of a normal carotid angiogram (courtesy of J Weir and PH Abrahams).

1 anterior cerebral artery
2 anterior choroidal artery
3 anterior communicating artery
4 cavernous portion of internal carotid artery
5 cervical portion of internal carotid artery
6 ethmoidal branch of ophthalmic artery
7 middle cerebral artery
8 ophthalmic artery
9 pertrous portion of internal carotid artery
10 posterior cerebral artery
11 posterior communicating artery

Advantages of MRI:
- Absence of ionizing radiation
- The ability to obtain images in coronal, sagittal, as well as axial plains
- More sensitive to the pathological changes in the brain tissues.

Disadvantages:
- Cannot be used for patients with pacemakers (the magnetic field interferes with their function)
- Cannot be used for patients with ferromagnetic intracranial aneurysmal clips or implants (they distort the images and could be displaced by the strong magnetic field)
- Claustrophobia.

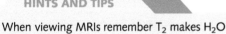

HINTS AND TIPS

When viewing MRIs remember T_2 makes H_2O brighter.

Myelography

A water-soluble iodine-based medium is injected in the subarachnoid space through a lumbar or a cervical approach. This outlines the spinal canal and nerve root sheaths, allowing the assessment of the spinal canal and the nerve roots.

Cord compression caused by extra- or intramedullary lesions is identified as a compression or interruption of the column of contrast. Post-myelographic CT scanning allows further assessments to the nerve roots within the theca.

Angiography

Serial cranial radiographs are taken after the injection of an iodine-containing contrast agent into a large artery (aorta, carotid, vertebral) to allow the identification of cerebral vessels (Fig. 17.59). Simultaneous digital subtraction of the surrounding soft tissues and bony structures allows the use of more dilute contrast and shorter procedure time, although the spatial resolution of the images will be compromised.

Venous digital subtraction angiography is possible, but the quality of the images obtained is distinctly inferior to those obtained through the arterial route.

The indications for angiography are:

- Extracranial atherosclerotic cerebrovascular disease (stenosis, particularly carotid), lumen irregularities or occlusions)
- Aneurysms and arteriovenous malformation
- Assessing cerebral vessel anatomy and tumour blood supply before neurosurgery
- Interventional angiography: embolization of angiomas.

Duplex sonography

This technique offers a combination of real time and Doppler flow ultrasound scanning, allowing a non-invasive assessment of extracranial arteries. It is particularly helpful as a screening test for lesions at the carotid bifurcation which avoids the need for angiography in many patients. The quality of this technique depends on the experience and skill of the operator.

Cerebral ultrasonography

This technique is used in newborn babies, as other imaging requires sedation and/or high radiation doses. The ultrasound is performed through the sutures and fontanelles, which have not fused. It is particularly useful for detecting the presence of hydrocephalus and intraventricular haemorrhage in premature babies.

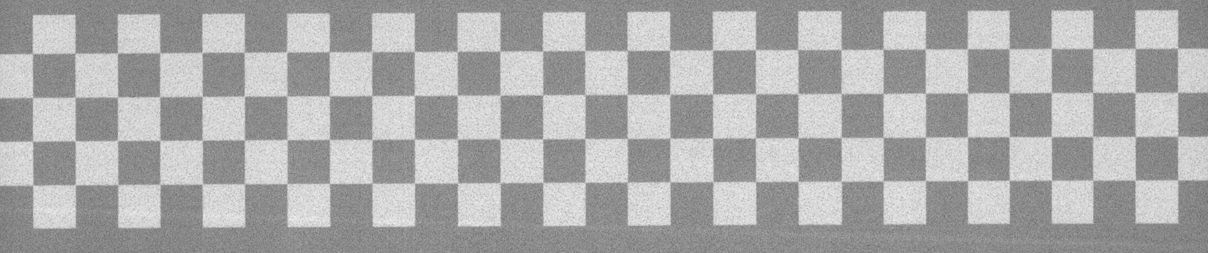

SELF-ASSESSMENT

Single best answer questions (SBAs)

For each of the following questions, choose the single best answer.

Chapter 1 Introduction and overview of the nervous system

1. Which ONE of the following is false concerning the coverings of the central nervous system?
   a. The brain and spinal cord are surrounded by dura mater.
   b. The cranial compartment is divided by sheets of dura mater called the falx cerebri and tentorium cerebelli.
   c. The subdural space is the primary site for circulation of cerebrospinal fluid.
   d. The cranial dura splits to contain the venous sinuses.
   e. The pia mater is closely applied to the surface of the brain and spinal cord.

2. Which ONE of the following is true concerning the coverings of the brain and spinal cord?
   a. Rupture of the middle meningeal artery following skull fracture results in haemorrhage into the subdural space.
   b. Rupture of a berry aneurysm in the circle of Willis typically results in an intracerebral haemorrhage.
   c. Cerebrospinal fluid circulates in the extradural space.
   d. A fall in the elderly tearing bridging veins results in a subdural haemorrhage.
   e. Meningeal irritation may cause neck flaccidity.

3. Which ONE of the following is TRUE? One characteristic of the meninges of the spinal cord is:
   a. A real epidural space between the dura and the vertebral periosteum.
   b. A potential epidural space between the dura and the vertebral periosteum.
   c. No subarachnoid space.
   d. A real subdural space.
   e. A specialized outgrowth of the dura called ligamentum denticulatum.

4. Which ONE of the following is true? Ependymal cells:
   a. Are responsible for myelin formation in the spinal cord.
   b. Occur only in individuals under the age of 10 years.
   c. Are primarily responsible for secretion of cerebrospinal fluid.
   d. Line the ventricular system and central canal of the spinal cord.
   e. Have important phagocytic properties.

5. Which ONE of the following is true? Astrocytes:
   a. Are involved in the synthesis of myelin in the brain.
   b. Are postmitotic cells.
   c. Line the ventricular system.
   d. Are involved in the secretion of cerebrospinal fluid.
   e. May proliferate in response to brain injury.

6. Which ONE of the following statements is true? Oligodendrocytes:
   a. Are responsible for myelination in the peripheral nervous system.
   b. Are postmitotic cells incapable of division.
   c. Are a major component of the blood–brain barrier.
   d. Are essential for saltatory conduction in the central nervous system.
   e. Are increased in number in demyelinating disorders.

7. Which ONE of the following is true? The temporal lobe of the brain:
   a. Contains the primary somatosensory cortex.
   b. Has no direct relationship to the hippocampus.
   c. Is seldom the site of epileptiform discharges.
   d. Contains the primary auditory cortex.
   e. Contains the secondary visual cortex.

8. Lesions of the parietal lobe can result in which ONE of the following?
   a. Anosmia.
   b. Aphasia.
   c. Contralateral hemianopia.
   d. Contralateral deafness.
   e. Contralateral sensory neglect.

9. Which ONE of the following is associated with temporal lobe trauma?
   a. Sensory loss.
   b. Anosmia.
   c. Visual impairment.
   d. Complex partial seizures.
   e. Dysphagia.

10. Which ONE of the following is true concerning the major functions of different areas of the brain?
    a. A brain tumour in the cerebellum may result in hearing defects.
    b. A frontal lobotomy results in major sensory defects.

c. Parkinson's disease is primarily a defect of the cerebellum.
d. Dyspraxia characteristically arises in the frontal lobe.
e. Hearing defects may arise due to a lesion in the temporal lobe.

11. Which ONE of the following is true? Following damage to the middle meningeal artery:
a. A subdural haematoma is produced.
b. A lucid interval may occur.
c. There is tachycardia and a rise in blood pressure.
d. The uncus of the temporal lobe herniates through the falx cerebri.
e. The pupil dilates on the side of the lesion, due to compression of the abducens (VI cranial) nerve.

12. A patient with a large ischaemic stroke affecting most of the territory supplied by the left middle cerebral artery would be expected to have which ONE of the following features?
a. Weakness of the left arm and leg.
b. Ataxia.
c. Loss of right visual field in both eyes.
d. Weakness of the right arm and leg.
e. Double vision and rotational vertigo.

13. A man aged 70 years develops a cerebral infarct in the region of the left internal capsule of the brain. In this location, which of the following is least likely to be the mechanism?
a. Myocardial infarction followed by mural thrombosis of the left ventricle and embolism to the brain.
b. Atheroma causing narrowing of the left internal carotid artery near its origin from the common carotid artery.
c. Atheroma of the left carotid artery with embolism of small platelet thrombi.
d. Episode of hypotension (shock) lasting 2 hours.
e. Thrombosis of the left middle cerebral artery.

14. Which ONE of the following is true? Intracerebral haemorrage:
a. Is the commonest cause of stroke in adults.
b. Typically results from a rupture of an aneurysm on the circle of Willis.
c. Occurs most frequently in the occipital lobe.
d. Is universally fatal in the elderly.
e. Is typically accompanied by raised intracranial pressure.

15. Which ONE of the following is true of the middle cerebral artery?
a. It arises from the middle menengeal artery.
b. It supplies the visual cortex.
c. It supplies the motor cortex.
d. It travels mainly in the subdural space.
e. It is at risk of compression by midline shift and uncal herniation.

16. Occlusion of the main trunk of the left middle cerebral artery may cause which ONE of the following:
a. Loss of vision in the left eye only.
b. Weakness of the right face, arm and leg.
c. Damage to the cerebellum.
d. Tremor at rest.
e. Weakness of the left face, arm and leg.

17. ONE of the following is true. The blood supply to the occipital cortex is principally from:
a. The posterior cerebral artery.
b. The middle cerebral artery.
c. The internal carotid arteries.
d. The middle meningeal artery.
e. The circle of Willis.

18. Which ONE of the following is false? Cerebrospinal fluid normally:
a. Is produced at a greater rate during the day than during the night.
b. Contains over 100 neutrophil polymorphs per ml.
c. Is resorbed via the arachnoid granulations.
d. Circulates from the lateral ventricles to the cisterna magna.
e. Is crystal clear.

19. Which ONE of the following is true? Raised intracranial pressure:
a. Results only from rapidly expanding brain lesions.
b. Commonly presents with visual loss.
c. If untreated can result in deafness.
d. Commonly presents with headache.
e. Involves the cerebellum, resulting in nausea and vomiting.

20. Which ONE of the following is a sign of raised intracranial pressure?
a. Tachycardia.
b. Systemic hypotension.
c. IVth nerve palsy.
d. Photophobia.
e. Papilloedema.

21. Which ONE of the following is NOT true? In bacterial meningitis:
a. The concentration of glucose in the cerebrospinal fluid is reduced.
b. *Streptococcus pneumoniae* is a typical causative organism.
c. Neutrophil polymorphs are found in the cerebrospinal fluid.
d. Adrenal haemorrhage is a recognised complication.
e. Infection is characteristically transmitted by blood transfusion.

22. Which ONE is true of cerebrospinal fluid?
a. It is produced in all the cerebral ventricles.
b. It is absorbed by the choroid plexuses.
c. It contains the same level of protein as blood.

d. It decreases in volume with brain atrophy.
e. It normally contains polymorphonuclear leucocytes.

23. The following locations are involved in the circulation of the cerebrospinal fluid, but not in the order given. Which ONE is normally fourth?
a. Foramina of the Fourth ventricle.
b. Lateral ventricle.
c. Choroid plexus.
d. Arachnoid granulations.
e. Third ventricle.

24. A girl aged 19 years develops headache, neck stiffness and fever. A sample of cerebrospinal fluid withdrawn by lumbar puncture contains large numbers of neutrophil polymorphs and has a low concentration of glucose. Which ONE of the following is NOT a legitimate conclusion to draw?
a. She has acute meningitis.
b. A viral aetiology is likely.
c. The acute inflammatory response is in this case harmful to the patient.
d. *Neisseria meningitidis* would be a typical causative micro-organism.
e. Inflammatory mediators involved include pyrogens.

25. Which ONE of the following is true concerning cerebrospinal fluid (CSF)?
a. It is mainly produced by the ependymal cells which line the ventricles.
b. The biochemical composition is that of a plasma filtrate.
c. The glucose content is increased in bacterial infections.
d. Resorption occurs into the cerebral veins.
e. Resorption occurs into local lymphatic channels.

Chapter 2 The development of the nervous system and disorders of development

26. Which ONE of the following is true in brain development?
a. Development of the brain is complete at 22 weeks' gestation.
b. The spinal cord develops only after the brain is fully formed.
c. Myelination of the brain is incomplete at birth.
d. Anencephaly is compatible with life.
e. Spina bifida is one of the rarest developmental abnormalities of the nervous system.

27. Which ONE of the following is true. The neural tube:
a. Gives rise to microglia.
b. Is derives from the endoderm.
c. Closes at the end of the fourth month of gestation.
d. Gives rise to pia mater and arachnoid mater.
e. Gives rise to the eyes as outgrowths from the forebrain.

Chapter 3 Cellular physiology of the nervous system and introduction to pharmacology

28. Which ONE of the following statements regarding neuronal structure and function is true?
a. The output of a neuron is a binary signal.
b. Projection neurons typically have short axons.
c. The resting neuron contains a lower concentration of potassium within the cell compared with the outside.
d. The equilibrium potential for potassium is −74.8 V.
e. The smaller the axonal diameter, the faster an action potential travels along the axon.

29. Which of the following proteins is NOT found within the neurone?
a. Neurofilament protein.
b. Tau protein.
c. Glial fibrillary acidic protein.
d. Microtubule associated protein (MAP) 2.
e. Tubulin.

30. Which ONE of the following is NOT true? Dendrites typically:
a. Are myelinated.
b. Have an arborizing (branching) pattern.
c. Carry impulses towards the neuronal cell body.
d. May have spines which increase their receptive area.
e. Receive synaptic inputs from axons.

31. Which ONE of the following statements about synapses is NOT true?
a. Synapses may be electrical or chemical.
b. The action potential triggers release of neurotransmitter from the postsynaptic membrane.
c. The neurotransmitter acts at a specific receptor.
d. Re-uptake or enzymatic degradation may be involved in the inactivation of a neurotransmitter.
e. Acetylcholine is the neurotransmitter at the neuromuscular junction.

32. Which ONE of the following statements about axons is correct?
a. They are always myelinated.
b. Axons within the central nervous system are myelinated by Schwann cells.
c. Neurofilament proteins are present in the cell body but do not extend into the axon.

d. The action potential is generated in the region of the axon hillock.
e. The major intracellular ion within the axon is sodium compared to potassium in the extracellular fluid.

33. Which ONE of the following is true? Acetylcholine:
a. Slows the heart by activating ionotropic receptors.
b. Is deactivated by choline acetyl transferase.
c. Depolarizes skeletal muscle via metabotropic receptors.
d. Can depolarize neurones by closing potassium channels.
e. Neurons degenerate in Parkinson's disease.

34. Which of the following substances is NOT a recognized neurotransmitter?
a. Glutamic acid.
b. Gamma-aminobutyric acid.
c. Glutathione.
d. 5-hydroxytryptamine (5-HT).
e. Substance P.

35. Which ONE of the following is true? At the mamalian neuromuscular junction:
a. Acetylcholine opens metabotropic sodium channels.
b. Acetylcholine opens fast ionotropic mixed cation channels.
c. The action of acetylcholine is opposed by GABA.
d. Transmission is generally rather slow.
e. The action of acetylcholine is terminated by choline transferase.

36. Acetylcholine is the transmitter at which ONE of the following?
a. Sympathetic but not parasympathetic ganglia.
b. The radial muscle of the iris.
c. Arrector pili muscles in the skin.
d. Apocrine sweat glands.
e. Nerve endings of sympathetic fibres causing vasodilatation of thoroughfare channels in skeletal muscle.

37. Which ONE of the following is the major excitatory neurotransmitter in the brain?
a. GABA.
b. Glycine.
c. Glutamate.
d. Dopamine.
e. 5-Hydroxytryptamine.

Chapter 4 The spinal cord and peripheral nerves

38. Which ONE of the following statements concerning the spinal cord is true?
a. The spinothalamic tracts carry ipsilateral sensory information.
b. The dorsal columns carry contralateral sensory information.
c. The lateral corticospinal tracts carry crossed fibres.
d. The tectospinal tract carries information to the midbrain.
e. The dorsal columns carry information about pain and temperature.

39. Which ONE of the following statements is true regarding the spinal cord?
a. In adults, the cord ends at the level of L3.
b. The dorsal tract columns decussate in the cord.
c. Tabes dorsalis leads to a loss of pain and temperature.
d. Right or left hemisection of the cord (Brown–Séquard syndrome) leads to contralateral sensory loss.
e. The grey matter lies peripherally.

40. Which ONE of the following is true? Dorsal column nucleus projection neurons:
a. Receive nociceptive spinal afferents.
b. Project in the ipsilateral medial lemniscus.
c. Project in the contralateral lateral lemniscus.
d. Project to the contralateral ventroposterior thalamus.
e. Project to the contralateral somatosensory cortex.

41. Which ONE of the following is false? In the spinal cord:
a. The ventral horn contains large motor neurons.
b. The dorsal columns are major ascending tracts.
c. Most of the blood supply is derived from the anterior spinal artery.
d. Touch sensation is transmitted by fibres in the spinothalamic tracts.
e. The anatomical segments of the spinal cord are located in the corresponding vertebral bodies.

42. Which ONE is of the following is not true? Nerve fibres of the corticospinal tracts:
a. Run from the precentral gyrus.
b. Cross over to the opposite side of the body.
c. Run in the pyramids.
d. Synapse in the anterior horns of the spinal cord.
e. Are predominantly sensory.

43. Which of ONE of the following is true of the descending corticospinal fibres?
a. They terminate on both interneurons and alpha motor neurons in the spinal cord grey matter.
b. All of the fibres from the left motor strip cross to the right in the medulla.
c. It has purely excitatory influence on the spinal alpha motor neurons.
d. They terminate on the alpha motor neurons of only the cervical spinal cord.
e. They originate in the red nucleus.

44. Which ONE of the following is true of the descending corticobulbar fibres?
a. All of the fibres to the VII nucleus are crossed.
b. All of the fibres to the V nerve nucleus are crossed.
c. They originate in the basal ganglia.
d. A lesion in their course causes a lower motor neuron facial weakness.
e. They enable cortical control of the cranial musculature.

45. Each of the following lesions is matched to a clinical manifestation. Which ONE pair is incorrectly matched?
a. Lower motor neuron lesion: hyporeflexia.
b. Upper motor neuron lesion: hyperreflexia.
c. Cerebellar lesion: dysphasia.
d. Lesion of the basal ganglia: rigidity.
e. Spinal cord lesion: dissociated sensory loss.

46. Which ONE of the following patterns of sensory impairment is most suggestive of a polyneuropathy?
a. Confined to the 4th and 5th digits of the right hand.
b. Confined to both upper limbs and the upper trunk.
c. Affecting the left side of the body and face.
d. Affecting the lateral aspects of both distal arms.
e. Affecting the legs up to the knees and both hands.

47. Which ONE of the following is true regarding injury to the ulnar nerve?
a. Most commonly seen after fracture of the mid-shaft of the humerus.
b. Results in sensory loss over the lateral surface of the palm of the hand.
c. Commonly associated with wasting of the muscles of the thenar eminence.
d. Seen in carpal tunnel syndrome.
e. Results in 'claw' hand deformity.

48. The long ascending fibres in the dorsal columns of the spinal cord convey impulses concerned with which ONE of the following:
a. Temperature.
b. Muscle contraction.
c. Blood pressure regulation.
d. Sense of position.
e. Pain.

49. The lateral spinothalamic tract conveys impulses of which ONE of the following:
a. Pain.
b. Proprioception.
c. Light touch.
d. Pressure.
e. Deep touch.

50. Which ONE of the following is not carried in the spinothalamic tracts?
a. Pain.
b. Proprioception.
c. Touch.
d. Pressure.
e. Temperature.

51. Which ONE of the following is not true? The spinothalamic tract:
a. Consists of second order neurons.
b. Synapses to afferent fibres in the dorsal horn.
c. Forms the spinal lemniscus.
d. Carries sensation from the opposite side of the body.
e. Runs in the posterior columns.

52. Which ONE is true? Dorsal column nucleus projection neurons:
a. Receive nociceptive spinal afferents.
b. Project to the ipsilateral medial lemniscus.
c. Project to the contralateral lateral lemniscus.
d. Project to the contralateral ventroposterior thalamus.
e. Project to the contralateral somatosensory cortex.

Chapter 5 Somatosensation and the perception of pain

53. Which ONE is false concerning the sensory system?
a. Important sensory ascending tracts are in the dorsal columns.
b. Sensation of position is typically initiated in muscle spindle receptors.
c. The back has a small representation on the somatotopic map.
d. Ascending sensory pathways run via the ventral posterior nucleus of the thalamus.
e. Pain and crude touch fibres are typically situated in different tracts.

54. Which ONE of the following statements concerning nociception and pain is not true?
a. Pain information is transmitted to the brain in the spinothalamic tracts.
b. Primary hyperalgesia occurs in undamaged tissue surrounding the originally damaged area.
c. The co-transmitter substance P causes a very long-lasting excitatory postsynaptic potential, thereby helping to sustain the effect of noxious stimuli.
d. The central nervous system is unable to accurately distinguish between superficial pain from cutaneous structures and pain from the viscera.
e. Inflammation affecting the diaphragm is felt in the tip of the shoulder.

55. Which ONE of the following is true? Pain:
   a. Is felt as a result of stimulation of encapsulated receptors.
   b. Information is carried via A delta and C fibres ascending in the dorsal columns.
   c. Arising in viscera causes reflex contraction of striated muscle via a monosynaptic reflex.
   d. Sensation is modulated at the dorsal horn by beta endorphin released from nerve endings of substantia gelatinosa cells.
   e. Impulses from the face enter the spinal nucleus of the trigeminal nerve (V).

56. Which ONE of the following is true? Meissner's corpuscles and Merkel's receptors:
   a. Are cutaneous thermoreceptors.
   b. Have large, diffuse receptive fields.
   c. Are found in large numbers all over the hand.
   d. Are found in large numbers at the tips of the fingers.
   e. Are found deep in the dermis of the skin.

57. Which ONE of the following statements regarding the regulation of pain is not true?
   a. Morphine is a μ-receptor agonist.
   b. Naloxone is μ-receptor antagonist.
   c. Opioid analgesics act by reducing the production of inflammatory mediators.
   d. Opioids cause pupillary contriction.
   e. Co-codamol is a combination of codeine and paracetamol.

58. Regarding the presentation and management of opioid overdose, which ONE of the following statements is true?
   a. Naloxone is a long-acting μ-receptor antagonist.
   b. Naloxone acts more rapidly than naltrexone.
   c. Opioid overdose causes hyperventilation.
   d. With repeated administration of opioids and consequent tolerance, pin-point pupils (characteristic of overdose) become less obvious.
   e. Opioid overdose causes increased P_aO_2

59. Which ONE of the statements below regarding opioid drug is incorrect?
   a. Morphine is less effective when given orally.
   b. Morphine has a half-life of approximately 12 hours.
   c. Codeine exhibits high oral bioavailability
   d. Pethidine does not cause miosis.
   e. Methadone has a half-life exceeding 24 hours.

60. Concerning non-steroidal anti-inflammatory drugs (NSAIDs), which ONE of the following statements is correct?
   a. Cyclo-oxygenase metabolizes arachidonic acid to leukotrienes.
   b. NSAIDs upregulate cyclo-oxygenase.
   c. Gastric ulceration is an important side effect of NSAID use.
   d. Reye's syndrome is associated with aspirin use in the elderly.
   e. Tranexamic acid is an NSAID.

61. Which ONE of the following statements is not correct? Local anaesthetics:
   a. Block the ability of axons to conduct action potentials.
   b. Block NA^+ channels in the axonal membrane.
   c. Are weak bases.
   d. Can pass straight through the lipid membrane of the axon when in the hydrophilic state.
   e. At low concentrations affect only small-diameter myelinated and unmyelinated fibres.

62. Which ONE of the following statements is true concerning somatosensation:
   a. The sensory homunculus is organized such that a given area of the body has a proportionate area of cortex responsible for its processing, regardless of the density of sensory receptors in that area.
   b. The sensory cortex is located in the frontal lobe.
   c. C type sensory afferent fibres are unmyelinated.
   d. Fibres signalling thermal information travel in the dorsal column of the spinal cord.
   e. Slowly adapting receptors are particularly adept at signalling the rate of change and duration of a stimulus.

Chapter 6 Motor control

63. Which ONE of the following is true concerning motor function?
   a. The temporal cortex receives afferent information from muscle receptors.
   b. Skeletal muscle is almost devoid of sensory receptors.
   c. Spinal interneurons can act to produce repetitive movements such as chewing and stepping.
   d. Spinal neural networks are under descending control through the hippocampus.
   e. A motor unit comprises the muscle cells innervated by a single motor neuron.

64. Which ONE of the following is true concerning the motor system?
   a. The major descending tracts are the corticospinal pathways.
   b. The extrapyramidal system affects visual pathways.
   c. Lesions of the parietal lobe may devastate the motor system.
   d. A patient with Huntington's disease has hypokinetic movements.
   e. A patient with Parkinson's disease suffers hyperkinetic movements.

65. Which ONE of the following is true concerning reflexes?
  a. Stroke patients who have sustained an upper motor neuron lesion typically show an upgoing plantar response to stroking the sole of the foot (Babinski reflex).
  b. Reflexes typically involve conscious thought.
  c. Coma patients typically show normal reflexes.
  d. The spinal reflex arc consists of four neurons.
  e. Reflexes are not affected by disease states.

66. Which ONE of the following is true? In Parkinson's disease:
  a. There is reduced activity of subthalamopallidal neurons.
  b. There is reduced activity of pallidothalamic and nigrothalmic neurons.
  c. Symptoms can be relieved by lesions of an overactive internal pallidum.
  d. There is massive degeneration of striatonigral neurons.
  e. Tremor results from an overactive thalamus.

67. Which ONE of the following is true concerning Parkinsonism?
  a. About 20% of cases in the UK are due to idiopathic Parkinson's disease.
  b. Patients with idiopathic Parkinson's disease do not respond to L-dopa.
  c. Idiopathic Parkinson's disease never occurs below the age of 40 years.
  d. May be caused by drugs.
  e. May be secondary to carbon dioxide poisoning.

68. Which ONE of the following is true concerning the treatment of idiopathic Parkinson's disease:
  a. L-dopa has been shown to slow disease progression.
  b. About 80% of patients will develop motor complications following treatment with L-dopa.
  c. Dopamine agonists are superior to L-dopa.
  d. Treatment should begin as soon as the diagnosis is considered.
  e. Stereotactic neurosurgery should be considered early in the course of the disease.

69. In a classic reflex, such as the knee jerk, the following events occur. Which ONE is fourth?
  a. Contraction of muscle.
  b. Stimulation of extrafusal fibres.
  c. Afferent nerve impulses.
  d. Impulses cross synapses with alpha motor neurons.
  e. Activation of intrafusal fibres.

70. Which ONE of the following is not true? The knee jerk is:
  a. Dependent on the presence of alpha motor neurons.
  b. Polysynaptic.
  c. Exaggerated if there is an upper motor neuron lesion.
  d. Important in control of posture.
  e. A myotatic reflex.

71. The following are locations in the motor pathway. Which ONE is normally fourth in the firing of a nerve impulse?
  a. Lateral corticospinal tract.
  b. Internal capsule.
  c. Decussation.
  d. Betz cell.
  e. Pyramid.

72. A patient has a slowly growing lesion in the internal capsule. Which ONE of the following would not be an expected consequence?
  a. Atrophy of nerve fibres in the corticospinal tracts.
  b. Loss of coordination.
  c. Loss of motor power on the opposite side of the body.
  d. Atrophy of the pyramids.
  e. Wallerian degeneration of involved nerve fibres.

73. Which ONE of the following is not an integral component of the knee jerk?
  a. Corticospinal tracts.
  b. Intrafusal fibres.
  c. Muscle spindles.
  d. Stretch receptors.
  e. Extrafusal fibres.

74. Which ONE of the following is true of the basal ganglia?
  a. Afferent fibres project to the putamen and caudate nucleus.
  b. The globus pallidus is closely related to the function of hippocampus.
  c. They have no direct effect on the motor pathway.
  d. They are primarily concerned with the processing of sensory information.
  e. They have a major output to the occipital cortex.

75. Which ONE of the following is true concerning Parkinson's disease?
  a. It results in loss of dopaminergic neurons in the basal ganglia.
  b. It commonly presents with ataxia.
  c. It occurs most commonly in adults under the age of 50 years.
  d. Rigidity and bradykinesia are common complications.
  e. Its symptoms can be relieved by treatment with acetylcholine agonists.

76. Which ONE of the following statements is true regarding the basal ganglia?
  a. The striatum consists of the putamen and globus pallidus.

b. Dopamine is the key neurotransmitter involved in the nigrostriatal pathway.
c. Neuroleptic drugs cause parkinsonism by inducing dopaminergic neuronal cell death.
d. A destructive lesion of the unilateral basal ganglia may lead to an ipsilateral hemi-parkinsonian syndrome.
e. The basal ganglia communicate with the motor cortex only.

77. Which ONE of the following statements about the thalamus is correct?
a. It contains two main nuclei.
b. It has no main sensory function.
c. It has its only input from the limbic system.
d. It has a role in motor regulation.
e. It is involved in the regulation of body temperature.

78. Which ONE of the following statements about the basal ganglia is correct?
a. The output from the basal ganglia is largely excitatory.
b. The basal ganglia have no role in cognitive or emotional aspects of behaviour.
c. The discharge of many basal ganglia neurons correlates with sensation.
d. Most direct outputs terminate in the spinal cord.
e. Most inputs originate in the cerebral cortex.

79. Which ONE is true concerning the cerebellum?
a. The cerebellum receives inputs only from the motor system.
b. The cerebellum helps to coordinate the actions of many muscles that move the skeleton.
c. The cerebellum sends out control signals to the sensory system.
d. The cerebellar structure is complex and markedly variable between species.
e. Lesions of the cerebellum result in paralysis and weakness.

80. The cerebellum does NOT receive afferent information from which ONE of the following parts of the nervous system?
a. Joint position receptors.
b. Pain receptors.
c. Vestibular apparatus.
d. Pons.
e. Cerebral cortex.

81. A man aged 65 years collapses with weakness down the left side of the body. Which ONE of the following is the most likely location of a lesion?
a. Cerebellum.
b. Corticospinal tracts.
c. Spinal cord.
d. Corticobulbar tracts.
e. Spinocerebellar tracts.

82. Which ONE of the statements below concerning the vestibular system is incorrect?
a. The otolith organs detect head position.
b. The vestibulospinal tracts influence antigravity muscles.
c. The vestibular nuclei project to cranial nerve nuclei controlling eye position.
d. The horizontal vestibulo-ocular reflex uses complementary information from both VIIIth cranial nerves.
e. Proprioception is mediated only by sensation from the musculoskeletal system.

Chapter 7 The autonomic nervous system

83. Which ONE of the following is true of the parasympathetic division of the autonomic nervous system?
a. Preganglionic neurons are located in the brain stem and spinal cord.
b. The major neurotransmitter released is noradrenaline (norepinephrine).
c. The effects of parasympathetic activity are most apparent under conditions of fear and stress.
d. It acts to cause pupillary dilation.
e. It decreases gastrointestinal mobility.

84. Which ONE of the following is true? Impairment of sympathetic nervous system function is suggested when there is:
a. Loss of vibration sense over the medial epicondyle of the humerus.
b. Shortening of the RR interval on the ECG accompanying a deep inspiration.
c. Pupillary constriction on shining a light in the eye.
d. A fall in systolic blood pressure greater than 30 mm Hg on assuming the erect from the supine position.
e. An extensor plantar response (positive Babinski reflex).

85. Which ONE of the following is true of the pupillary light reflex?
a. It is integrated in the occipital cortex.
b. There is a direct and consensual response.
c. Parasympathetic fibres are conveyed in the IV (trochlear) nerve.
d. The efferent limb of the reflex relays in the otic ganglion.
e. The circular muscle of the iris is caused to contract by noradrenaline (norepinephrine).

86. With respect to the autonomic nervous system, which ONE of the following is true?
a. Cranial nerves II, VII, IX and X contain parasympathetic fibres.

b. The transmitter released at post-ganglionic sympathetic endings is adrenaline (epinephrine).
c. Noradrenaline (norepinephrine) is a more effective bronchodilator than adrenaline.
d. The pupillary light reflex is integrated in the midbrain.
e. In accommodation for near vision, sympathetic stimulation causes contraction of the ciliary muscle.

87. Which ONE of the following statements is true? The parasympathetic division of the autonomic nervous system:

a. Leaves the CNS via the thoracolumbar outflow.
b. Has the ganglionic synapse in the majority of instances at a distance from the viscus being innervated.
c. On stimulation, increases the conduction velocity of the cardiac impulse through the atrioventricular node of the heart.
d. Causes relaxation of the detrusor muscle of the urinary bladder.
e. Utilizes acetylcholine as the neurotransmitter at the junction of postganglionic endings with effector cells.

Chapter 8 Vision

88. Which ONE of the following is true? In the eye:
a. The sclera is continuous with the arachnoid layer.
b. The cornea has no sensory innervation.
c. Ciliary muscles are responsible for altering the curvature of the lens.
d. The fovea contains rods and cones.
e. Branches of the central retinal artery do not pass over the fovea.

89. Which ONE of the following is true concerning phototransduction?
a. Photoreceptors are the most anterior structure of the retina.
b. Activation of the phototransduction cascade ends with the activation of transducin.
c. In conditions of darkness photoreceptors are hyperpolarized.
d. Cone photoreceptors require more to become fully activated and are therefore used for day vision.
e. Rod photopigments are involved in the transduction of colour.

90. Concerning the neural processing of light in the retina, which ONE of the following is false?
a. Bipolar cells synapse with ganglion cells which are the output cells of the retina.
b. ON bipolar cells contain a G-protein coupled receptor that hyperpolarizes the cell in the presence of glutamate.
c. The receptive surround of an ON cell is stimulated by the presence of light.
d. Magnocellular cells are large cells with a large receptive field.
e. Parvocellular cells can respond to either colour or fine detail.

91. Which ONE of the following is true concerning the central visual pathway?
a. The primary visual cortex is located in the temporal lobe.
b. The optic chiasma is a site of significant axonal decussation.
c. Optic tract axons end in the medial geniculate nucleus.
d. Its involvement is not typical in multiple sclerosis.
e. It contains only unmyelinated axons.

92. Which ONE of the following is correct? In the analysis of vision:
a. The magnocellular pathway is involved in the analysis of object detail.
b. The parvocellular interblob pathway analyses object detail and shape.
c. The koniocellular and parvocellular-blob pathways analyse object motion.
d. Visual analysis is completed in V1.
e. Perception relies solely on the occipital lobe.

93. Which ONE of the following thalamic nuclei is important in the visual pathway?
a. Ventral posterior nucleus.
b. Ventral anterior nucleus.
c. Medial geniculate nucleus.
d. Lateral geniculate nucleus.
e. Ventral lateral nucleus.

94. Which ONE of the following statements regarding eye movements is incorrect?
a. The vestibulo-ocular reflex may be impaired in IIIrd nerve palsies.
b. The frontal lobes have a role in saccadic eye movements.
c. Smooth pursuit eye movements hold images steady on the optic disc.
d. Vergence eye movements are important in accommodation.
e. Saccadic and smooth pursuit eye movement may alternate.

95. Regarding glaucoma, which ONE of the following is true?
a. Intraocular pressure should be below 5 mmHg.
b. Glaucoma is an uncommon cause of blindness.

c. Acute open-angle glaucoma is an ophthalmological emergency.
d. Tropicamide dilating drops should be instilled into the eye to examine extent of damage to the optic nerve.
e. Glaucoma may be caused by blockage in the scleral sinus.

96. Which ONE of the following is not a cause of acute visual loss?
a. Retinal detachment.
b. Amaurosis fugax.
c. Migraine.
d. Cataracts.
e. Optic neuritis.

97. Which ONE of the following is not a cause of optic disc papilloedema?
a. Raised intracranial pressure.
b. Venous obstruction.
c. Malignant hypertension.
d. Hypercapnia.
e. Cerebrovascular disease.

Chapter 9 Hearing, speech and language

98. Sensorineural deafness is not caused by which ONE of the following:
a. Lesions at the cerebellopontine angle.
b. Ménière's disease.
c. Advancing age.
d. Perforation of the tympanic membrane.
e. Lesions within the petrous temple bone.

99. Which ONE of the statements below regarding testing of cranial nerve VIII is false?
a. In conductive deafness bone conduction is louder than air conduction.
b. When there is conductive deafness in one ear, sound is heard louder in the *affected* ear when using Weber's test.
c. Unilateral vestibular dysfunction causes jerky nystagmus with the fast phase towards the unaffected side.
d. Caloric testing involves flushing the external auditory meatus with cold and hot water.
e. Syringobulbia is a peripheral cause of an VIIIth nerve lesion.

100. Dysphasia is due to impairment of which ONE of the following?
a. Muscles of the larynx.
b. Vocal cords.
c. Speech centre in the brain.
d. Vestibulocochlear (VIIIth cranial) nerve.
e. Comprehension mechanisms.

101. Dysarthria is due to impairment of which ONE of the following?
a. Muscles of the tongue.
b. Vocal cords.
c. Speech centre in the brain.
d. Vestibulocochlear (VIIIth cranial) nerve.
e. Comprehension mechanisms.

102. ONE of the following is true. Receptive aphasia:
a. Is caused by a lesion in Broca's area.
b. Frequently follows a stroke in the right cerebral hemisphere.
c. Leads to production of fluent but nonsensical speech.
d. Is the inability to form new memories.
e. Is tested for using a tuning fork.

Chapter 10 Olfaction and taste

103. Which is true concerning the olfactory system?
a. The olfactory nerve is commonly involved in multiple sclerosis.
b. The primary olfactory cortex is located in the parietal lobe.
c. The olfactory nerves enter the cranial cavity via the sphenoid sinus.
d. Preliminary processing of olfactory information occurs in the olfactory bulbs.
e. Anosmia is a rare complication of head injury.

104. Regarding olfaction and gustation, which ONE of the following statements is incorrect?
a. Hydrophobic compounds reach taste receptors on the epithelial layers of the tongue, palate and pharynx by dissolving in mucus.
b. The sensation of sourness is caused by H^+-ion production by acids.
c. Cranial nerve I passes through the cribriform plate.
d. Taste signals from the posterior one-third of the tongue are transmitted in the chorda tympani (cranial nerve VII).
e. The cerebral hemispheres have ipsilateral gustatory perception.

Chapter 11 The brainstem

105. Which ONE of the following statements is true? The medial lemniscus is in part derived from fibres of the:
a. Gracilis cuneatus nuclei of the same side.
b. Gracilis and cuneatus nuclei of the opposite side.
c. Gracilis nucleus of the same side and the cuneatus nucleus of the opposite side.

d. Gracilis nucleus of the opposite side and the cuneate nucleus of the same side.
e. Ventral posterolateral nucleus of the thalamus.

106. Which ONE of the following patterns of weakness is most suggestive of a left-sided pontine lesion?
a. Proximal weakness of all four limbs.
b. Weakness confined to both legs.
c. Weakness of the left side of the body including the face.
d. Weakness of the left side of the face and the right limbs.
e. Weakness confined to the right leg.

107. Which ONE is true concerning sleep, consciousness and coma?
a. Sleep is characterized by an initial phase with rapid eye movements.
b. The Glasgow Coma Scale is useful for defining conscious level.
c. Medical students deprived of sleep show improved motor coordination and verbal fluency.
d. Coma is always followed by death.
e. Brainstem death may be reversed after oxygen therapy.

108. Which ONE of the following is true? During REM sleep:
a. Systolic blood pressure falls by approximately 50 mm Hg.
b. Desynchronized activity is seen on the EEG.
c. The threshold for arousal is decreased.
d. Growth hormone secretion is markedly increased.
e. There is increased tone in the neck, trunk and limb muscles.

109. Which ONE of the following is not one of the recognized indicators of brain death?
a. Pupils fixed and non-reactive to light.
b. Plantar responses extensor.
c. Corneal reflexes absent.
d. Vestibulo-ocular reflexes absent.
e. Reflex response to suction catheter in the trachea absent.

Chapter 12 Neuroendocrinology

110. Which ONE of the following is true concerning the limbic system?
a. The hippocampal formation has an efferent connection via the fornix to the mamillary bodies.
b. The amygdala receives a major input from the optic pathway.
c. The hippocampal formation has a major projection to the cerebellum.
d. Dysfunction results in sensory abnormalities.
e. Function is enhanced by a high alcohol intake.

111. Which ONE of the following statements about the hypothalamus is correct?
a. It has an important role in movement co-ordination.
b. It has a major vascular connection to the pineal gland.
c. It releases melatonin in a circadian rhythm.
d. It has little influence on the function of the autonomic nervous system.
e. It has a role in the regulation of body water content.

112. The cingulate gyrus receives most of its arterial supply from the branches of which ONE of the following?
a. Middle cerebral artery.
b. Posterior cerebral artery.
c. Superior cerebral artery.
d. Anterior choroidal artery.
e. Anterior cerebral artery.

113. Which ONE of the following statements about the limbic system is correct?
a. It connects the cingulate gyrus with the hypothalamus.
b. It is connected between the cerebral hemispheres by the corpus callosum.
c. It is principally involved in motor function.
d. It is normal in Wernicke's encephalopathy.
e. It has major projections to the cerebellum.

Chapter 13 Memory and the higher functions

114. Which ONE of the following is true concerning memory function?
a. Alzheimer's disease commonly results in a loss of long-term memory.
b. Damage to the medial temporal lobe results in profound loss of recent memory.
c. The amygdala plays a key role in long-term memory.
d. Lesions of the frontal lobe may impair long-term memory.
e. The mamillary bodies and thalamus are involved in short-term memory recall.

115. Which ONE of the following is true in coma?
a. The patient has a normal response to internal stimuli.
b. Coma is caused by damage to selected regions of the cerebral cortex.
c. Neuronal hypoxia is a common cause of coma.

d. Large space occupying lesions are unlikely to result in coma.
e. There is little evidence for involvement of the brainstem in coma.

116. Which ONE of the following is true? In the assessment of a patient's level of consciousness using the Glasgow Coma Scale (GCS):
a. The overall score can vary between 0 and 15.
b. The pupillary response to light is assessed.
c. Patients with a GCS score of 12 are in coma.
d. The best verbal response is assessed.
e. A change in score of 3 points between two consecutive observations is not significant.

117. A major site of damage in Korsakoff's disease is which ONE of the following?
a. Dorsomedial hypothalamus.
b. Hippocampus.
c. Amygdala.
d. Fornix.
e. Mamillary bodies.

Chapter 14 Basic pathological processes within the nervous system

118. Transtentorial herniation as a result of a lateralized cerebral hemisphere bleed most characteristically leads to which ONE of the following?
a. Ipsilateral VIth nerve palsy.
b. Contralateral hemiparesis.
c. No change in conscious level.
d. Backache worse on straining.
e. Sneezing.

119. Which ONE of the following is TRUE of multiple sclerosis?
a. The Schwann cell is primarily involved.
b. The grey matter of the brain is never involved.
c. Optic neuritis is a common presenting feature.
d. Significant disability is inevitable at 10 years from onset.
e. The detection of oligoclonal bands in the cerebrospinal fluid is definite proof of the diagnosis.

120. Which ONE of the following statements about Alzheimer's disease is correct?
a. It is completely untreatable.
b. It is never inherited.
c. It usually presents with memory complaints.
d. It most often presents with visual hallucinations.
e. It progresses rapidly to death over the course of a year.

121. Which ONE of the following statements about Alzheimer's disease is correct?
a. The limbic system is the first region of the brain to be involved in Alzheimer's disease.
b. Visual abnormalities are common in the early stage of the illness.
c. The temporal lobes may enlarge toward the final stage of the illness.
d. Spinal cord lesions are common in elderly patients.
e. Neurofibrillary tangles are prominent in astrocytes.

122. Which ONE of the following is false? Carbamazepine:
a. Is the drug of choice for typical absence seizures.
b. Affects the efficacy of combined oral contraceptives.
c. Has a recognized tendency to lead to leukopenia.
d. Is a recognized effective treatment for primary generalized epilepsies.
e. Is of value in treating partial seizures.

123. Regarding brain tumours, which ONE of the following statements is true?
a. Brain tumours are responsible for approximately 15% of all childhood malignancies.
b. In adults over three-quarters of brain tumours are located infratentorially.
c. In adults, the commonest primary tumours of the brain are astrocytomas.
d. Meningioma is the commonest malignant tumour of children aged 4–8 years.
e. Meningioma is typically a malignant tumour that rapidly invades neural tissue.

Chapter 15 Neurogenetics

124. Which ONE of the following is true regarding neurodegenerative diseases?
a. They never occur in childhood.
b. They are always associated with dementia.
c. They are the result of loss of astrocytes.
d. They are due to trauma.
e. They are sometimes the result of genetic mutations.

125. Whcih ONE of the following conditions is dominantly inherited?
a. Alzheimer's disease.
b. Multiple sclerosis.
c. Parkinson's disease.
d. Epilepsy.
e. Huntington's disease.

126. Which ONE of the following statements about Huntington's disease is incorrect?

a. It is characteristically associated with caudate atrophy.
b. It is inherited as an autosomal recessive condition with low penetrance.
c. It characteristically causes dementia and involuntary movements.
d. It is an example of a CAG repeat disorder.
e. Men and women have an approximately equal risk of developing the disease.

Chapter 16 Pharmacology of the central nervous system

127. Which ONE of the following statements about anxiolytics is incorrect?
a. Benzodiazepines block γ-aminobutyric acid (GABA) action by binding to the GABA receptor.
b. Benzodiazepine actions can be prolonged by active metabolites.
c. Benzodiazepines raise the seizure threshold.
d. Buspirone may act on presynaptic 5-hydroxytryptamine (5-HT) receptors to decrease endogenous 5-HT release.
e. Dependence occurs easily with benzodiazepines.

128. Which ONE of the following statements regarding antidepressants and antipsychotics is true?
a. The cheese reaction occurs because of inhibition of cerebral monoamine oxidase by monoamine oxidase inhibitors.
b. Tricyclics show an antimuscarinic and anti-adrenergic sideeffect profile.
c. 'Typical' antipsychotic potency is proportional the D_4 blocking ability.
d. The motor side effects of antipsychotics are due to effects on the pyramidal system.
e. Clozapine blocks the D_2 receptor preferentially.

129. Which ONE of the following is true of CNS transmitters?
a. Anxiety is controlled by serotonin reuptake inhibitors.
b. Alzheimer's disease is controlled by atropine-like compounds.
c. Schizophrenia is controlled by dopamine antagonists.
d. Depression is controlled by GABA agonists.
e. Insomnia is controlled by tricyclic antidepressants.

130. Which ONE of the following groups is the most widely used class of drug for treatment of depression?
a. Serotonin receptor agonist.
b. Serotonin re-uptake inhibitor.
c. Dopamine receptor antagonist.
d. GABA receptor agonist.
e. Glutamate (NMDA) receptor antagonist.

Chapter 17 Clinical assessment of the nervous system

131. Which ONE of the following best describes the characteristic gait caused by a common peroneal nerve lesion?
a. Wide-based, unsteady and associated with erratic body movements.
b. Shuffling and slow with a small stride length, flexed posture and decreased arm swing.
c. Overflexion of the hip and the knee on one side, giving a high stepping appearance.
d. 'Waddling', tilting from one side to the other with an exaggerated lumbar lordosis.
e. The erect moving body is supported by just one leg at a time and only one foot is firmly on the floor at any time.

132. Which ONE is true concerning the cranial nerves?
a. The oculomotor nerve is the second cranial nerve.
b. Testing the function of the cranial nerves tests the autonomic nervous system.
c. The optic nerve is compressed by an enlarging pituitary tumour.
d. Eye movements are controlled by the optic nerve.
e. The IXth cranial nerve is involved in hearing and position sense.

133. Which ONE of the following is true? The oculomotor nerve:
a. Contains both sympathetic and motor fibres.
b. Innervates the superior oblique extraocular muscle.
c. Has a motor nucleus located in the medulla.
d. Contains sympathetic motor fibres arising from the Edinger–Westphal nucleus.
e. Is involved in the accommodation reflex.

134. Which ONE of the following is true? The facial nerve:
a. Contains only sensory components.
b. Supplies the muscles of mastication.
c. Is responsible for taste and sensation on the posterior third of the tongue.
d. Innervates the submandibular and sublingual salivary glands.
e. Has three major divisions which supply sensation to the face.

135. Which ONE of the following is true of cranial nerves?
a. The olfactory (I) and optic (II) nerves are motor in function.
b. The trigeminal (V) nerve is attached to the medulla oblongata.
c. The oculomotor (III) nerve carries parasympathetic and motor fibres.
d. The glossopharyngeal (IX), vagus (X) and accessory (XI) nerves are demyelinated in multiple sclerosis.

e. The facial (VII) nerve supplies taste fibres to the posterior one-third of the tongue.

136. Which ONE of the following is true? The trigeminal (V) nerve:
a. Carries motor and autonomic fibres.
b. Deals with taste and facial sensation.
c. Innervates the muscles of facial expression.
d. Supplies the muscles involved in chewing.
e. Innervates the salivary and lacrimal glands.

137. If the trigeminal (V) nerve was damaged, which ONE of the following would you still be able to do without impairment?
a. Feel someone stroking your face.
b. Have toothache.
c. Chew food.
d. Produce saliva.
e. Feel a warm breeze caressing your cheek.

138. Which ONE of the following is true? The abducens (VI) cranial nerve:
a. Controls most of the extraocular muscles.
b. Has the longest intracranial course of all the cranial nerves.
c. Arises from a nucleus in the midbrain.
d. Has a sympathetic component.
e. Innervates the conjunctiva.

139. In the activation of the light reflex, the following are involved. Which ONE is fourth?
a. Oculomotor nerve.
b. Sphincter pupillae muscle of the iris.
c. Edinger–Westphal nuclei.
d. Optic nerve.
e. Pretectal area, rostral to the superior colliculus.

140. The oculomotor (III), trochlear (IV) and abducens (VI) nerves run together in the cavernous sinus. If a brain tumour pressed on them, which ONE of the following would be the LEAST likely to have consequence in the ipsilateral eye?
a. Ptosis.
b. Blindness.
c. Dilatation of the pupil.
d. Loss of the light reflex.
e. Paralysis of eye movements.

141. Bell's palsy is an acute inflammatory condition of the facial (VII) nerve. Which ONE of the following would not be a predicted effect?
a. Pain around the ear.
b. Paralysis of the facial muscles.
c. Loss of sensation over the cheek.
d. Absence of the corneal reflex.
e. Loss of taste in the anterior tongue.

142. Which ONE of the following is not a function of the vagus (X) nerve?
a. Parasympathetic fibres to the heart.
b. Swallowing.
c. Sensation from the face.
d. Motor fibres to the larynx.
e. Sensory fibres from aortic baroreceptors.

143. A pituitary tumor is most likely to cause which ONE of the following visual field defects?
a. Left homonymous hemianopia.
b. Right homonymous hemianopia.
c. Central scotoma.
d. Left upper quadrantanopia.
e. Bitemporal hemianopia.

144. In the neurological context, which ONE of the following is the *best* definition of a stroke?
a. Infarction of the territory of the middle cerebral artery.
b. Loss of consciousness.
c. Weakness of the muscles of both lower limbs.
d. Sudden loss of muscle power on one side of the body.
e. Difficulty in coordination.

145. Which ONE of the following is the *best* definition of hemiparesis?
a. Infarction of the territory of the middle cerebral artery.
b. Complete loss of power in one arm and leg.
c. Weakness of the muscles of both lower limbs.
d. Partial loss of muscle power on one side of the body.
e. Difficulty in coordination.

146. Which ONE of the following is the *best* definition of paraplegia?
a. The consequence of a tumour in the spinal cord.
b. Loss of muscle power in both lower limbs.
c. Weakness of the muscles on one side of the body.
d. Loss of power in all four limbs.
e. Loss of sphincter control in the bladder.

147. Which ONE of the following clinical signs would NOT be associated with an upper motor neuron lesion?
a. Hypertonia.
b. Fasciculations.
c. Clonus.
d. Brisk reflexes.
e. Positive Babinski sign.

148. Which ONE of the following is NOT a cause of mixed upper and lower motor neuron signs?
a. Motor neuron disease.
b. Acquired immune deficiency syndrome (AIDS).
c. Guillain–Barré syndrome.
d. Syphilis.
e. Chronic upper motor neuron weakness causing 'disuse atrophy'.

149. Which one of the following statements is false? MRI:
  a. Is the best imaging technique for the spinal cord.
  b. Is unsafe for patients with cardiac pacemakers.
  c. Uses radio waves and magnetic fields to produce images.
  d. Is a faster examination technique than CT.
  e. Does not use X-ray.

150. Which ONE of the following blood test abnormalities increases a patient's risk of stroke?
  a. Polycythaemia.
  b. Hyponatraemia.
  c. Hypernatraemia.
  d. Elevated urea.
  e. Low thyroid-stimulating hormone (TSH).

Extended-matching questions (EMQs)

For each scenario described below, choose the single most likely option from the list of options.

Each option may be used once, more than once or not at all.

1. Cortical localization

A. Left cerebral hemisphere
B. Right cerebral hemisphere
C. Frontal lobe
D. Parietal lobe
E. Temporal lobe
F. Occipital lobe
G. Broca's area
H. Prefrontal cortex
I. Wernicke's area
J. Hippocampus

Instruction: Match one of the options listed above to the descriptions given below.

1. Essential for the comprehension of speech.
☐
2. Usually the dominant hemisphere.
☐
3. Damage here may result in personality changes.
☐
4. Contains the primary somatosensory cortex.
☐
5. Where the muscle movements that articulate speech are determined.
☐

2. The blood supply to the central nervous system

A. Middle cerebral artery
B. Transverse sinus
C. Vertebral artery
D. Posterior cerebral artery
E. Anterior communicating artery
F. Internal carotid artery
G. Superior saggital sinus
H. Anterior cerebral artery
I. Basilar artery
J. Cavernous sinus

Instruction: Match one of the options listed above to the descriptions given below.

1. Gives rise to the middle cerebral artery.
☐
2. Supplies the medial side of each hemisphere.
☐
3. Supplies the medulla, pons, and cerebellum.
☐
4. Supplies the occipital lobe.
☐
5. The primary site of venous drainage from the cortex.
☐

3. Cerebrovascular disease

A. Completed stroke
B. Capsular haemorrhage
C. 54 mL/100 g per minute
D. Stroke in evolution
E. Vasculitic stroke
F. Thromboembolic stroke
G. Ischaemic penumbra
H. 28 mL/100 g per minute
I. Haemorrhagic stroke
J. Transient ischaemic attack

Instruction: Match one of the options listed above to the descriptions given below.

1. Normal rate of cerebral blood flow.
☐
2. Surrounds the central necrotic zone of an infarct.
☐
3. Stroke that occurs secondary to atheroma or cardiogenic emboli.
☐
4. Focal neurological deficit of presumed vascular origin from which a full clinical recovery occurs within 24 hours.
☐
5. Constitutes approximately 15% of all strokes.
☐

4. Glial cells

A. Schwann cells
B. Astrocytes
C. Choroid plexus cells
D. Bergmann glia
E. Müller's cells
F. Microglia
G. Radial glia
H. Satellite cells
I. Oligodendrocytes
J. Enteric glial cells

Instruction: Match one of the options listed above to the descriptions given below.

1. Secrete CSF.

☐

2. Myelinate axons in the peripheral nervous system.

☐

3. Provide the framework for surrounding neurons and capillaries.

☐

4. Capable of antigen presentation.

☐

5. Glial cell found in the retina.

☐

5. The development of the nervous system and disorders of development

A. Endoderm
B. Mesoderm
C. Ectoderm
D. Diencephalon
E. Holoprosencephaly
F. Anancephaly
G. Spina bifida
H. Neural crest
I. Neuroblasts
J. Heterotopia

Instruction: Match one of the options listed above to the descriptions given below.

1. Embryological layer forming the nevous system and skin.

☐

2. Neuronal migration disorder.

☐

3. Congenital disorder in which the forebrain of the embryo fails to develop into two hemispheres.

☐

4. Gives rise to most of the cells in the peripheral nervous system.

☐

5. Differentiates into the neurons of the grey matter of the spinal cord

☐

6. Neurophysiology of synaptic transmission

A. Glutamate
B. Quantum hypothesis
C. γ-aminobutyric acid (GABA)
D. Noradrenaline (norepinephrine)
E. Calcium ion
F. Calcitonin
G. Spatial summation
H. Sodium ion
I. Metabotropic
J. Inotrope

Instruction: Match one of the options listed above to the descriptions given below.

1. Influx of this ion leads to liberation of vesicles from their presynaptic actin network.

☐

2. Theory of small identical excitatory postsynaptic potentials (EPSPs), each corresponding to individual vesicle release.

☐

3. Type of receptor that is coupled to a G-protein.

☐

4. Principal excitatory neurotransmitter of the brain.

☐

5. Principal inhibitory neurotransmitter of the brain.

☐

7. Spinal tract

A. Upper motor neuron (UMN)
B. Ventral corticospinal tract
C. Reticulospinal tract fibres
D. Medulla
E. Lower motor neuron (LMN)

F. Tectospinal tract
G. Ventral spinocerebellar tract
H. Corticobulbar fibres
I. Medial longitudinal fasciculus
J. Gamma motor neurons

Instruction: Match one of the options listed above to the descriptions given below.

1. This is the site of the decussation of the pyramidal tracts.

☐

2. Spasticity, brisk reflexes and extensor plantar responses are signs of this lesion.

☐

3. Hypotonia, hyporeflexia and atrophy are signs of this lesion.

☐

4. These fibres do not decussate.

☐

5. Tract with efferent fibres that help maintain the control of posture.

☐

---

8. Somatosensation and pain

A. Meissner's corpuscles
B. Substance-P
C. Morphine
D. COX-1
E. Pacinian corpuscles
F. COX-2
G. Lidocaine
H. Fentanyl
I. Nociceptors
J. Glutamate

Instruction: Match one of the options listed above to the descriptions given below.

1. Inhibition of this enzyme is thought to be responsible for the desirable analgesic effect of NSAIDs.

☐

2. Causes a very long-lasting excitatory postsynaptic potential, helping to sustain the effect of noxious stimuli.

☐

3. Polymodal varieties (attached to C fibre afferents) are sensitive to temperature in excess of 46 °C.

☐

4. Blocks the ability of axons to conduct action potentials by blocking Na^+ channels in the axonal membrane.

☐

5. Sense vibration.

☐

---

9. Reflexes

A. Deep tendon reflexes (e.g. knee jerk and ankle jerk)
B. Gag reflex
C. Corneal reflex
D. Plantar reflex
E. Flexion withdrawal reflex
F. Cough reflex
G. Doll's eye reflex
H. Pupillary reflex
I. Oculocephalic reflex
J. Autonomic nervous system reflexes

Instruction: Match one of the reflexes listed above to the reflexes described below.

1. This reflex utilizes the sensory nucleus of the trigeminal nerve and the motor nucleus of the facial nerve.

☐

2. This reflex utilizes the sensory nucleus of the glossopharyngeal and vagus nerves and the motor nuclei of the glossopharyngeal, vagus and accessory nerves.

☐

3. This reflex is responsible for Babinski's sign when spinal pathology is present.

☐

4. This reflex has a polysynaptic pathway in the spinal cord.

☐

5. Lower motor neuron lesions result in dulling of this reflex.

☐

---

10. Neuropathies

A. Lateral cutaneous nerve of the thigh
B. Ulnar nerve
C. Carpal tunnel syndrome
D. Erb's palsy
E. Klumpke's palsy
F. Radial nerve
G. Median nerve
H. Common peroneal nerve

I. Prolapsed intervertebral disc
J. Sciatic nerve

Instruction: Match one of the options listed above to the statements below.

1. This disease is associated with thenar wasting.

☐

2. Numbness of the little finger and half of the ring finger and weakness of the intrinsic muscles of the hand indicate a lesion of this nerve.

☐

3. This nerve may be damaged by a posterior fracture of the acetabulum.

☐

4. Avulsion of the C5/6 nerve root causes this palsy.

☐

5. Avulsion of the C8/T1 nerve root causes this palsy.

☐

11. The autonomic nervous system

A. Acetylcholine
B. Noradrenaline
C. Prazosin
D. Adrenaline (epinephrine)
E. Salbutamol
F. Atenolol
G. α_1 adrenorecptor
H. α_2 adrenorecptor
I. β_1 adrenorecptor
J. β_2 adrenorecptor

Instruction: Match one of the options listed above to the statements below.

1. The neurotransmitter released by sympathetic postganglionic neurons.

☐

2. The neurotransmitter released by parasympathetic preganglionic neurons.

☐

3. Selective β_1 adrenorecptor antagonist.

☐

4. Agonists acting at this adrenoreceptor cause smooth muscle relaxation.

☐

5. Activation of this adrenoreceptor results in increased heart rate and force of contraction.

☐

12. Vision

A. Giant cell arteritis
B. Age-related macular degeneration
C. Acute closed angle glaucoma
D. Primary open angle glaucoma
E. Posterior cerebral artery occlusion
F. Diabetic retinopathy
G. Retinitis pigmentosa
H. Pituitary adenoma
I. Neurofibromatosis
J. Multiple sclerosis

Instruction: Match one of the conditions listed above to the statements below.

1. Often presents with progressive night blindness.

☐

2. A patient presenting with a history of jaw pain on chewing and a raised erythrocyte sedimentation rate (ESR).

☐

3. Commonly presents with bitemporal hemianopia.

☐

4. A cause of homonymous hemianopia.

☐

5. May present with optic neuritis.

☐

13. Speech and language

A. Larynx
B. Cranial nerve VII
C. Dysphonia
D. Cerebellum
E. Wernicke's area
F. Dysarthria
G. Broca's area
H. Dysphasia
I. Arcuate fasciculus
J. Cranial nerve VIII

Instruction: Match one of the conditions listed above to the statements below.

1. Disorder characterized by abnormal articulation caused by upper motor neuron lesions of the cerebral hemispheres or lower motor neuron lesions of the brain stem.

☐

2. Disorder characterized by impaired ability to understand or use the spoken word caused by a lesion of the dominant hemisphere.

☐

3. Lesions here may caue deafness.

☐

4. Dysfunction here produces an altered quality in the tone of the voice.

☐

5. Damage here reduces motor output for speech which becomes effortful and dysfluent but with well-preserved comprehension.

☐

14. Cranial nerves

A. Optic nerve (II)
B. Oculomotor nerve (III)
C. Trochlear nerve (IV)
D. Trigeminal nerve (V)
E. Abducens nerve (VI)
F. Facial nerve (VII)
G. Vestibulocochlear nerve (VIII)
H. Glossopharyngeal nerve (IX)
I. Vagus nerve (X)
J. Accesssory nerve (XI)

Instruction: Match one of the conditions listed above to the statements below.

1. Provides parasympathetic innervation to the eye.

☐

2. Lesions of this cranial nerve may result in an afferent defect of the corneal reflex.

☐

3. Asking the patient to shrug their shoulders is a method of testing this cranial nerve.

☐

4. Innervates the superior oblique muscle.

☐

5. Is responsible for taste on the anterior two-thirds of the tongue.

☐

15. Neuroendocrinology

A. Antidiuretic hormone (ADH)
B. Corticotropin-releasing factor (CRF)
C. Oxytocin
D. Thyrotropin-releasing factor
E. Adrenocorticotropin hormone (ACTH)
F. Neuropeptide Y
G. Thyroid stimulating hormone
H. Prolactin
I. α-melanocyte stimulating hormone (α-MSH)
J. Cholecystokinin (CCK)

Instruction: Match one of the conditions listed above to the statements below.

1. Neurogenic diabetes insipidus results from a lack of production of this homone in the hypothalamus.

☐

2. This hormone increases the desire to eat.

☐

3. Released by the anterior pituitary gland, this hormone travels through the systemic circulation until it reaches the adrenals, whereupon it stimulates release of cortisol from the adrenal cortex.

☐

4. This hormone is synthesized and secreted by the anterior pituitary gland and regulates the endocrine function of the thyroid gland.

☐

5. This hormone is responsible for the letdown reflex in breastfeeding mothers.

☐

16. Higher functions

A. Declarative memory
B. Korsakoff's syndrome
C. Coma
D. Working memory
E. Attention
F. Executive function
G. Non-declarative memory
H. Dyspraxia
I. Persistent vegetative state
J. Neglect

Instruction: Match one of the options listed above to the statements below.

1. The retention of information needed to guide ongoing behaviour.

☐

2. May be mediated by top-down or bottom-up mechanisms.

☐

3. The inability to perform skilled actions despite intact basic motor and sensory abilities.

☐

4. This disorder is typically caused by a right parietal lobe lesion.

☐

5. Condition in which there is a non-functional cortex with a functional reticular activating system.

☐

17. Demyelinating disease

A. Interferon β
B. Intravenous methylprednisolone
C. Carbamazepine
D. 70+ years
E. Lhermitte's sign
F. Dysmyelination
G. Babinski's sign
H. Multiple sclerosis
I. 20–40 years
J. Azathioprine

Instruction: Match one of the options listed above to the statements below.

1. Disorder in which myelin is inherently abnormal and does not form appropriately.

☐

2. Peak incidence of multiple sclerosis.

☐

3. Electric-shock-like sensation extending down spine into limbs on neck flexion.

☐

4. Reduces relapse rates in multiple sclerosis.

☐

5. Treatment of choice for acute relapse of multiple sclerosis.

☐

18. Neoplasms of the central nervous system

A. Medulloblastoma
B. Lymphoma
C. Metastatic brain tumour
D. Craniopharyngioma
E. Astrocytoma
F. Meningioma
G. Oligodendoglioma
H. Pituitary adenoma
I. Schwannoma
J. Ependymoma

Instruction: Match one of the options listed above to the statements below.

1. The commonest malignant solid tumour of childhood (4–8 years).

☐

2. A benign, slow-growing tumour that commonly develops in cranial nerve VIII.

☐

3. Accounts for up to 10% of central nervous system complications in AIDS patients.

☐

4. Bitemporal hemianopia may be a presenting feature of this tumour.

☐

5. The commonest primary tumour of the brain.

☐

19. Degenerative disease

A. Tau protein
B. Parkinson's disease
C. Haloperidol
D. Vascular dementia
E. Alzheimer's disease
F. Transmissible spongiform encephalopathies (TSEs)
G. α-synuclein
H. Anti-cholinesterase inhibitor
I. Aspirin
J. Prion protein

Instruction: Match one of the options listed above to the statements below.

1. Disorder typified by the inability to form new memories due to the deposition of neurofibrillary tangles and ß-amyloid plaques in the parahippocampal areas.

☐

2. May slow cognitive decline in some patients with Alzheimer's disease.

☐

3. Deposition of amyloid containing this protein is a histopathologial characteristic of variant CJD (vCJD).

☐

4. Intracellular fibrillary aggregates of this protein are implicated in the pathogenesis of dementia with Lewy bodies.

☐

5. Disorder characterized by a step-wise deterioration in cognitive function.

☐

20. Neurogenetics

A. von Hippel–Lindau syndrome
B. Charcot–Marie–Tooth type I
C. Iatrogenic Creutzfeldt–Jakob disease
D. Prader–Willi syndrome
E. Becker's muscular dystrophy
F. Angelman's syndrome
G. Huntington's disease
H. von Recklinghausen neurofibromatosis
I. Kaposi sarcoma
J. Gerstman–Straussler–Scheinker (GSS) disease

Instruction: Match one of the neurogenetic diseases listed above to the statements below.

1. A trinucleotide repeat disorder.

☐

2. Inherited muscle wasting disease.

☐

3. A neurocutaneous syndrome.

☐

4. An inherited spongiform encephalopathy.

☐

5. Inherited peripheral neuropathy.

☐

21. Neuropharmacology

A. Diazepam
B. Amitryptyline
C. Lithium
D. Clozipine
E. Flumazenil
F. Risperidone
G. Ondansetron
H. Chlorpromazine
I. Fluoxetine
J. Domperidone

Instruction: Match one of the neurogenetic diseases listed above to the statements below.

1. May be used in the treament of a benzodiazepine overdose.

☐

2. Most likely to cause extrapyramidal side effects.

☐

3. 5-HT_3 receptor antagonist.

☐

4. Dysrhythmias are potentially fatal consequences of overdose.

☐

5. Selectively blocks seritonin (5-HT) reuptake.

☐

22. Pupil and eye movement disorders

A. Abnormal doll's eye movement
B. Intranuclear opthlmoplegia (INO)
C. Disconjugate eye movement
D. Holmes–Adie pupil
E. Large fixed pupils
F. Conjugate gaze to one size
G. Horner's syndorme
H. Pin-point pupils
I. Nystagmus
J. Unilateral dilated fixed pupil

Instruction: Match one of the neurogenetic diseases listed above to the statements below.

1. Associated with loss of deep tendon reflexes and pupil constriction to 0.1% pilocarpine.

☐

2. Seen in opiate overdose.

☐

3. Indicates a supratentorial mass lesion.

☐

4. Involuntary rhythmic oscillation of the eyes.

☐

5. Seen following administration of atropine eyedrops.

☐

23. Neurological examination

A. Slurred speech
B. Dyspraxia

C. Dyscalculia
D. Ataxia
E. Bulbar palsy
F. Ask patient to interpret common proverbs
G. Ask patient what time of day it is
H. Ask patient to spell WORLD backwards
I. Ask patient to draw clock, put hours on, and set to 3 o'clock
J. Agnosia

Instruction: Match one of the options listed above to the statements below.

1. May indicate a cerebellar lesion.
☐
2. May indicate motor neuron disease.
☐
3. Means of assessing a patient's attention.
☐
4. Means of assessing a patient's abstract thinking.
☐
5. The inability to recognize sensory input in the absence of primary sensory pathway dysfunction.
☐

24. Abnormal movement (dyskinesia)

A. Tic
B. Physiological tremor
C. Dystonia
D. Clonus
E. Chorea
F. Essential tremor
G. Myoclonus
H. Intention tremor
I. Resting tremor
J. Athetosis

Instruction: Match one of the options listed above to the statements below.

1. Usually inherited in an autosomal dominant fashion and may involve the head (titubation).
☐
2. May be caused by Huntington's disease.
☐
3. Brief, shock-like muscle contractions.
☐
4. Sustained muscle contraction causing unusual postures.
☐
5. Commonly seen in Parkinson's disease.
☐

25. Investigations

A. Alzheimer's disease
B. Acoustic neuroma
C. Pituitary stalk lesion
D. Intracerebral abscess
E. Multiple sclerosis
F. Cerebral contusions
G. Diffuse traumatic axonal injury
H. Neurosarcoidosis
I. Anterior cerebral artery territory infarction
J. Raised intracranial pressure

Instruction: Match one of the options listed above to the statements below.

1. This disease is associated with periventricular white matter lesions.
☐
2. What might an MRI of a patient with a history of bitemporal hemianopia show?
☐
3. Widened sulci and enlarged ventricles may be seen on a CT scan of this disease.
☐
4. This condition is one of the causes of ring-enhancing lesions on CT.
☐
5. A cerebellopontine mass on MRI and a history of a deafness (determined sensorineural by an audiogram) includes this differential diagnosis.
☐

Chapter 1 Introduction and overview of the nervous system

1. C
2. D
3. A
4. D
5. E
6. D
7. D
8. E
9. D
10. E
11. B
12. D
13. D
14. E
15. C
16. B
17. A
18. B
19. D
20. E
21. E
22. A
23. A
24. B
25. D

Chapter 2 The development of the nervous system and disorders of development

26. C
27. E

Chapter 3 Cellular physiology of the nervous system and introductions to pharmacology

28. A
29. C
30. A
31. B
32. D
33. D
34. C
35. B
36. E
37. C

Chapter 4 The spinal cord and peripheral nerves

38. C
39. D
40. D
41. E
42. E
43. A
44. E
45. C
46. E
47. E
48. D
49. A
50. B
51. E
52. D

Chapter 5 Somatosensation and the perception of pain

53. B
54. B
55. E
56. D
57. C
58. B
59. B
60. C
61. C
62. C

Chapter 6 Motor control

63. E
64. A
65. A
66. C
67. D
68. B
69. B
70. B
71. C
72. B
73. A
74. A
75. D
76. B
77. D
78. E
79. B
80. E
81. A
82. E

Chapter 7 The autonomic nervous system

83. A
84. D
85. B
86. D
87. E

Chapter 8 Vision

88. C
89. D
90. C
91. B
92. B
93. D
94. C
95. E
96. D
97. E

Chapter 9 Hearing, speech and language

98. D
99. E
100. C
101. B
102. C

Chapter 10 Olfaction and taste (gustation)

103. D
104. D

Chapter 11 The brainstem

105. B
106. D
107. B
108. B
109. B

Chapter 12 Neuroendocrinology

110. A
111. E
112. E
113. A

Chapter 13 Higher functions

114. B
115. C
116. D
117. E

Chapter 14 Basic pathological processes within the nervous system

118. B
119. C
120. C
121. A
122. A
123. C

Chapter 15 Neurogenetics

124. E
125. E
126. B

Chapter 16 Pharmacology of the central nervous system

127. A
128. A
129. C
130. B

Chapter 17 Clinical assessment of the nervous system

131. C
132. C
133. E
134. D
135. C
136. D
137. D
138. B
139. A
140. B
141. C
142. C
143. E
144. D
145. D
146. B
147. B
148. C
149. D
150. A

1. Cortical localization

1. I
2. A
3. C
4. D
5. G

2. The blood supply to the central nervous system

1. F
2. H
3. I
4. D
5. G

3. Cerebrovascular disease

1. C
2. G
3. F
4. J
5. I

4. Glial cells

1. C
2. A
3. B
4. F
5. E

5. The development of the nervous system and disorders of development

1. C
2. J
3. E
4. H
5. I

6. Neurophysiology of synaptic transmission

1. E
2. B
3. I
4. A
5. C

7. Spinal tract

1. D
2. A
3. E
4. B
5. C

8. Somatosensation and pain

1. F
2. B
3. I
4. G
5. E

9. Reflexes

1. C
2. B
3. D
4. E
5. A

10. Neuropathies

1. C
2. B
3. A
4. D
5. E

11. The autonomic nervous system

1. B
2. A
3. F
4. J
5. I

12. Vision

1. G
2. A
3. H
4. E
5. J

13. Speech and language

1. F
2. H
3. J
4. A
5. G

14. Cranial nerves

1. B
2. D
3. J
4. C
5. F

15. Neuroendocrinology

1. A
2. F
3. E
4. G
5. C

16. Higher functions

1. D
2. E
3. H
4. J
5. I

17. Demyelinating disease

1. F
2. I
3. E
4. A
5. B

18. Neoplasms of the central nervous system

1. A
2. I
3. B
4. H
5. E

19. Degenerative disease

1. E
2. H
3. J
4. G
5. D

20. Neurogenetics

1. G
2. E
3. H
4. J
5. B

21. Neuropharmacology

1. E
2. H
3. G
4. B
5. I

22. Pupil and eye movement disorders

1. D
2. H
3. J
4. I
5. E

23. Neurological examination

1. D
2. E
3. H
4. F
5. J

24. Abnormal movement (dyskinesia)

1. F
2. E
3. G
4. C
5. I

25. Investigations

1. E These are usually seen on magnetic resonance imaging, but not always.
2. C Likely to be a pituitary adernoma.
3. A Remember definitive diagnosis only comes from post-mortem pathology; one must be guided by signs clinically.
4. D Usually a sign for urgent neurosurgical removal.
5. B These can be removed via surgery. However, surgery may lead to other iatrogenic cranial nerve palsies (e.g. facial nerve palsy).

Glossary

Agnosia Loss of ability to recognize objects/people/sounds/smells/shapes while the specific sense is not defective (*gnosis* = knowledge).

Akinesis A state whereby an individual is unable to produce movement (*kinesis* = movement).

Amnesia Partial or total loss of memory (*amnestos* = not remembered; *mne* = to remember).

Anaesthesia Total or partial loss of sensation, especially tactile sensibility (*aethesis* = feeling).

Anorexigenic Having or causing a reduction in feeding behaviour.

Aphasia Impairment of the ability to produce or comprehend language (*phatos* = to speak).

Apraxia Loss of ability to execute learned (familiar) movements, despite the desire and physical ability to do so (*praxis* = to do).

Ataxia Unsteady and clumsy movement of the limbs/trunk due to failure of fine coordination of muscle.

Autonomic Relating to the autonomic nervous system, which controls those body functions that are not under conscious control (e.g. heart rate, breathing, sweating) (*autos* = self).

Axon Part of the neuron that conducts an action potential.

Bradykinesia Slowing down and loss of spontaneous and voluntary movement (*brady* = slow, *kinesia* = movement).

Bulbar Relating to or involving the medulla.

Cerebrum The large, rounded structure of the brain which occupies most of the cranial cavity and is divided into the two cerebral hemispheres.

Circadian From Latin *circa* = around and *dies* = day, meaning literally 'around a day'.

Chorea Rapid, irregular, involuntary jerking/twitching movements (from the Greek 'to dance')

Cognition The mental process of knowing, including aspects such as awareness, perception, reasoning and judgment (incorporates gnosis).

Coma State of deep, often prolonged unconsciousness, usually the result of injury, disease, or poison, in which an individual is incapable of sensing or responding to external stimuli and internal needs (*koma* = deep sleep).

Contralateral Occurring on or acting in conjunction with a part on the opposite side of the body (*contra* = in contrast or opposition to; *lateralis* = side).

Coronal Plane that is parallel to the surface of the face.

Decerebrate The characteristic of an individual who has suffered a brain injury that results in almost no neurological function.

Dendrite Specialized neuronal cell body extensions which receive messages from other neurons.

Depolarization Change in membrane potential towards a more positive potential.

Diencephalon The posterior part of the forebrain that connects the midbrain with the cerebral hemispheres, encloses the third ventricle, and contains the thalamus and hypothalamus.

Diplopia Visual disorder that results in double vision.

Dorsal Posterior.

Dyscalculia Difficulty understanding/manipulating numbers.

Dysgraphia Impaired ability to learn or to write (*-graphia* = writing).

Dyslexia Impaired ability to learn to read (*-lexis* = words).

Dysphasia Impairment of speech and verbal comprehension.

Dyspraxia Partial loss of the ability to coordinate purposeful movements in the absence of motor or sensory impairments.

Endocytosis Uptake of materials from outside a cell in vesicles that arise by inward folding of the plasma membrane.

Endothelial cell Thin flattened cell, a layer of which lines the inner surfaces of body cavities, blood vessels and lymph vessels.

Equilibrium potential Membrane potential at which there is no net passive movement of ion species into or out of a cell.

Fasciculation An involuntary coarser form of muscular contraction than fibrillation, consisting of involuntary contractions or twitchings of groups of muscle fibres.

Fenestration Natural or surgically created opening in a surface.

Foramen Communication between two cavities.

Ganglion Mass of nervous tissue composed mainly of neuronal cell bodies, usually lying outside the central nervous system. Plural = ganglia.

Grey matter Grey nervous tissue containing cell bodies as well as unmyelinated fibres; forms the cerebral cortex.

Hemiparesis/hemiplegia Total or partial paralysis of one side of the body that results from disease of or injury to the motor centres of the brain *(hemi-* = half; *-paresis* = to let fall, paralysis).

Hypersomnia A condition in which one sleeps for an excessively long time but is normal in the waking intervals *(huper* = above, beyond; *somnia* = sleep).

Iatrogenic Illness caused by medical treatment.

Idiopathic Occurring without known cause.

Infra- Prefix meaning inferior to, below or beneath.

Infratentorial Below the tentorium cerebelli and within the posterior cranial fossa.

Inotropic A substance that affects the contraction of muscle, especially heart muscle *(ino* = muscle/sinew).

Insomnia Chronic inability to fall asleep or remain asleep for an adequate length of time *(in* = not, *somnia* = sleep).

Ipsilateral Located on or affecting the same side of the body.

Leptomeninges The pia mater and the arachnoid mater considered together as covering the brain and spinal cord.

Meatus Opening or passageway in the body.

Meninges Plural of meninx; a membrane, especially one of the three membranes enclosing the brain and spinal cord (dura mater, arachnoid mater and pia mater).

Myopathy Disease of skeletal muscle not caused by nerve disorders. Cause the skeletal or voluntary muscles to become weak or wasted.

Neuroblast Cell of early embryonic life which later develops into a neuron.

Neuropathy Disturbance of function or pathological change in a nerve.

Neurotransmitter Chemical released by nerve cells at synapses that influence the activity of adjacent cells.

Neurulation Embryonic formation of the neural tube by closure of the neural plate.

Nucleus A group of specialized nerve cells or a localized mass of grey matter in the brain or spinal cord.

Ophthalmoplegia Paralysis of eye muscles.

Orexigenic Having a stimulating effect on the appetite.

Paraesthesia A sensation of pricking, tingling or pain on the skin having no objective cause and usually associated with injury or irritation of a sensory nerve or nerve root *(para* = incorrect in this context and *aesthesis* = feeling).

Paraneoplastic Symptom that is the consequence of the presence of malignancy, but that is not due to the local presence of cancer cells.

Parasomnia Any of several disorders that frequently interfere with sleep, occurring especially among children and including sleepwalking, night terrors and bed-wetting.

Photophobia Abnormal sensitivity to light.

Proprioception The unconscious perception of movement and spatial orientation arising from stimuli within the body itself *(proprius* = one's own; -ception from *recipere,* to receive).

Ptosis Drooping of the eyelids (Greek for fall).

Saccade Normal (largely unnoticed) rapid darting of the eyes from one fixed point to another.

Sagittal Vertical plane dividing body into right and left portions.

Spasticity Increased muscular tone where abnormal stretch reflexes intensify muscle resistance to passive movement.

Supra- Prefix meaning above.

Supratentorial Located above the tentorium cerebri.

Synapse Functional connection between a nerve cell axon and target cell (e.g. other nerve cells, muscle cells or gland cells).

Telencephalon The anterior portion of the forebrain, constituting the cerebral hemispheres and related parts.

Tract A bundle of nerve fibres having a common origin, termination and function.

Ventral Anterior.

Vertigo Illusion of movement.

White matter White nerve tissue consisting chiefly of myelinated nerve fibres.

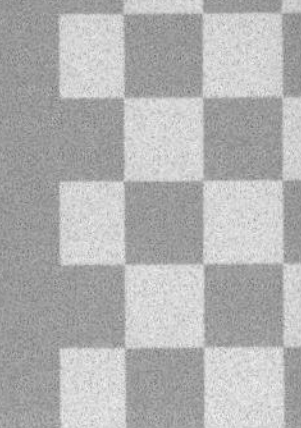

Index

Note: Page numbers followed by *f* indicate figures and *ge* indicate glossary term.

D

E

F

G

M

N